Overcoming Anxiety in Sex and Relationships

T0372874

This book gives readers an accessible and comprehensive understanding of how anxiety, stress, and pressure can have a profound impact on pleasure, connection, and sexual functioning, offering practical tips and techniques for resolving common sexual struggles.

Anxiety can influence a multitude of aspects that make us who we are, changing how we move through, make meaning of, and interact with the world around us. Paula Leech begins by defining anxiety and how it affects our physiology before guiding readers to identify some of the primary sources of anxiety in their lives, such as family, gender, culture, religion, relationship dynamics, and sexual trauma. Encouraging clients to take responsibility, she offers alternative ways of conceptualizing and defining sex, sexuality, sexual values, and a client's ongoing sexual development as a way of addressing some of the emotional, social, and psychological barriers to intimacy. Practical and engaging, this book includes mindfulness and embodiment exercises to help clients release stored tension, work through specific sexual struggles and "dysfunctions," and deepen their connections with their body.

This guide is essential reading for established and training sex therapists as well as for those who experience anxiety-based sexual challenges with their partner.

Paula Leech, LMFT, CST-S, is a certified sex therapist who has worked with individuals, relationships, and families in private practice for over ten years. She mentors sex therapists in training, and teaches at various institutes across the USA and Canada.

Overcoming Anxiety in Sex and Relationships

A Comprehensive Guide to Intimate and Emotional Freedom

Paula Leech

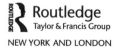

Routledge
Taylor & Francis Group

NEW YORK AND LONDON

Designed cover image: Brian Leech

First published 2025
by Routledge
605 Third Avenue, New York, NY 10158

and by Routledge
4 Park Square, Milton Park, Abingdon, Oxon, OX14 4RN

Routledge is an imprint of the Taylor & Francis Group, an informa business

ISBN: 978-1-032-43840-5 (hbk)
ISBN: 978-1-032-43839-9 (pbk)
ISBN: 978-1-003-36908-0 (ebk)

DOI: 10.4324/9781003369080

Typeset in Sabon
by SPi Technologies India Pvt Ltd (Straive)

Additional Support Material can be found at www.routledge.com/9781032438399

Contents

Interviewees

Candice Hargons (she/her) is an award-winning associate professor of counseling psychology at the University of Kentucky, where she studies sexual wellness and liberation. She is the host of "F*ck the System: A Sexual Liberation Podcast and How to Love a Human," a liberation podcast that asks people with multiple marginalized identities what the world would be like if it loved them. She has published over 50 research articles and has been featured in The Huffington Post, the APA Monitor, Good Housekeeping, Women's Health, Blavity, Cosmopolitan, and the New York Times.

Serina Payan Hazelwood, MAIS, CSE (she/her/ella) is a queer, Indigenous-Chicana, scholar, author, educator, and community gatherer. She is a certified holistic sexuality educator and yoga teacher dedicated to liberatory praxis through Indigenous Knowledges. Her work is rooted in the cosmologies of the land. Reclamation, ritual, and renewal are the guiding value systems that inform the human experience of her work.

Israel Martinez, LCSW, CST (he/him) is a gay man, a sex and relationship therapist, and an author who has been working with the LGBTQ+ community on a professional basis for close on 20 years. This background has provided him with unique expertise on issues that tend to be a part of the lesbian, gay, bisexual, transgender, and queer experience.

Abbie Nederhoed, LCSW (they/them) is a licensed clinical social worker and a therapist who specializes in kink, non-monogamy, and alternative relationship styles. As an educator, Abbie seeks to share from lived experience, bringing additional insight from their mental health and sex therapy training. One of their passions in mental health and kink is to create and hold space for others to explore their authentic self while honoring the fact that many have to mask their identities so as to keep themselves safe within the systems they navigate.

Michelle Thibeault, PT (she/her) is the founder and owner of Diversified Physical Therapy (DPT). In 1998 she graduated with a B.S. in physical therapy from the University of Hartford. In 1999 Michelle opened DPT, specializing in treating pelvic floor dysfunction, although she treats all types orthopedic diagnoses. In 2012 she graduated from the Sex Therapy Postgraduate Institute of New York as a sex counselor. She is also an energy medicine practitioner using various modalities of healing. In addition to her practice, she teaches workshops on a variety of topics.

Positionality Statement

The information I share with you has been accrued through the lens of a white, straight-presenting, cisgender woman moving through the world armed with the privilege inherent in these identities alongside my history, the identities of my family, and my financial and community status. What I find interesting, my curiosities, and the information my working memory retains is all inherently connected to all the parts of who I am, how I move through the world, and what my life has offered me in terms of growth and learning, struggle, and confusion. All information passes through my psychology, positionality, memory, and emotionality, and onto these pages in a way that is personal and unique to all the aspects of me, and therefore may be problematic to some. My proximity to power has gotten me here, and has caused harm to others, including communities, something I continue to reflect on in my learning.

In this sense the writings here reflect the places my inner world takes me, the areas my life and relationships have challenged me to explore, alongside my blind spots and hang-ups with the content areas I feel are not mine to speak to or that I do not have an evolved relationship with. The content is a developmental snap-shot of what I have studied as me, with the clients and therapists I have had the privilege to work with and learn from, within the cultures and societal structures I am embedded. I will miss the opportunity to speak to and represent communities, identities, experiences, and to draw from teachings that would provide a richness and critical perspective to the material, to our understanding of sex, of what it means to be human. I am hopeful that if this book is a starting point for some, it may inspire further learning and exploration, an ongoing befriending of this vast and complex part of who we are, and that the journey may lead you toward the multitude of brilliant voices that occupy this profession and those adjacent (sex educators and counselors).

What I bring to these pages is an understanding that I am and have benefitted from systems of power that have actively harmed my Black,

Indigenous, and People of Color (BIPOC) peers. I understand the privilege of being me, and the role it has played in my being here today (as much as I can). What I appreciate about the work of therapy and have come to understand about the enormous potential it holds for therapists and clients alike, is that it challenges us to constantly learn about ourselves, no matter the cost. It is the ultimate mirror, and there is no greater catalyst for growth and change, individually and therefore collectively. I'm looking forward to whatever continues to show up in my desire to understand the enormity and complexity of what sex is and can be and the many ways it may inform how I can continue to step into accountability, connection, and the kind of embodied understanding that creates lasting, profound change.

It's an honor to be growing alongside you.

Support Material

Additional material, including extended interviews and exercises, can be accessed online. Please go to routledge.com/9781032438399 and click on the link labeled Support Material. A link to the supplementary material will appear.

Introduction

What Sex Asks from Us

Do you like to dance? Do you enjoy the adrenaline that builds as you step out onto the floor? The weightlessness that is born from shedding the noise of the day, releasing tension as you catch up with the rhythm, eventually surrendering to the music, transported by the freedom that comes with pure, unbound movement, emotion, and energy? Some of us have had, or even do have, that kind of relationship with dancing. When *that* happens, it's pure magic. But how often is that your experience? How easy or challenging is it to step out on that dance floor, in the presence of others, maybe even in the presence of a particular other, and just dance despite the fact that we might be concerned about how our body looks to those around us as it moves, how our steps may or may not be out of synch, how challenging it is to let go of control, how safe or unsafe we may feel in our own skin or surroundings, how to choreograph our movements so that we look like we _____ (are confident, are "good" at dancing, are having fun, can blend in, are kind of sexy but not too sexy, and so on)? Fairly quickly something as inherently abstract, emotional, and primal as dancing can go from transcendent and liberating to uncomfortable and restrained with the simple introduction of our own complex, never-resting, self-aware, self-conscious brain and its "what ifs?" Sex is the same.

As a sex therapist, clients present in my office with a wide variety of sexual struggles, yet often also very narrow ideas about what to expect from therapy. Frequently, the impression is that I will hand them a few new positions to reignite the spark, strategies for initiating to "break through" the awkwardness, or that I will simply "fix their partner" (aka, make their partner what they would like them to be in order to enjoy the kind of sex they imagine they want) without digging into their lives, who they are, and how they see themselves outside of the bedroom in any meaningful way. These ideas, and others like them, reflect the ways we treat sex in our society: as an aspect of human life that is distinctly separate, compartmentalized, or walled-off from the other realms of who we are and how we navigate life and relationships. In this separate arena, sex gets reduced into

DOI: 10.4324/9781003369080-1

a series of behaviors that we move through in ways that we judge as skillful or not. It becomes something to fail or succeed at, largely dependent upon our technique, amount of experience, and ability to magically intuit how to pleasure others. Within this framework, sexuality and desire impossibly exist independently of mood, the goings-on in the life of the person and their relationship(s), the past, their present, sense of self-esteem, and so on. "Shoulds," expectations, performance, and control in the face of an experience that asks us to let-go over and over again in the midst of our own vulnerability is contradictory, and confusing, and the perfect breeding ground for anxiety; a feeling completely at odds with sexual arousal and functioning, and therefore a feeling we want to take very seriously.

If sex therapy lived up to its reputation by "staying in its lane," and addressing solely what lives on the surface of who we are sexually and how it manifests, we would be neglecting the critical role anxiety plays in our challenges, bypassing *the* primary barrier to pleasure, sensation, arousal, learning, connection, play, and fun. We would be missing the most vital aspects of the work that lead to meaningful, lasting change and a dynamic and ever-evolving sexual life (e.g. *I should be blowing their mind, I should cum from this, I should be better at* _____). The kind of sexual life that doesn't allow itself to get stale and perfunctory with time. The kind of sexual space that is dynamic and therefore adaptable to the ceaseless stream of changes that inevitably happen in the life of the individual or relationship. Without casting a wide net, and addressing the stew of emotion, psychology, and relationships that sexuality and sexual functioning is built from and of, the client with erectile dysfunction will continue to worry about whether their erections will last or show up at all. The client with performance anxiety will still be confronted with overwhelm and stress as they set about employing that new technique or position. And the client who has experienced sexual pain will still navigate the kind of tension that lives in the body as it braces for another potentially uncomfortable experience with sex, regardless of style.

Sex is endlessly more complex than we give it credit. We are endlessly more complex. The struggles that we encounter in the bedroom are made of so much more than meets the eye. Our anxiety, stress, worry, and fear (and therefore aversion, erectile dysfunction, early ejaculation, vaginismus, delayed ejaculation, etc.) are manifestations of our history and relationship to ourselves and others, connected in the present by a desire to step into an experience that asks us to risk, let-go, trust, and surrender. It also asks that we share, reveal, play, connect, express, attune, and respect and exercise boundaries. It requires us to be vulnerable, even with a stranger. These elements aren't optional: our physiological response, our arousal and pleasure, depends on a level (albeit never perfect) of comfort in our relationship to them both in and out of the bedroom. Anxiety can be found lurking within and among these elements as aspects of our humanity that we all struggle with to varying degrees, translated and manifest in sex. Addressing anxiety in the body and mind directly correlates to more freedom in the bedroom; it's that simple.

Who Am I?

As a young person, I studied sex to appear "cool" and "experienced," masking how frozen and stiff I felt when approaching the actual experience of it with others. I fantasized that friends and potential partners might imagine I was amazing in bed and that I clearly must be with my knowledge and comfort with the topic (keyword being *topic*). I studied sex because of how uncomfortable it made me, how completely disconnected I felt from my body and sensuality, and how entirely overcome with anxiety I felt trying to navigate it with partners. I did sex to get love, without ever understanding what my wants and desires were, how to speak to them, how to let-go in my body, how to be OK with my very small breasts and lanky physique. I was, and very much still am, the person very reluctantly and self-consciously stepping out onto the dance floor.

As an adult, I continue to study sex, not only because studying and working with sex is in-and-of-itself healing, but because the curiosity and fascination I began this journey with as a child expands with time. I'm a terribly anxious person with a complex and evolving relationship to my sexuality, and I help people navigate the same. I am in the same boat as my clients, which is inevitable, as we all are. I have the privilege of talking about sex all day: as a therapist with clients; as a supervisor, mentoring therapists on their path to sex therapy certification; and as an instructor of sex therapy. My familiarity with anxiety has enabled me to see the profound impact it has on our sexuality in every arena (understanding and living our gender expression, sexual orientation, our kinks, relationship structures, etc.), and it has revealed itself as the primary cause of the common sexual "dysfunctions" we've grown so familiar with (barring any medical or physiological diagnoses). Sex therapy is anxiety therapy.

How to Use This Book

Part I of the book will define anxiety, both in terms of our experience of it as an emotion and quality of thought, and as a physiological process. We will take a look at how it operates, how we succumb to its influence, and how and when it's useful. We will examine the physiology of anxiety and the ways it interrupts our sexual functioning directly, impeding the unfolding of arousal and our arousal processes in ways that we inadvertently reinforce.

In Part II, we will investigate the question "What is my anxiety trying to teach me?" by looking at common elements of socialization, upbringing, and culture that contribute directly to our experience of ourselves as sexual beings and inform our sexual behavior and experience in ways that are restrictive. By delving into areas including: our family of origin; race, religion, gender, sexual orientation; sexual trauma, sex and aging; and the ways in which sexual behavior and preference is pathologized, we come to understand how the ideas and values we've carried interfere with what sex asks of us (letting-go, surrender, vulnerability, sharing, revealing, connection, play), and how to relinquish them in favor of an embodied understanding of sex that is of our conscious choosing today.

With the sexual self-knowledge gained from Parts I and II, we jump into practice in Part III. We will learn through practical, actionable exercises and techniques how to minimize or even completely eliminate the influence of anxiety on our sexual experience and functioning, tapping into the ongoing learning, pleasure, and potential that can be found when we address its message. Specific sexual challenges will be addressed, in addition to a general framework for coming into a more intimate, embodied sexuality that allows for significantly greater ease in sexual interaction, both with one's self and others.

Moving Forward

What happens when we stay on the dance floor rather than listening to our anxiety and shuffling off? What happens sexually when we make different choices from greater insight, communicating different messages to the body, enabling an inner freedom that no longer depends on a lengthy list of requirements from our external context (aka: *I need to be in this kind of mood, with this kind of stimulation, avoiding these parts of the body, focusing on this particular thing, with this amount of control*)? What happens when we get out of our own way? This book *is* that exploration: a way to help you understand sex, help you understand yourself, in order to get you and your body on the same page, and out from underneath anxiety's grip. You will be picking up where you left off, or never even really began, in terms of evolving your understanding of yourself as a sexual being, with sexual values, wants, and desires that move and shift alongside you, because forging an intimate, accepting relationship with your sexuality is *the* gift that keeps on giving.

We all deserve a space where we can show up, let go, and connect – in a way that feels true to us now, in this moment, given the day we had, the feelings we're feeling, and what we're needing from sex right now. Can we give that to ourselves? *Letting-go* of the performance, *releasing* the fear, and *surrendering* to what is, at its core, an expansive, wild, and boundless love for self and others.

* * *

Who are we talking about when we refer to "we" in terms of the origins and ongoing influence of funky ideas and values around sex? Larger systems of oppression, colonialism, white supremacy, and religious ideology, among many others. And ourselves! We have carried forward and embodied harmful and limiting ideas, an inescapable consequence of being a human embedded in context. All of that and more is connected to sex, and all of it will surface as you read. The book is meant to reveal the questions; you get to determine the answers.

This is not a research essay, and I am not a researcher in a traditional sense (I simply don't have the brain for it). Nor does this book cover the vast array of cultural, societal, and historical influences on our ongoing sexual development as they interact with anxiety. The information contained in this book is the very condensed result of many years of conversation and learning with and from clients, students, and fellow therapists who have trusted me to journey alongside them and to oversee their cases.

Part I

Anxiety and Sex

When learning a new skill or trick or hobby, we are required to thoroughly think each step of it through so as to grasp it. Like learning how to drive: turning the car on, adjusting the mirrors, preparing to reverse out of the parking spot, checking the blind spots; it all feels so coordinated and complex as a beginner. The mind must diligently consider every aspect, including how to maneuver the body and navigate emotional experience, to assure our safety and move us along towards progress and proficiency. Gradually, complexity and stress turn into simplicity and ease, which transforms into instinct. Unless something interrupts that evolution, a scary close call or an actual accident that keeps us stuck in hyper vigilance. Sex is the same.

Getting to know the ins and outs of another person's body, of our own inclinations, or of the mechanics of our sexual functioning can feel as intimidating as getting behind that wheel as a rookie, perhaps even more so. The awkwardness, overwhelm, and insecurity inherent in those formative experiences are often buffered by the excitement and curiosity that grows in proportion to the increased comfort with ourselves, our process, those instincts. Once the manual-less logistics are no longer so foreign, so new and in need of our brain's thorough analysis and processing, higher-order thinking steps aside in favor of immersion into the emotional and sensory landscape, arousal and excitement emerging as defining characteristics rather than vague elements encouraging the continued, often clumsy, learning process. We begin to understand how to experience and express our sexuality rather than trying to interpret or strategize our way through it – if all goes as planned.

Sex is particularly susceptible to developmental interruption, to confusion that rolls itself into shame, anxiety, or even trauma as we struggle to meet its asks and bump into all the ways others struggle as well. With sex being primal, intuitive, and emotional at its core, when anxiety, panic, or

DOI: 10.4324/9781003369080-2

fear take hold as co-passengers in the experience, our thinking brain comes online, urgently directing our attention into "human cerebral" zone to make sense of the feelings. We can (and often do) get stuck here, calling upon the kind of logical problem-solving methods we might employ in the workplace to address our abstract sexual complexity. The difference between clumsy and nervous but excited exploration, and frantic problem solving, is meaningful to our sexual functioning. A "stress mind" is a place where sex refuses to live. Why?

In Part I of our journey, we will get clear on our understanding of anxiety, the physiology of it, and how it is at odds with the unfolding of our sexual arousal and functioning. We will turn to the body to understand what is actually required in order to access pleasure, orgasm, and a meaningful sense of maneuverability within our experience of arousal. This part of the book allows us to grasp the role that emotions play in our sexual struggles from a physiological perspective (spoiler alert – they are everything).

Nothing kills the mood like anxiety; and it turns out, for very real, very biological reasons.

1 What Is Anxiety?

Uncertainty, unknown, unpredictability – we grab for these words frequently to describe the most thrilling elements of life, like an adventure movie, a psychological thriller, or a real coming-of-age tear-jerker. Conversely, we can find these words in reference to the discomfort inherent in risk-taking (which can be found in nearly every decision we make in the absence of a guaranteed outcome) which for many of us might be more like an edge-of-your-seat, jump-scare horror film. Anxiety is what haunts us about that scary movie, the impression it left behind that appears and reappears as we lay our heads down to sleep (*What if an axe wielding maniac breaks into my home?*). Anxiety's "What ifs?" are *the* major inhibiting force in life, love, and intimacy, often found as the emotional outcome of hiding (sometimes of our own choosing, other times out of necessity) from ourselves and others.

Anxiety's stories, predictions, and physiological arrest can make a mess of our sex, obstructing any real view of the complexity of who we might be sexually, what our likes, dislikes, and desires are and (often very importantly) are not made of, impeding any real sense of trust in ourselves in our interactions, and completely derailing or interfering with our sexual functioning. It keeps us at the edge of our seat in our own bedrooms, even when *we know* the scary killer clown is dead.

So, what are its constituents? Why does it surface? And how does it operate? How might it be holding us back in ways that are not, or at least no longer, invited? To understand anxiety's unique hold on us sexually, we need to understand how to define it, understand our history with it, and bring awareness to the quality of our relationship to it in our everyday lives. Why? Because what we feel, how we think, relate, work, play, and rest inform our sexual wants, needs, and desires, and how we go about navigating these elements within ourselves and with others. Concurrently, how we "do" anxiety and what it's made of at the workplace, among peers, and out in the world lends itself to how we

DOI: 10.4324/9781003369080-3

experience and react to anxiety sexually. Our relationship to anxiety holds the key to understanding how this emotion has the potential to make (yes, that's possible) or break a sexual experience; how to go from sexually inhibited and under anxiety's thumb, to sexually liberated and able to spot, manage, and learn from the feeling when it shows itself (because it will, we're human).

Anxiety's Behavior and Reputation

Anxiety in the Body, Anxiety in-and-on the Mind

Anxiety describes both a physiological (sensory and nervous system reaction in the body) and neurological process that directly informs a quality and method of thinking and behavior, like all emotions do. I can feel anxious in my body without any thoughts accompanying the sensation, and/or I can find myself in an anxious pattern of thought that inspires physiological processes in the body that we can and often do grow accustomed to, and therefore miss. The psychology of anxiety often looks as follows. This emotion likes to:

1 Take a situation in the present (approaching a group of people you don't know well at a conference).
2 Reference the past in order to gain some sense of knowing or control over what might happen (*when I approached the "cool" kids in high school at lunch, they mocked me*).
3 Project an ominous prediction about what might happen onto the future (*I'm likely to say something awkward*).
4 Which then directly influences our behavior (*I'll just hang back*).

In other words, anxiety will draw inspiration from experiences in the past of a similar or relating nature to one we may be experiencing in the present, to alert us to the potential of harm in the sometimes very near, other times far-off, future. It reaches back into memories that were challenging, negative, or that felt like they were unsuccessful at best, to traumatic or humiliating at worst, as inspiration to create and cast its prediction. Consequently, the quality of the emotion tied to the memory is almost never proportionate to the current situation or scenario. It creates stories about what might happen that are all fairly, if not completely, catastrophic in nature, failing to reveal the often much-more-likely positive or neutral outcomes. We react to these predictions, the stories our anxiety creates for us, as if they're real rather than considerations, opportunities to think about if or how we might move forward and take care of ourselves at the same time. Our fear (the base feeling from which anxiety arises) overtakes our logic. Consequently, it can, and often does, immobilize us, preventing us from taking the necessary, healthy risks life requires for ongoing growth and momentum to unfold.

Anxious Thoughts Elaborated

"*You always* _____!" "*You never* _____!" Anxiety is invested in our immobility long-term, communicating that we should not only reject this risk now, but always. One strategy it employs towards this end is to erase the gray, in favor of entirely black-and-white, broad-stroke thinking. In fact, whenever we are in a heightened state of affect, this happens. The world we're dealing with, our ideas about what is transpiring or likely to take place, become win/lose, pass/fail, right/wrong, all or nothing. The enormity of the thoughts match the intensity of the feeling: anything less would be swallowed up, overlooked, or even completely unable to get through the physiological barrier the anxiety creates.

"You always let me down on our anniversary" – *so I'll resign to disappointment rather than putting myself out there and articulating my wants clearly, **risking** trusting that you may surprise me with more defined information.*

"You never stand up for me with your family" – *and I have this idea that I'm not good enough or worth fighting for, so instead of risking letting you see that insecurity and opening up about why this is so hurtful to me, I will wall myself off and distance from you.*

Do I risk movement, get brave and speak to the larger fear, or do I stay where I am? Which one is ultimately riskier? Ultimately scarier? Anxiety is directly tied to risk, to our perception of risk, and therefore it points us towards the places we experience the least amount of trust. Cornered, we have three options:

1 Seek to control;
2 Investigate what the lack of trust is ultimately made of and take action accordingly;
   and/or
3 Risk trusting.

Most of us reluctantly choose #3 every time we board a plane, whereas many of us default to #1 when dealing in romantic and sexual partnerships. The ways we navigate #1 are born from the anxious internal dialogue of the moment, and therefore often lack relational input, communication, or connection, placing us at greater risk of further challenges. For example:

A person with a penis loses their erection with a new partner, putting a complete halt to the encounter as they immediately launch into frustration and apologies whilst moving away physically. What are they assuming here? That the sexual interaction was a complete failure because of this one aspect of the experience? That the partner is disappointed, maybe even angry and in need of an explanation, totally averse to moving-on and playing in other ways? They're guessing that the erection is central to any pleasure that might've been had (a product of socialization) and therefore the experience must be over. Concluding the absolute worst.

Anxiety makes it so that we are quite literally unable to recognize or even notice the nuance, the possibilities that live in between "success" and "failure" (because there are so many!). It express routes us straight to the furthest ends of defeat (in this case), with all of the assumptions and stories that live there. What could an alternative scenario look like for this person and their erection? How would they even access ideas or conceive of options? If they were to visit the range of possibilities and their potential outcomes in the same way that we visit ideas for dinner, in an exploratory, curious, even-handed way, the situation may have looked entirely different. An even hand, though, requires an even temperament, that is our nervous system must be attended to first, something we practice doing in the moment, and creating room for with partners. Then, by bringing in a little honestly and curiosity alongside an adventurous spirit, we eliminate any jumping to conclusions that might have impeded further pleasure and fun. We quit trusting our own head and interact, despite how risky, or how scary, that might feel.

When under anxiety's influence relationally, our behavior at the status quo is riskier, if not far riskier, than communicating openly and honestly, centering reward that can include comfort, exploration, and/or connection as the goal, and attending to any feelings that come up on the part of the partner *if* and when they show up. So much more information surfaces as a result, information that we can use and work with rather than trusting our very rigid, black-and-white thinking and shutting the whole thing down – the ultimate act of control. We will talk explicitly about how to do this and not kill the mood, later.

On the Other Side of the Anxiety Wall

As a "heavy weight" emotion, anxiety squashes the more nuanced feeling states that live underneath it, keeping us from the necessary wisdom they bring. As an internal compass, emotions suggest our likes, dislikes, areas of curiosity, danger, our level of comfort, degree of trust, our yes's, no's, and maybe's. They are a primary means of learning about ourselves, every day all day; and the degree or level of intensity matters as additional information for understanding and considering. The difference between

I'm a little nervous about hooking up with this person and *I'm very nervous about hooking up with this person* may be a critically important distinction, helping us better serve or protect ourselves, make more informed decisions or risks, and assist in the determination of a "right course." Walking around with anxiety as our baseline creates a barrier to noticing "a little nervous," or accessing feelings that lack the intensity required to be identified, consequently inhibiting us from behaving according to these lesser degree feeling states, express routing us from what might have been slight frustration to big anger because where do we go from anxious? To volatile, as anxiety will add a charge to emotions powerful enough to get through the barrier it creates (ever get irrationally angry over something insignificant when anxious?). Lessening anxiety's influence or presence opens the door for expansive learning and discovery, on a much more minute, nuanced level, moment-by-moment. This learning is invaluable both in terms of what we come to understand about ourselves sexually, but also in terms of what we learn about ourselves in a general sense, strengthening and adding to our evolving sense of self. As an added bonus, by opening the door for more moderate feeling states, we make it easier to communicate, problem solve, and access creative solutions and ideas.

Our relationship to our feelings has a direct influence over the comfort we experience with sex – sex being an expression of feeling. Ever heard the saying, "*If you push an emotion down, it's in the basement lifting weights*"? When we try to separate ourselves from our feelings, they don't simply evaporate over time, they remain, accumulating and acquiring greater magnitude and intensity as they are joined by other unprocessed, unfelt emotions and the messages they carry. Anxiety, therefore, can also be a manifestation of a collection of feelings. That is, *if I don't acknowledge, process, and feel my grief, rage, confusion, it will collect in my body and psyche and bleed out as anxiety.* This anxiety is ultimately alerting us to distrust and/or threat in the face of our own emotional complexity because we've internally communicated and reinforced the message that our feelings are not safe to feel in a general sense, that they're a disturbance and not to be let in. When we distrust our own emotions, or feel we need to wall them off from ourselves and others, we will inevitably struggle letting-go into an experience characterized and built by emotional expression – we will struggle to enjoy sex. Unless sex is the exception, the only or primary place where I allow myself to feel my feelings, it *is* that simple.

Anxiety as Diagnosis

Historically, we've talked about anxiety as pathology. You "have" anxiety like you "have" chronic migraines, an unwelcome struggle (often thought of as primarily medical in origin) that some, but not everyone, has to interact or cope with on a regular basis. Anxiety has distinguished itself as one of the few emotions deserving of being recognized as a diagnosable disorder, a curious aspect of our relationship to it culturally. Many people find themselves plagued by feelings like anger and grief, and yet these feelings are not given the status of a diagnosis, as conditions we can or should treat with medication. And yet, anxiety *can* be paralyzing, interfering with our ability to take necessary steps in life: ask that person out, go for that new job, and even at its most severe, leave the house. It can become a feeling that walks around with us all day, becoming so practiced that we can no longer identify its presence, influence, or even the sensations that accompany it in the body. It can begin to feel like the anxiety *is* us. In this way anxiety, like some of its siblings and cousins, can be thought of as existing on a spectrum both in terms of the actual experience of the emotion in relation to other higher/lesser degree feeling states (from nervousness to anxiety to panic and/or paranoia), and in terms of its influence (from an occasional visitor that we recognize in terms of accompanying thoughts and feeling sensations in the body, to *the* driving presence in our lives, completely at the wheel, informing every move we make throughout our day, week, lives). That's powerful stuff! Still, the unintended consequence of creating a disorder out of a human emotion is that it introduces the misguided idea that anxiety is not normal, and certainly never helpful; that we don't all suffer under the enormity of the feeling, the hold it can have on our thoughts, the influence it has over our decisions and behavior, the consequences it can have on our physical health. Without exception, no one is exempt. We all struggle here. Acknowledging the struggle allows us to get to know our anxiety more intimately. Getting to know it more intimately paradoxically creates a separation from it. Within that separation lies the ability to make different choices, act with intentionality, extract the useful information from it (because it always illuminates important information), and take back control so that we can then let go of control, when and where it matters most.

All in the Family

"I have anxiety, my Dad had it too. It runs in the family." Anxiety is often contextualized as something that is "handed down" the family line, which can be accurate, but like everything it's complicated. It's true that anxiety is part of what it means to be alive and aware, but we are not *necessarily* destined to be a particular caliber of anxious because of any biological predisposition to the feeling. Feelings simply do not operate that way. There is no research to indicate an "anxiety gene," rather a combination of genetic factors that interplay to increase susceptibility. It feels fair to call this combination of factors "our temperament." Temperament plays a role in how we relate to the world around us, how we experience emotion, including the intensity of feelings. That intensity or sensitivity directly influences how reactive we are to our emotional experience, to anxiety producing thoughts, experiences, or situations. But anxiety needs content to work with in order to *be* anxiety, just as anger needs experience of violation or harm in order to be anger. We are not always able to identify its story, but it works with one or some in order to exist.

On the "nurture" side of the nature vs. nurture pie, anxiety can be identified as a family process, a feeling that gets embedded in the system and organizes the players accordingly. One person feels particularly anxious, which then influences their behavior, which then informs how others interact with and behave around them, and thus the family orients itself around the anxiety; a process we become familiar with and can carry forward into our adult relationships. To identify this process more acutely in our own lives, it is meaningful to recognize the many faces anxiety can take on as it manifests. Anxiety doesn't always look anxious, it can look like chronic agitation, a temper, worry, reactivity, volatility, hyperactivity, under-functioning, over-functioning, controlling, mistrust (of self and others), selfishness, and/or emotional shut-down. So hypothetically, if we have an uncle with a temper who can be experienced by those around him as frightening when his temper flares, holidays look a lot like the family tip-toeing around him, acquiescing to his point of view, accommodating or shrugging off his monologues about politics in the name of peace. To manage our own anxiety about Uncle's behavior, we attempt to control or contain his, which is an anxiety-inducing endeavor.

Coping and Adaptation

Control, Control, Control

How do we react to anxiety? What is our most common, go-to strategy? We reach for control where and when we can get our hands on it in our immediate environment, and then white-knuckle our grip (or double-down). While it can feel like relief in the moment, it does nothing to address the information that inspired the feeling in a way that effectively resolves the worry, heartache, or trauma long-term, as we are looking in the wrong direction (i.e. *I'm reading through your emails and texts multiple times a day but I must continue to do it daily because it's not answering the question of why you strayed, it is doing nothing to address my insecurities about who I am in this relationship, who I am to you*). Answers to the wrong or misplaced questions only bring more questions, and the anxiety becomes a bottomless pit. It inadvertently keeps the anxiety comfortably in place. How do we sniff out where anxiety has taken up the most space in your life? Where do you exercise or feel inclined to exercise the most control? What lives underneath that inclination? What are you actually reacting to?

Putting Out Fires

> Notice how fear itself does not equal anxiety. Fear is an adaptive learning mechanism that helps us survive. Anxiety, on the other hand, is maladaptive; our thinking and planning brain spins out of control when it doesn't have enough information.
>
> (Brewer, 2022, p. 17)

Life is one series of unknowns after another, on a minute-to-minute, day-by-day basis. Very rarely do we have adequate information and learning from the past to help us understand what similar situations in the present might mean. Despite never experiencing the same exact situation twice, living an identical moment, we are constantly drawing from and relying on past experience to help us determine relative safety, understand our options, and make informed or advantageous choices moment-by-moment. When a situation *feels* safe based on the memories and associations it brings forward from the past (very often found in lower-stake scenarios that we experience with greater regularity), we risk with greater ease! For example, *when I went to the restaurant I frequent last week, it wasn't super crowded so I think I have a decent shot at grabbing a table again.* However, the ability to play-out scenarios when planning for the future becomes compromised, the missing and limited information and therefore lack of trust boldly present, when the situation feels more high-stakes and exceptional; anxiety understands this. *When I went to that restaurant last week, it wasn't super crowded, but what if it is tonight and I have to stand there awkwardly, trying to make a good impression on my date?* Both examples reference the past, but the second scenario contains more unknowns, limited information to draw from, and a higher investment in outcome: *if I go on my own and don't get a table, no big deal, I'll just leave or look at my phone while I wait. If I go with my date and we have to wait, I might have to deal with discomfort that could look like grasping for shallow small talk, difficulty knowing how to respond or what questions to ask, awkward attempts at eye contact.* Consequently, we can find ourselves responding to its stories with problem solving, focusing on the object of our anxiety, and working to find a solution, only to find another anxiety story/dilemma eagerly waiting in the wings:

- *If there's a wait, we can go outside.*
  - *If we go outside, we might miss our name being called.*
- *While we wait inside, I could ask about their day.*
  - *It might be too loud to hear if its crowded and people are piling in.*
- *I could go grab us a drink while they stay back to wait for our table to be ready.*
  - *Will they think I drink too much if I rush off to the bar?*

Anxiety is parasitic, latching onto the next best target (sex is an incredibly easy one, by the way!). We will put out fires one after the next, on a loop, until we shift our focus from the thing in our immediate environment, the target object or scenario, to the feeling itself. Dr. Siggie Cohen, a child development specialist, demonstrates this process when working with children (i.e. in interaction with an adult):

> I can see you're feeling scared right now (not scared of this ... or that ... just scared). I know being scared doesn't feel good at all, it's actually quite terrible. And when we're scared, all of us, we want the fear to go away. And it can! If we stand up to it from the inside. We tell ourselves, "I'm scared, and I don't like it. But I am also safe. I am going to be ok."
>
> (Cohen, 2024)

Our internal dialogue (because we can do this for ourselves) will look the same or similar. Take the following example when working with anxiety that surfaces sexually:

> I am feeling anxious right now. I can feel tension in my chest and my heart is beating fast. I am also safe. I am safe and will continue to stay here. It's ok for me to release, I'm letting go of tension in my body.

Anxiety vs. Stress

We simply cannot talk about anxiety without talking about stress, as the distinctions between them are hard to pin down. They can present similarly, often nearly identically physiologically, and when it comes to your sexual arousal and functioning, your body doesn't differentiate between the two. Both register a lack of safety; both can derail sexual functioning. In terms of our own working definition, the major distinction has to do with our conceptualization of the stressor; it has to do with our relationship to what is known versus the unknown future, be it immediate or far off. As mentioned, anxiety is born from the possibilities that exist that have yet to be determined. It attempts to fill in the void. Stress, on the other hand, is a reaction to a known event or situation, a perceivable threat. *How will we make it to the airport on time when we forgot to get gas and it's 15 minutes out of the way? How will I make that 3 p.m. deadline when I still have so much work to do?* In this way, stress is often triggered by something external and known and in need of management, versus anxiety which is often born from internal dialogue and storytelling in the presence of possibility, the trigger of which *can be* elusive or harder to identify. Management of known variables versus storytelling and catastrophizing about the unknowns.

The two can exist alongside one another in addition to dancing together in a complex interplay. Anxiety can take the stressor (that 3 p.m. deadline) and run with the potential consequences of falling short or elaborating on the things that could go wrong when trying to get there. Quite the dynamic duo.

Upsides to Stress? Positives to Feeling Anxious?

Can stress be useful? Can anxiety be useful? People are often reluctant to work on their anxiety or stress in any meaningful way, crediting it for their productivity, upward mobility at work, or ability to keep the house and family running smoothly and efficiently. It seems our anxiety about lessening anxiety's influence takes us to the opposite side of the spectrum, moving us from feeling overrun by anxiety to imagining the complete and utter absence of it. Don't be fooled, there is no such thing as eliminating anxiety or stress. There *is* such a thing as managing and transforming our relationship to it. Motivated, hard-working, diligent, organized: these are qualities that can exist underneath anxiety for the hypothetical person above that can fan the flames of the feeling. Qualities that suggest an investment in the outcome of our work that can make it all feel high-stakes, which anxiety loves. Changing our relationship to anxiety doesn't take away these important and useful qualities, just as it doesn't take away the anxiety. You are still you, just with a different perspective, armed with different tools, more at the wheel in terms of how you relate to your feeling states, anxiety included.

Anxiety and stress, like all emotions, are useful information, important to our experience and learning insomuch as they flow through us, passing as we see the feeling, feel the feeling, receive its message, and then let it be/ go. Easier said than done. Moving through our feelings is something we have to practice with ourselves and partners, it is a muscle to exercise, a skill to build, and it can look different every time as certain emotions require more attention, more processing, more feeling into. The ability to recognize anxiety and stress, for example, and to understand what it is alerting us to, accurately and proportionately, requires substantial and deliberate self-attunement and awareness, the ability to notice/witness one's own experience unfold, just as we practice in meditation.

This tightening in my chest and jaw is anxiety, I'm feeling anxious.
   What am I responding to?
      I perceive my partner acting strangely and I'm worried they've been drinking.
         What would it mean to me if they had been drinking?
            That they don't have any regard for my feelings and would rather risk our relationship than adhere to our boundaries.
               What needs to be communicated? What questions do I need to ask before trusting my anxiety?
                  What does my body need from me right now?

It is when our feelings get stuck, hung-up on, or suppressed that they become problematic, spiraling into frenzied thoughts, controlling behavior, reactivity, and restless nights; and this often happens in an "unconscious" or disconnected state. Feelings that begin as something else entirely, such as sadness, disappointment, grief, or anger, transform into anxiety when held in the body, "swallowed" or "pushed down," unable to be processed, felt, released. One way or another, they demand our attention; and we want them to! The challenge is in understanding how to extract the meaningful information they carry, how to locate it to allow the feeling to move through. This requires that we come closer, slow down, feel, and get curious, which is a counter-intuitive move, particularly with anxiety.

Wrapping Up

Our anxious thoughts will always be compelling: it's something we should expect. Anxiety draws inspiration from the most challenging experiences we've collected, the most meaningful material. When powerful enough, it can feel like its tactic is to bully, wear down, but in clever and often creative ways. It can dress itself up as instinct, intuition, or insight; as *the* master of disguises. Anxiety gives us information, it points us toward our bruises, wounding, barriers to intimacy, areas in need of healing. When it isn't given the power to be the big bully, anxiety is a concerned co-passenger asking you to consider putting on your seatbelt in case of an accident. Anxiety and stress alert us to areas of caution in life, granting us forethought, promoting planning and safe and responsible behavior. It is trying to tell us why we struggle, but it shows us in movies of thing right in front of us rather than giving us their origin story, or the collection of themes the stories touch upon that have less to do with the current situation and more to do with our relationship to ourselves.

Let's end with Carly's story, to put it all together:

> *I start to feel really anxious when my partner starts trying to make me cum. I imagine her disappointment when it doesn't happen, thinking she'd done something wrong, wondering if we're even compatible … at least sexually. My last partner just got so frustrated and took it so personally. So, I just fake it. I check out and pretend.*

Present-moment situation: Partner trying to make me cum.

Past reference: Ex's frustration and taking my inability to reach orgasm personally.

Projected prediction: My partner is going to be disappointed when I don't cum when or how she thinks I should or ought to, or at all.

Action taken: Fake orgasm, pretend enjoyment, check out of experience.

What anxiety could be illuminating: Performance narratives, difficulty communicating, lack of connection to body, difficulty letting-go, challenges with trust (self and/or other), "trying" too hard (tension in the body).

Sexually, the anxiety we experience is completely connected to larger ideas and beliefs we carry about who we are, who we ought to be, what we should be feeling, how we need to be experienced, and what our worth is made of. What is your sex-related anxiety showing you that has nothing to do with sex whatsoever? What's under the hood of your car?

*

Anxiety is a pain, a barrier, an immobilizing force, and also a great teacher. Let's get to know how it operates physiologically, the effect it has on our sexual functioning, and where to begin building an understanding of how to work with your body to cultivate trust, ease, access to sensation, and the sense of control it steals away.

2   Sex as a Natural Function

If we want to jump higher, we try harder. If we want to run faster, we push harder. If we want to feel stronger, we work harder. What we understand our relationship to our bodies to mean when we want them to do something for us is frequently tied to effort, control, focus, and strategy. And yet, if we place what sex asks of us (letting go, vulnerability, expression, sharing, revealing, connection, play) at one end of the spectrum, the elements of striving, powering through, working, controlling, and managing live solidly at the opposing end. Attempting to get our bodies to experience pleasurable sensation, orgasm, and arousal while the heart and mind are endeavoring toward a specific outcome and/or interacting with challenging thoughts and emotions that send a general message of lack of comfort or safety to our systems is a losing game; much like trying to enjoy a dinner out when you've landed the extra chatty, won't-leave-your-table server. There's no room for pleasure to emerge within the tension resistance brings in that space between "what I want" and what is actually happening. But how do we free ourselves of that tension, and the "strive" mentality we often default into with sex when we've been told our sexuality is something we need to "do" in a particular way (gender specific) with a particular level of skill, according to a particular script? We identify and address barriers, risk, and let go. Sounds simple, but what are we letting go *of* exactly? Precisely why is this element so critically important to the unfolding of arousal? And what are the prerequisites?

When anxiety surfaces in the face of the unknown, we reach for control. This can look like the active pursuit of information (from simple answer seeking to obsessive digging), taking action according to anxiety's agenda (e.g. *I better work harder towards orgasm or my partner will think I'm not having a good time*), and/or looking to substances, ritualized behaviors, and escapism (which can be as simple as distraction, or as severe as reckless and dangerous acting out). When we get anxious during a sexual experience, or when we perceive that we want the situation to look or feel different, we attempt to manage or control our bodies, physiology, and our

DOI: 10.4324/9781003369080-4

sexual functioning much as we attempt to control other aspects of life. This logic makes sense (*I was able to get myself to run faster to win the race, so I can most assuredly make my orgasm happen in synch with my partner*) if sex were a submissive partner. Very fortunately, it is not.

Natural Functions

Most of us have heard of Bill Masters and Virginia Johnson, the gynecologist and his assistant who formed a research team in the late 1950s dedicated to the study of human sexual response and to the treatment of sexual dysfunctions. Yet, despite their fame, what can most of us identify in terms of what their contributions to the field actually looked like? Actually meant? Although their work has been critiqued and expanded upon with time, they were pioneers, and their partnership has given us so much in terms of our understanding of how sex operates and how our bodies respond to sexual stimulation. One take-away of particular importance has to do with control and our sexual physiology, namely the business of *natural functions*.

What is a natural function? It is a neurophysiological process with which:

- One is born;
- Cannot be taught;
- Is not under our direct voluntary command/control (i.e. we cannot make or prevent it from happening).

(Weiner & Avery-Clark, 2017)

Processes that fall under this category include digestion, bladder and bowel function, respiration, and – our sexual functioning.

Natural processes involved in sexual functioning include:

- Erection;
- Lubrication;
- Orgasm;
- Arousal at large.

We cannot make digestion happen or not happen any more than we can force arousal to do or not do the same. *Our sexual functioning is not under our direct voluntary control.* "Conscious demand to directly control a natural function creates anxiety, and anxiety interferes with the expression of any natural function" (Weiner & Avery-Clark, 2017, p. 12). That is, attempting to intervene and exert control is the number one cause of sexual dysfunction. One example of how this can unfold is:

- We begin engaging sexually with a partner.
- Anxiety surfaces as the experience moves along and we begin to worry or even just "think" about how things will go, forecasting the likely events, anticipating any difficulties.
- Anxiety and/or lack of presence (being in our head/thinking through sex rather than "in" our bodies, sensation, the experience itself) introduces tension into the body and we begin to "try" or "work" at having sex.
- The harder we try, the more swiftly our bodies shut arousal down, the more we guarantee arousal (lubrication, erections, ejaculatory control, heightened sensation) will not return in this particular interaction.

So how much control *do* we have over how our bodies behave sexually? If we can't stop or interrupt when our bodies are doing something we don't want them to do like preparing to ejaculate earlier than we'd like, or taking too long to get there, can we encourage along things like arousal, orgasm, and erections?

Head Games

When I want to get myself turned-on, I like to focus on my partner's jawline. I know it sounds weird, but when he wants me, he sort of clenches his jaw in a way that makes me crazy. I'll look for it on him, or I'll imagine it. It just feels like he's containing his desire, that there's this power in him that is trying to burst out. I feel simultaneously intimidated yet protected and safe. It's a small thing, but so hot.

(Steph)

Who knows what that "clenching" actually *is* for her partner, and who cares? Steph has created a story about what that visual may mean that brings excitement and anticipation to the experience, heightening her arousal, bringing her deeper into the fantasy element of the interaction, furthering her connection to sensation. If Steph attempted to find that feeling but got caught up on if or how much her armpits smelled from the day, which then moved into what her partner might think if he caught a whiff of any body odor, informed by what that has represented for her and in her social/cultural context (i.e. unhygienic, sloppy, unclean, lacking self-awareness), we're no longer working with desire and arousal whatsoever, just like that distracting dinner. Emily Nagoski, author of *Come as You Are: The Surprising New Science that Will Transform Your Sex Life* (2015), discusses this effect our thoughts have on our desire and arousal, specifically our brain's tendency to sort sexually relevant stimuli and/or aspects of our context and environment into two categories that either heighten desire and arousal (our accelerators), or dampen and extinguish desire and arousal (our brakes). What content or information (visual, thought, sensation, fantasy) do we attend to and attach meaning to that accelerates or amplifies our desire and arousal, versus pumps the brakes on these internal and physiological experiences and processes? The brain is at the helm here with both, but its role shifts and evolves throughout the experience, often leading us in one of two directions:

- The brain can assist the body in an ongoing way as it moves into total absorption in sensation, connection, and potentially orgasm, weaving thought and fantasy throughout, in a sort of back and forth dance toward surrender and/or climax; or
- It can lead us further into focused thinking, detached from the body and sensation entirely, away from connection and orgasm, working hand-in-hand with anxiety.

Interacting with and focusing on sensation in an intentional way can be one powerful exit out of the kind of mind chatter that feeds our breaks and inhibits the natural function of sexual response from unfolding. Coming deeper into our sensory experience challenges us to let go of (as opposed to "resist," which only creates tension) the thoughts that threaten submersion in our experience, in pleasure. We will practice this in Part III.

Letting Go vs. Surrender

Sexual experience can be thought of as a sort of "shedding," whereby we're asked to release layers upon layers of our conditioning, our armor, our defenses, our performance, the many scripts we carry with us that we've collected over the years, all with instructions about how to be something or someone else "better" than who we perceive we are. It asks us to let go of the stronghold we have on our external environment and the control we attempt to maintain over how it operates (which is only possible with the ability to exercise, respect, and negotiate boundaries). It asks us to trust sensation, our bodies, our instincts, emotions, and other elements (if present), and immerse ourselves in an experience beyond ourselves.

Relationally, we release or let go of unwanted or uninvited intellectual content, physical tension, or mental state in the presence of a degree of trust (or when deliberately and knowingly risking trusting ourselves or partners even when it's hard – this doesn't have to be perfect). Letting go is something we do, all at once or over-and-over again as we move through a sexual experience; surrender is the outcome, the breakthrough. It is the point at which we are no longer tethered to any particular aspect of our experience: we are being carried through it. When people describe a transcendent or even spiritual experience of sex, they have broken through into surrender.

> When we surrender we give up, but not in the way we think giving up means. We don't give up to or on the situation, but rather, we give up the notion that we should be able to or can manage the situation, that we can control any of it. We give up the belief that we can make reality different than what it is. As much as we are conditioned to never give up, in the case of surrender giving up the mistaken belief that we are in charge offers a profound relief.
>
> (Colier, 2016)

Getting out of the Way

We feel safer being in control, we feel more powerful with control. Without it we can feel lost, insecure, irresponsible, small, unproductive, disoriented, vulnerable. We lean into control when we want people to be and do and behave in ways that make us comfortable; we lean into control when we want situations to be what we want them to be to assure a good time, impress others, hide our insecurities. This is human nature, an unavoidable characteristic of what it means to be in relationship with others, to want comfort while minimizing pain.

When it comes to sex, we lean into control when we want the experience to be what we need it to be to get the love we crave, fit the story of the "ideal sex life," satisfy the ego, avoid our trauma. Over time we trick ourselves into believing that more control in the face of our anxiety equals less anxiety, less potential for disaster, when control begets control. We must work harder to maintain it as the anxiety that inspired it goes undigested, undealt with in a meaningful way, avoided but still there; its message of catastrophe waiting in the wings, organizing our experience, exerting powerful influence. Control disguises itself as the answer to our sexual anxiety when it is a day-old band aid that we must continuously press back on, each time with less and less success. When our sexual functioning necessitates release and risk, we are faced with the dilemma of confronting what control helps us hide. Sex asks many things of us, one being honesty.

When we think about breathing, it often makes it harder to breathe. Sex is the same.

3   Our Physiology and Sexual Functioning (Vaguely Defined)

> Is this the right time to have sex? Am I safe emotionally, physically, psychologically? Is this a task to complete, something to manage, or work at? I'm in my head about this, it must not be the time to play, connect, and share intimate parts of who I am and how I love. I will manage our physiology accordingly.
>
> (Your nervous system)

In sex therapy, we listen to what the conscious mind can process, interpret, and make meaning of, while concurrently zooming-in on what the body is communicating both in the therapy room and in the bedroom, and why and how it *always* makes sense. Even in the midst of very real medical concerns that are known to impact sexual functioning such as diabetes or multiple sclerosis, the client's psychological relationship to their medical diagnosis, the anxiety that accumulates around it, and its role in whatever is going on sexually is teased out and differentiated from the issue itself as far as is possible with an in-depth look at behavior, physiology, relationality, thought, and feeling. The ways in which the body is behaving – leading up to, at the beginning of, in the middle, and at the concluding phases of arousal (if we move through all three) or sexual experience – illuminates the impact of the medical diagnosis versus where the thoughts and feelings of the person themselves are directly dictating a physical response.

Collectively, we have grown to appreciate that the mind and body work together in this way, informing one another and potentially wreaking havoc on our immune system, relationships, and sexual lives – if we ignore the signs and signals they give us. Yet even the notion that they are connected somehow misrepresents how deeply they affect and influence one another, how profoundly attuned they are to each other, and how they are truly parts of a whole, complete, and cohesive system.

Precisely how attuned is the mind to the body and vice versa when it comes to your sexual functioning and the processes that unfold alongside

DOI: 10.4324/9781003369080-5

the moving and shifting of your emotional states? Why is this question important? Because with this knowledge comes the ability to start working with your body and what it is communicating moment-by-moment rather than working against it without even knowing that's what you're doing. The sabotage stops here.

Sympathetic vs. Parasympathetic Nervous Systems

Our nervous system is a system of systems, like our body at large. It is a complex control center responsible for transmitting signals from the brain to the body via the spinal cord. There are parts and subparts involved in this complex operation, but what we will focus on is the branch of the nervous system that is directly responsible for sexual arousal or lack thereof: our autonomic nervous system and, more specifically, the sympathetic and parasympathetic nervous systems that are housed within it.

The autonomic nervous system (or the involuntary nervous system) regulates physiologic processes that are not under our direct or voluntary control (our natural functions). It provides nerves to your internal organs such as your heart, diaphragm, intestines, stomach, and genitals. Their activities are largely reflexive. The presence of food in the stomach, for example, triggers a series of reflexes that cause digestion. We can't make it stop or cause it to happen any faster. The same thing is true of the genitals. A touch on the penis can trigger a reflexive erection, or a touch to the opening of the vagina can trigger reflexive vaginal lubrication (Keesling, 2006, p. 30).

The sympathetic nervous system is responsible for the rapid spread of energy in the body. It initiates our fight, flight, freeze, and overall stress response. When activated, our heart rate picks up, eyes dilate, muscles tighten, breathing becomes rapid and shallow. Blood moves away from the genitals and the surface of the skin and toward our large muscle groups (flight or fight), or our vital organs (freeze).

The parasympathetic nervous system, on the other hand, is responsible for the conservation of energy or our rest/digest response. When active, our heart rate, breathing, and blood pressure slow and blood moves freely throughout the body. It helps the body restore and find homeostasis after a stressful or high energy event, or simply at the end of each day while in rest or sleep.

Our sexual arousal cycle gets activated, lives, and thrives under the para-sympathetic nervous system response. This is why people with penises experience nocturnal erections or emissions and some people with vulvas describe waking-up to or experiencing profound sexual arousal during sleep or just after waking. By and large, when one system is on the other is off. There is a complex interplay between the two, but the excitation associated with sexual arousal that gets kicked up in the body is predicated on a foundation of release or comfort. Despite how contradictory it sounds, the body is very capable of remaining released and at ease while also welcoming arousal, excitement, and the progressive build of energy and tension that moves us toward and culminates in orgasm. It can maintain both ends of this spectrum at the same time: our body's sexual stirrings while in slumber prove this to be true. Release in the body is the prerequisite. Without the intervention of our conscious mind and any emotional, physical, or psychological worry-or-stress-based tension that accompanies it, our bodies are naturally released, relaxed, and know what to do to carry us along.

The Critical Sleep Link

Sleep is a natural function governed by our parasympathetic nervous system. Falling asleep is a process of letting-go, moment-by-moment, eventually breaking through into surrender, as is sexual responsiveness. Falling asleep and sleep itself connects us deeply with the fantasy realm (that we are always in touch with to significant degrees throughout our day) as we rewind and replay the events of our day or create stories that invite release. Our sexuality does the same, thrusting us into a fantasy realm, into the power of the stories we imagine, react to, and potentially play out (of or related to our partner in the moment, or connected to erotic visualizations and story) that deepen immersion in sensation and connection. When we are in fantasy space, we are walking that line between conscious storytelling and subconscious working through and processing of our lived realities. With sexual arousal and surrender, our fantasy experience deepens further into the control of our subconscious brain as we are "taken" by emotion, sensation, and connection. With sleep, our fantasy experience deepens further into the control of our subconscious brain as we are "taken" by release, rest, and our physiology. Why are these parallels important? They help us understand why the way we approach sex *has* to be different from how we approach the vast majority of other aspects of our lives, as an experience made from and characterized by letting go and trusting your body and mind to do the rest. Sexual functioning and sleep are siblings.

Sleep:

- As I *"fall" asleep I begin to* **let go** *of the stressful parts of the day, the argument I got into with my spouse, that 3 p.m. deadline tomorrow, that tense encounter with my boss.*

- *I increasingly bring forward imagery and stories that allow me to fall deeper into a trance state. I let go into* **fantasy**.
- *As I continue to let go, deeper and deeper into fantasy and sensation, I* **surrender** *to sleep.*

Arousal:

- *As I* **let go** *into sensation and emotion, I compartmentalize or let go of the stressful parts of the day, the argument I got into with my partner, that 3 p.m. deadline tomorrow, the tense encounter with my boss.*
- *I increasingly sink into imagery or visuals (of the person with me, via the workings of my imagination, or explicit media) that envelop me in* **fantasy**, *taking me deeper into a trance state.*
- *As I continue to let go, deeper and deeper into sensation, emotion, and arousal, I* **surrender** *to orgasm, or pleasure, or release.*

Releasing and relinquishing control can be challenging. Yet, if we can "fall" into sleep, we know how to let go into parasympathetic response, even if this is the only place we can identify doing so in our lives. It's a starting point we have access to. Rest, digest, restore – our sexual functioning is restorative, a version of rest (even when it's wild), a way of rediscovering and clearing the emotional, psychological, and physiological tension via connection and catharsis; a regaining of homeostasis, a coming back to "center." This journey our sex can take us on when real surrender is present is not one-dimensional; rather it offers a wide range of emotional experience and physical sensation to bring us back to center. Do we dare let it be complex? Do we have an option?

So, let's pick our poison:

- Partner A, who is in their body, who comes alive through sex, and who passionately cries for more or produces intense tears and shaking right after orgasm, depending on the day.
- Or Partner B, who is not in their body, who is clinically, quietly, and stiffly moving through technique they learned in a book about how to "pleasure their partner," in the same way they might inspect your body for an ingrown hair or apply medicine to a wound.

The reality is that these *are* our choices ultimately, or at least we should expect them to be. If we're not hiding, holding back, or performing, we are disarmed, truly naked in all senses of the word: raw, exposed, vulnerable. Our physiology asks us to step in and allow the body to do the rest, we have to step into bravery and risk in order to trust and jump. We do a version of this every night as we lay our heads down alongside our fears, and sleep.

Activating the Sympathetic Nervous System with Ease

Therapist: You've described noticing that you lose your erection predictably in the moments just prior to penetration. Do you ever lose your erections on your own? When engaging in self-touch?

Client: Sometimes, but not as predictably. I get a little stressed even on my own. I was raised to believe you aren't supposed to masturbate, let alone think about anyone outside of your partner while doing it. I always feel slightly guilty or wrong or something every time. I'm also never really able to get rid of the worry that I might lose my erection and there's something wrong with my body, even by myself, so I can get in my head a little there too.

Therapist: Do you ever wake up with an erection? Experience them in the morning or middle of the night?

Client: I do, the very early morning is when I can usually maintain my erections with the greatest ease.

Playing stress detective, where can you spot some sources of it? We know right away with this client that anxiety, stress, and perhaps guilt and shame follow him into his solo sexual life. How challenging might it be for him to feel at ease in his body while contending with "slightly guilty" or "wrong"? Can he even recognize the tension when it's likely been with him his entire adult life, perhaps even longer?

By digging into his words, we begin to confront and break down the stress itself. His physiology will yield to his psychology every time, so this is a must. This might look like the following:

1 *"Raised to believe you aren't supposed to masturbate"* What were the sexual values you were exposed to? Beliefs around sex and sexuality from family, culture, religion of origin? How do you feel about these ideas now, as an adult? Do your beliefs and values differ? If so, what's that like?

2 *"Let alone think about anyone outside of your partner while doing it"* What does your fantasy life look like? What exactly are the "shoulds" you hold in relation to it? Let's list them out and get really clear about what rules are at work behind the curtain.

3 *"I always feel slightly guilty or wrong or something every time"* How does that manifest? Are these feelings with you throughout the entire experience, or do they show up immediately after? How do you give yourself permission to move into sensation? What thoughts attempt to take it away?

Like a surgeon, the client and therapist go in as deeply as they can into the anatomy of the anxiety this person is experiencing sexually in order to understand what is influencing and triggering the activation of the sympathetic nervous system. If we want lasting change, the slower we go in this process, the more quickly progress is felt and observed. Rushing means missing vital clues and learning while simultaneously undermining the foundation of release characteristic of the parasympathetic nervous system response and required for our sexual functioning to come online. We want to identify and address as many sources of stress and anxiety in the body and mind as are reachable, exorcising the tension, and opening as many pathways to ease and absorption as possible.

Wrapping up the Nervous System

The second a palpable moment of stress comes to life, your brain registers a lack of emotional safety (sex as performance, *my needs don't matter*, self-criticism, shame, and so on) and we switch over from our parasympathetic nervous system (rest, digest, restore) to our sympathetic nervous system response (fight, flight, freeze). When the slightest bit of cortisol, or stress hormone, hits our bloodstream, the body is trying to understand what kind of threat it is working with and how to overcome or bypass it, which can translate as emotionally shutting down, getting overwhelmed, "powering through," or getting in our heads and trying to think through the experience. All the while, blood is on the move and very quickly away from all the places we need it to be in order for lubrication to happen with vulvas, erections to last with penises, and sensation to be accessible enough to access pleasure and excitement (moving us out of delayed ejaculation territory). When we don't have blood flow, we don't have lubrication, that is we don't have optimal sensation throughout the surface of the skin and in our genitals and the ability to comfortably accommodate penetration. We can pave the way for meaningful blood flow to travel towards or away from our genitals. How? This brings us to another major player in the mix: your pelvic floor.

The Pelvic Floor

In Chapter 21, we will delve into the details of the pelvic floor and how to partner with it towards the resolution of sexual "dysfunctions." In the meantime, it is important to know that our pelvic floor (or the muscles that stretch like a hammock from our pubic bone to our tailbone that support vital organs in our pelvis including the bladder, bowels, and reproductive organs) acts as a sort of central command station for our sexual functioning. *By and large it comes down to this: pelvic floor muscles released = blood flows in, pelvic floor clenched = blood flows out.* This is a simplification as obviously some blood flows in or else we'd have more serious problems, but meaningful blood flow to the places we want it to go (i.e. our genitals) is compromised when tension enters our musculature, signaling stress or lack of safety to the body. What are some specific consequences of a clenched or tense pelvic floor? A few of the primary "sexual dysfunctions" as they relate specifically to pelvic floor engagement (as opposed to psychological or emotional causes) will give us clues. We will break down these challenges *and more* in greater detail in Chapter 5.

Painful Sex. Lubrication is the name of the game when it comes to comfortable penetrative sex with a vagina; and without meaningful blood flow, it will be lacking, if available at all. Blood flow is responsible for genital swelling (engorgement) and lubrication, not to mention what we've already covered in terms of sensation. Penetrative sex can also be made painful by hypertonic and/or a clenched pelvic floor, often associated with stress, panic, recoil, lack of comfort or felt sense of safety, or even shame.

Note: the causes of sexual pain can be complicated and are often misdiagnosed. It is important to get a thorough work-up from a qualified medical professional and even seek a secondary opinion if pain is dismissed as psychological. Psychologically induced pain is common, but the ability to uncover any biological contributors to pain sensation in the body is vital, both to our ongoing relationship to our sexuality, but also to our experience of learning that comes with comfortable embodiment and exploration.

Erectile Dysfunction. Clenching the pelvic floor by moving into a "strive" or "power through" mindset causes the blood that was already in the shaft and beyond the pelvic floor muscle to be pushed further into the penis, creating a harder erection momentarily, while the tension introduced in the pelvic floor creates a sort of "seal" at the base, preventing easy blood flow from continuing to move into, fill, and flow through the penis – and the erection is lost.

Early Ejaculation. When the pelvic floor is released, the muscles involved in ejaculation are held back or reserved. Tension builds in the body, and in these muscles naturally, as we approach orgasm. When we introduce access or additional tension, it furthers this process along, triggering ejaculation earlier on in the experience than might be optimal or anticipated.

Getting in touch with this muscle group and becoming intimately familiar with sensation in the pelvic floor can help us identify when tension has entered into this part of the body, often as a reaction to the quality of the mind, allowing us to move the other way (i.e. release the tension), paving the way for easy and optimal blood flow and an overall greater sense of ease as release in the body tends to slow the mind. Practicing pelvic floor exercises will also allow us to understand what full release in the pelvic floor feels like, something many of us are unfamiliar with as we contend with the anxiety of modern life and familiarity with a level of anxiety as our baseline for moving through the world.

*

A Word about the Word "Safety"

Safety is referenced as a key ingredient in the emotional, psychological, and physiological unfolding of arousal and desire throughout this book. If we zoom in, this is a subjective and abstract idea, and therefore a subjective and abstract determination informed by lots of complexity. Like trust, our sense of safety in all areas can move around, shifting and changing with the forward movement of our relationships and own personal evolution. Sometimes our assessment of safety can be unreliable given our history, traumas, and lessons in intimacy and closeness. Safety is also a privilege, our relationship with and understanding of it profoundly influenced by race, class, gender, ability, and who and how we love.

We will intentionally address and discuss how to identify and cultivate a sense of safety within ourselves and our relationships in Part III. In the meantime, when we talk about the body receiving the message of a lack of safety, we are speaking to any incoming information via our feelings, thoughts, or sensations that suggest the time is not right to rest, play, and surrender. We are referring to the message that there is something to attend to or worry about. The emotions that can signal a lack of safety can be conceptualized on a spectrum:

Concerns – worries – fear – anxiety and stress – panic

Dissociation and checking out in order to achieve safety (e.g. comfort, peace, stability, rest, regulation) can occur at any place on the spectrum and is also informed by our history and the extent to which our bodies have registered threat in the face of sexual stimuli, feelings of vulnerability, and/or lack of control.

Safety is not black and white, and nothing in life is completely safe, therefore we are looking for the "*safe enough to risk letting go*" spot, the "*I'm OK right now*" feeling. This is evidence that we are in a context, individually and relationally, to be able to attend to and take care of ourselves with ease.

4   Performance, Goal Orientation, and the Striving Mindset

How Would You Describe Your Best Sexual Experiences?

In one word: connection. Like really being in synch.

It takes time getting to know your partner, getting comfortable being vulnerable with them, figuring out how your bodies work together. And for me it is "great" when we are in sync, super intimate, and close, like pressed against each other and breathing in each other's mouths close, breathing heavy and hands in hair. Eye contact and intense. Usually involves me having an orgasm but doesn't have to!

The first thing that comes to mind is when it's so passionate and you both are so into it, it's like it's the only thing happening in the world. Then the exhausted afterglow when all you can do is lay there all happy and sweaty for a while.

What makes "good" sex good? What *is* "bad" sex, exactly? We all have our likes and dislikes that we bring to the table, for example *"I love doggie-style sex,"* *"I'm not a fan of 69-ing,"* or *"I go crazy for a good hard yank of my hair."* As we collect these likes and dislikes via our experiences, the answer to the question can increasingly resemble the way we'd approach an inquiry around what makes for good or bad French toast; namely, as a list of fairly fixed characteristics or a recipe that we can generally agree on, execute with consistency, and that requires specific ingredients we all have access to. This way of thinking about good vs. bad sex can risk conveying a larger message that there is a way to "master" sex, become a "pro" if or when things are sexually dicey, challenging, or stale in our own lives and relationships. All that's required is a simple scroll through the internet to find articles with promises in lists like, "10 Key Components of Super Hot Sex," or "5 Ways to Blow Your Partner's Mind." The inventory of good or bad sex ingredients, we forget, is super subjective, sometimes even more so (arguably) than what makes for good or bad French toast. Following a generic recipe when it comes to sexual intimacy has consequences that are

DOI: 10.4324/9781003369080-6

important to bear in mind as it fails to capture the spirit of intimacy, and the magic of sharing ourselves, deeply and fully, in relationships. Our likes and dislikes are shaped by context: the person, place, scenario, nature of the relationship, and so on. We can land on them gently, knowing that they may not feel the same with someone else, under different circumstances, in a different brand of relationship. What makes for good sex with one person may make for an uncomfortable experience with another.

Let's talk about one version of this hypothetical "sex pro" scenario. Let's say we have a cisgender/heterosexual, 30-something-year-old, super handsome (whatever that looks like for you) man; he's charming, but with an edge. We'll call him Troy.

Troy has been with his fair share of cisgender women. His partners have traditionally described him as an exciting lover: attentive, passionate, adventurous, but also "proficient" when it comes to pleasuring a vulva. It's his thing. He begins gently; teasing his partners clit with the tip of his tongue, then slowly moves into long, slow strokes with the flat, soft middle, making sure to incorporate his warm breath into each stroke, pausing every few minutes simply to stare his partners in the eyes, feeling and communicating his power, then approaching and pulling away, teasing and playing with the mounting anticipation. He knows how to drive a collection of people wild, a badge he wears with honor.

Then Troy meets Celia. Celia is a cis/pansexual woman in her late 20s; charismatic but reserved, and deeply intelligent. He's into her in a way he's never experienced before: getting nervous and jittery before dates, feeling insecure and lost in conversation, reaching for something interesting to say or offer. After a few dates, Celia invites Troy back to her place (this is it! Finally, we'll be in my wheelhouse – I'll blow her mind). They chat for a bit, then move in closer to one another. Troy sees his opportunity and leans in, kissing Celia gently. He feels instant sparks as the kissing becomes more intense. Moving from kissing to making out, from the living room to the bedroom, from fully clothed to nothing on, Troy begins to make his way to her vulva, kissing her stomach, pressing into her thighs with the palms of his thumbs as he descends. Softly landing on her clit with the tip of his tongue, her legs jerk back. "I actually don't really like direct stimulation to my clitoris, it's too much. Can you apply just a little pressure right above it with your fingers? Just sort of ... lightly rub in small circles." Troy panics a little (right above the clit? What does that mean exactly? How far above?). As he attempts to interpret her feedback, he finds himself in a familiar place emotionally with Celia, but new territory entirely in terms of his sexual experience: nervous, tense, insecure, lost.

Let's pause with Troy for a moment and pan over to a different, and equally common, version of a similar struggle:

Jared (cis/gay/37-year-old white male) visits a couple's therapist for the first time with his partner of 5 years, Manny (cis/gay/29-year-old Hispanic male). The following is a brief window into their third session:

Jared (speaking to
the therapist):   It feels like we're so stuck and Manny just does nothing!
                         I'm the one at home reading books, purchasing webi-
                         nars, taking all the notes in our sessions, and he just sits
                         there. Like, I think he might actually be perfectly con-
                         tent to be in a sexless partnership. I was watching one of
                         said sad webinars that discusses the "Tell-tale Signs
                         Your Relationship Is in Trouble" and one of the main
                         threats to longevity is lack of investment in doing the
                         work! How will we ever get out of this rut if he doesn't
                         care about learning how!

As discussed, learning is our friend! And Jared is *the* super eager learner: taking notes each session and doing his due diligence to study up with a variety
of well-researched sex and relationship self-help books and popular podcasts
in between meetings. He's learned all the technique, watched a plethora of
both generic and educational porn, scoured the internet for every ounce of
learning and advice from the most highly regarded professionals and Ted
talks. He presents nearly as well-versed as the therapist in his understanding
of desire, intimacy, and sensuality. Despite the sex-savvy bootcamp he's put
himself through, things remain at a standstill in the bedroom.

*Therapist: Jared, what if I asked you to stop taking notes? Completely
           stop all research, reading, and at-home study? What if I told
           you that all of it actually takes you away from the most mean-
           ingful learning we want to access here: what your sexual strug-
           gles mean in* **this** *relationship, for you and Manny, rather than
           the rest of the world?*

What critical information are *both* "experts," Troy and Jared, missing?
What works and doesn't work for, or what might be happening with, *their*
partners specifically right now? For Jared (the "eager learner"), missing the
mark looks like searching for a map to reference in the universe that exists
outside of their unique, complex relationship; some generalized instruction
that is going to erase his confusion and feelings of vulnerability in the
face of sexual disconnection (which often means emotional disconnection),

information that simply doesn't exist for sexuality and intimacy. Troy (the "vulva pleaser") is relying almost entirely on data, or the "map" he's created from experiences with past lovers, to please the current one; leaning into and prioritizing feedback conjured up from memory space rather than getting curious about the experience, the body, the person right in front of him. How both manifest are versions of performance anxiety, a sympathetic nervous system response, and both lead to more trouble.

Performance and Anxiety, Performance-Anxiety

Performance isn't always a bad word as it relates to our sexual lives. People can find themselves exaggerating, adding to, or even completely acting out aspects of sexual experience, in terms of behavior, feeling states, and level of psychological arousal for themselves and/or their partners on a regular basis, adding dimension to the interaction. Some would argue that a degree of performance is present in most, if not all, sexual encounters, especially pronounced with newer partners or novel experiences. Performance can move our own arousal along, eliciting a state of mind. I can "perform" insatiable lust and longing, channeling what I know of those feelings to bring them forward, "acting" in order to give our body/heart/mind the message *"this is what I want, I welcome these feelings in."* A meaningful distinction is made, however, when someone is performing for themselves or others out of and with a foundation of comfort, openness, or pleasure (and with their own continued comfort and experience in mind), versus out of fear or obligation (e.g. *I need to orgasm or at least perform orgasm in order to bolster my partner's ego*). Driven by goal orientation and exacerbated by our inclination to "power through," the body switches gears as we "work" at playing a part or accomplishing a challenge as we would work to give a presentation to our colleagues.

If performance anxiety has its roots in fear, what exactly are we so afraid of? Why do we get anxious about our sexual prowess, competency, skill (i.e. performance)? What do we have to lose? This has everything to do with everything we think we are and are not; our self-esteem or sense of ourselves as worthwhile, capable, even lovable in a general way. *"If I can make you cum, I've validated my worth as a man,"* for example. Anxiety might take this further by adding, *"If I can't make you cum, I haven't distinguished myself as more capable, more deserving of your love and time than others, and I might lose you alongside my pride."*

(Exercising our therapist mind: Are there other aspects of the stories mentioned that are worthy of our attention, curiosity, and reflection? Aspects of the clients' identities that might play a role or exert influence on the challenges described? What areas might you want to explore?)

Sex and Intimacy, Sex vs. Intimacy, Sex *as* Intimacy

We refer to sex as "intimacy," using the two words interchangeably to reference the same thing despite their definitions being vastly different on paper. Does this impact our sexual mindset? Should it? Oxford Languages and Miriam-Webster provide the following distinctions (watch out, they bite!):

Sex (noun): sexual activity including specifically sexual intercourse (Oxford Languages).

Since this definition includes "specifically intercourse" (which, of course sex can involve, but is not by any means a required activity to still be considered "sex"), let's define that as well:

Sexual Intercourse (noun): Sexual contact between individuals involving penetration, especially the insertion of a man's erect penis into a woman's vagina, typically culminating in orgasm and the ejaculation of semen. (Oxford Languages)

Intimacy: 1. The state of being intimate: familiarity, 2. Something of a personal or private nature. (Miriam-Webster)

Stepping around these blatantly narrow and hetero-normative definitions (nearly all easily obtainable definitions of "sexual intercourse" involve a "man's penis" and a "woman's vagina," failing to capture how a hugely substantial portion of the population are engaging in sexual intercourse (anal, oral, manual, penetrative sex with sex toys, etc), people whose gender may not align with the sex they were assigned at birth, and those who have same-sex or intersex partners), what is clear is that these words are not encompassing identical or even similar content. Could this be a social strategy? A way to "put a robe on" a very naked concept, just a less X-rated way of referencing what goes on behind closed doors? Maybe. Or could this be a clue, pointing us towards the things we value, the needs and wants and desires we access through sex that have nothing to do with the dictionary version of "sex" whatsoever? To break it down for ourselves in a more expansive way:

- Sex (not as a noun in the "what's the sex of the baby" sense, but a noun in the "an event" sense, like "the circus") is a series of behaviors we engage in (individually or with partners) that kick up a physiological response in the body that we often experience in the form of pleasurable sensation and/or physical and emotional release.
- Intimacy, on the other hand, is the psychological and emotional pleasure or reward found in the sharing, revealing, and learning that goes on between people and within oneself.

What are the ingredients of intimacy?

- Sharing;
- Revealing;
- Authenticity;
- Vulnerability;
- Connection;
- *Risk*.

When we approach an intimate interaction, we are putting ourselves out there. We are risking being or feeling rejected, isolated, alone, and/or ashamed. And yet, we risk, often over and over again, as if knowing intuitively the healing that can live on the other side should we be met with acceptance, care, more or continued closeness, and understanding; feelings that cultivate a deep sense of connection, the antidote for the wounding that disconnection creates. There is no guarantee of safety in intimacy, as true "safety" would require psychological and emotional armor or lack of accessibility, walling us off from real sharing, meaningful revealing. We create as safe a context as we can for ourselves with the people we choose to be intimate with, and then jump.

Intimacy is only experienced if both parties understand that what is being revealed is private or personal for the individuals involved, therefore often not freely and readily offered to others, and is being revealed because each person chose that sharing rather than feeling obligated (or on the flipside, feeling entitled) to it. Familiarity becomes a consequence of intimacy on repeat, the ongoing learning that comes from ongoing sharing.

Sex *is* intimate, to varying degrees in just the same way as sex *is* vulnerable. What we understand these series of behaviors and their physiological response to mean, what adds to the sensory experience that can culminate in orgasm, *is* what we make up about why it is so important or impactful or meaningful that we are moving through these behaviors and experiences with another person(s) or even ourselves. We learn that being naked is private, our "private parts" are private, alongside arousal and desire and orgasm. If these things were not true, how erotic or intense might sex be? If sex were so completely normalized that there was no need for privacy whatsoever and we could masturbate while sipping coffee at a cafe in the same way we scroll through our phones, would it feel as profound? No (that's an easy one), because intimacy breathes life into sex.

If sex is intimate, if intimacy is at the heart of what makes sex rewarding, then treating sex as "performance" inspires emotional and psychological distance. Working at sex siphons the heat out of the exchange, if heat was permitted to build in the first place. "Striving" to be intimate feels like obligation rather than authentic offering. And yet, we have to acknowledge the world we're working with and the narratives we're given.

We must call a spade, a spade. With so many of us walking around having been handed performance as primary when it comes to sex, stepping outside of that idea or expectation can cause friction if the expectation is not met. If we don't *"make the other person cum," "have orgasms ourselves," "last long enough,"* or *"pleasure the other,"* we can invite in the potential for disappointment or frustration or worse (whilst weeding out some people in need of some growth themselves along the way). And yet, "trying" to do any of the above often leads to disappointment anyway. We are faced with two options: risk stepping into our eroticism, seeing where it takes us, where there is no agenda but we're emotionally online; or strive to make "good" sex happen, get it right, living in our headspace at the expense of emotional and bodily freedom and presence. Pick your poison.

Do Our Egos Have a Place in the Bedroom?

According to Eckhart Tolle, author of *The Power of Now*, the "ego" is the part of your mind that comments, doubts, and speculates on everything. It is driven by fear of being nothing, which it tries to alleviate through identification with material, thought, and emotional elements, giving rise to what we think of as our "self," and particularly our sense of self-importance. Sex can find itself grouped with other endeavors we turn to, to bolster an understanding of our story of ourselves *for* ourselves. It can be a mile marker of self-importance, a pivotal player in our (or many people's) quest to be "good enough," important, valuable. But is that so bad?

Sex *is* connection, and watching another person experience pleasure from their connection with, and experience of, who we are and how we interact sexually can fill us up emotionally. Some would argue there is no greater high, and our sense of self-worth can benefit. Where this becomes problematic is when our self-esteem is on the line each time we go to engage sexually, when we need to prove to ourselves that we are worthy of loving, by being _____ [fill in the blank] sexually. If the ego is driven by the fear of being nothing, then sex can risk becoming another way we prove we're something, someone, important, good, skilled, hot, capable, smooth. It becomes another badge we carry to let ourselves know we matter, rather than it being an expression of our inherent sense of self-worth, an expression for expression's sake, an experience. When we need it to feed our ego, the stakes are high. Our bodies understand this (high stakes = tension = anxiety), and our partners experience it (disconnection or very real, palpable anxiety). If we need it for our sense of value, we will work to accomplish sex in a predetermined way, approaching it as a challenge, culminating in clenching and tension (i.e. seeming "checked out" or distant) rather than letting go into ease, culminating in orgasm and release (i.e. being experienced as present, connected, free).

With egos on the line, and our sense of self-worth directly informing our mental and emotional health and well-being, each sexual experience becomes an anxious one as we work to avoid the shame that lives on the opposing end of the "self-important–I'm nothing" spectrum. What can often begin as a "high" from being in the presence of ourselves reflected back in a way that demonstrates pleasure and enthusiasm, becomes a challenge whereby we vanish increasingly into our anxiety and determination to access that experience over and over again to meet a need (or at least a strong want). The more we "perform" to appease anxiety, the more we lose ourselves, the more difficulty we have accessing pleasure and sexual functioning. It's a vicious, self-perpetuating cycle.

Sharpening Our Skill Set

What *can* we get "good" at when it comes to sex? We can become increasingly proficient in understanding our own bodies, communicating our wants and boundaries, exploring and getting to know our own desires, inviting-in emotion, and ultimately cultivating ease in a sexual experience. When we practice driving that car as a teen, we are gaining familiarity with our own instincts, with our own emotional experience at the wheel, with the coordination involved in becoming an extension of the machine. If we focused on what the engine was doing and if it was overheating and what it needed to operate at its ultimate performance as we cruise down the road, we are most assuredly setting ourselves up for a crash, or at least some irresponsible, reckless driving. Through deep attunement to self, eventually we find ourselves cruising with the windows down, a good playlist on, admiring the sky.

Sex Is Play

Of the things sex asks of us, play can feel off for some. But there's a meaningful distinction to be made here: not all sex is *playful*, but sex is a form of play. When we think about casting our egos aside, setting ourselves free from performance, striving, and controlling in an experience, what is left? Imagination/fantasy, expression, movement, and connection. Precisely the qualities that define play amongst children.

Our culture has determined that play in adulthood is no longer appropriate, no longer invited, not part of the script. Nearly every definition of the word includes "children" as the sole consumers of play, despite the most common definition itself being "to engage in activity for enjoyment and recreation rather than a serious or practical purpose" (Oxford Languages). In this sense, we play constantly, through humor, flirtation, socializing, through experiences with food, our hobbies, and so on.

Sex does offer a larger goal for some, namely procreation, but even with this centered, the assumption is that we are experiencing enjoyment or release or connection (i.e. reward) along the way. Taking it too seriously *will* zap the fun out of the experience and transform what was once a fun and freeing dance move into a series of robotic steps. As such, sex is play, kink is play, fantasy is play, role play is play, dirty talk is play, power exchange is play, dance is play. If sex isn't a form of play, it's – weird, hard to understand, logistically lawless. Does sex feel like play for you? If not, why?

Can the Degree of "Effort" be a Clue?

I like some parts of sex, but it just feels like a lot of work most days. For example, I'll start to go down on my partner, which I love, and then I'll be over it or start getting tired but feel obligated to keep going and doing a good job. Most days it's just easier for me to masturbate honestly, but my partner would take that personally if they knew. I wish sex was simpler.

When Bernard (cis, gay, 41-year-old) experiences that Leo (cis, gay, 46-year-old) is not gaining an erection in the course of their sex play (a fairly frequent occurrence), he panics, deciding he must be doing something wrong, Leo must not actually be attracted to him, or that Leo is bored. Consequently, Bernard shifts gears and begins ramping things up: more rigorous or "rough" stimulation, exaggerated performance (more dramatic facial expressions, louder noise making, more dirty talk), and incorporating more "moves" (primarily behaviors and techniques he learned from porn) into their interaction. This has the consequence of leaving Leo feeling unseen, disconnected, and under his own brand of pressure to be in the same place emotionally and physiologically as Bernard, creating a feedback loop that keeps the erectile dysfunction in place.

The "strive" mindset we often default to when sexual experiences are a struggle is an entire mode of functioning. The brain recognizes this "mode" and is trained to respond in the way it does when faced with answering questions in a job interview: in a focused, narrow, internal way rather than through reflective honesty, curiosity, and collaboration.

In a similar way, the degree of effort can let us know where we've left ourselves. If working hard is fun, then by all means keep working! For many of us, however, strenuous effort is fatiguing/exhausting, something we wish to leave behind in an experience of self-care. In order to protect our relationship to intimacy, to sex, we want to edit out aspects of the experience that feel like tiresome exertion and/or boredom in order to avoid creating that association. This means welcoming in (explicitly) disappointment, or even slightly frustrated (because we're grown-ups and we can handle it!). Giving our partners explicit permission to abandon mission and pivot when they grow fatigued makes it more likely they'll return to our shared sexual connection tomorrow, or the next day, or sooner than if they had exhausted themselves, and vice versa. If sex is associated with work, well then – who wants to "work" for fun? If exhaustion becomes the past experience the brain has to draw from to predict our current one, we've set ourselves up for low or no desire. When we find ourselves exerting significant effort in a sexual experience, a check-in can help us re-center: *Why am I working so hard? What do I hope to accomplish here? Is my ego invested in the outcome of this behavior? Do I fear my partner's reaction if I suggest a pivot? How might I return to sexual care for myself in this interaction?*

How awesome would it be to hear:

Thank you for touching me there, and I want you to know you can stop whenever you want to. Only do what feels good for you for as long as it feels good for you. I can take care of myself, there is no pressure here.

Seeking the "A"

We are placed in academic settings from the time we're three or four, taught to get good grades and to "out-smart" our peers in order to get into a decent college and win at life. Who are we if we're not the best at something? The most skilled? The coolest? The most popular? Who are we outside of our accomplishments when we have been defined by them since we were little? Play is the place where we understand how to let go of striving, endeavoring, impressing. Relationships (friendships, family, romantic and sexual partnerships) are what we turn to for connection based on who we are versus what we do, the respite from our training. If we find it challenging to understand or define who we are outside of our accomplishments, our relationships and sex lack intimacy, and become another test to pass.

How much value have you placed in how much you accomplish in life? In how much you achieve, produce, do? If our worth is defined by mastery, by doing things right and by-the-book, sex will challenge you to expand, to encounter yourself as who you are and not what you do, for how you feel and not what you think, for what your body experiences now rather than how to get to pleasure (theirs or yours) next. It offers respite, it is the exhale of our lived experience, if we can allow it to be the great teacher it is. If we can stop trying so hard.

5 Mind/Body Connection and Disconnection

Ever feel like you're having an easy conversation with a partner on a date and then become aware that your arms are folded across your chest, you're sort of angled away from the person, and making very little eye contact? The body is demonstrating a sort of closing off while you're trying to open up. What gives? A complex internal conversation, often a battle of opposing forces, affecting our bodies, our physiology, and sometimes in contradictory ways.

This might look like:

Immediate feelings and desires

I really want to give my partner oral sex, the thought of it is super-hot.
    Openness, arousal, excitement
I love watching my partners experience pleasure.

Just below surface consciousness

Am I going to be able to make that happen? (Introduction of anxiety/tension in the pelvic floor/sympathetic nervous system activation)
I don't think I really know what I'm doing.

A layer deeper: subconscious prediction

What if it becomes obvious that I don't know. (Further constriction in body, disconnection from sensation, disconnection from other, challenges with sexual functioning)
They'll think I look ridiculous.

Core belief

I'm an imposter. (Closing off emotionally, shielding self from vulnerability, moving into "head space," absence of arousal, "powering through")

DOI: 10.4324/9781003369080-7

Life doesn't give us the space to access all the layers of the onion all the time. While moving through a meeting or a social event, we aren't able to be attuned to all of the parts of the internal conversation as it unfolds; and thank goodness for that! Sometimes we need to hang out in a first-layer territory (*This is fine!*) to get through the date, the audition, the family holiday (*Whew! That was hard*). Too much depth threatens our attention, our relational attunement, our focus on the task at hand. And yet other times, we are called to slow down and begin to dissect so as to understand the complexity, and address why it's there. One or more emotional aspects of our experience have become intrusive or noticeable enough to merit our time and investment. The body lets us know when a meaningful theme, belief, or part of who we are is calling for our attention, in need of healing. Sex does the same.

Good Parts/Dirty Parts

Client: *I don't really touch or interact with my vulva. I masturbated more when I was younger, but not so much as an adult. I don't really care to; it feels yucky or something.*

Therapist: *Have you ever looked at your vulva up close? Taken a mirror to understand where parts are or what they look like?*

Client: *No. I've never bothered to look, I have no desire to see any of it. I know what the outside looks like and that's enough. I've probably seen a diagram in high school at some point, so it's not like I don't know what's there.*

Our bodies are our bodies first and foremost, a collection of parts with important roles and functions, all sources of learning and information, all incredible in their own ways. We treat our "sexual" anatomy, or the parts of the body considered "erogenous zones," differently, frequently separating them off from the rest of who we are, working with them in isolation and sometimes in shame. Yet what inherent qualities or meaning does a vulva, a penis, breasts, or intersex genitals have outside of their functionality? These are parts of the body, just like an elbow or chin; they are aspects of our anatomy that have been linked to ideas, values, morality, rules, judgment (like the other parts but in their own unique way), fear and taboo in a way that creates or reinforces a separation and/or fans the flames of a conflicted relationship. How confusing is it, for example, that we've decided parts of the body are "dirty" or "bad" to interact with and yet we marvel at their magic when they create and/or birth children? Shameful one day and sacred the next.

These parts, all the parts, *are* us. Intimate familiarity with our musculature while doing a yoga pose is no more or less important than intimate familiarity with sensation around our nipples, in the pelvis, the shaft of the penis. What makes the information that the vulva communicates – when we experience discomfort around the vaginal opening, or tightening, or pleasure – any more or less important, more or less worthy of our attention, than what the stomach has to say when it's hungry or tied in knots when we're nervous? More importantly, we turn to the body (whether we know it or not) all day every day for information about our experience, our instincts, for cues about our needs, wants, likes, dislikes, desires. We understand when something is wrong with a part of the body by noticing how it feels, how it looks, how it might be responding differently than how we know it each day. Without that information, we can easily find ourselves in the midst of panic regarding infections or changes, of the sexually transmitted kind and beyond (*Is this how my skin usually feels here? Are there usually these tiny red bumps?*).

Our sexual struggles are fueled by the disconnection we experience from our own genitals (i.e. our own body). The answer to many sexual difficulties that people stumble upon online, or what seems to make the most sense according to our rational minds, has been to separate, to move away from sensation, to distract. This is an unfortunate and harmful idea that is not only (i) ineffective, but also makes room for (ii) more disconnection in all areas of sex – with fantasy, with emotion, with a partner, if present.

Familiarity is the answer, even with difficulties like early (or premature) ejaculation. Self-connection proficiency is our way into more satisfying, embodied, sexual and intimate experiences. What can you identify as a barrier to this level of attunement with yourself? With all parts? What ideas block full body knowledge? Full body love? How might feeling into more of our physicality, our physical and sensory selves, inform a deeper connection to who we are in a more holistic way? All information from all the parts can be invited as intimate channels of learning, wisdom, direction. They are all connected and all sexual in their own way, all participants in our sex if we have it.

"No" but "Yes": Boundary Check

In therapy we appreciate boundaries and yield to them when they're exercised or presented. The felt experience of effective boundaries is critical in cultivating safety and trust, two ingredients that act as antidotes to anxiety. This can be an overt expression of a boundary, or it can look like "*I don't really feel like going there today,*" or "*Yeah, that part of my life is fine,*" and/or emotional shutdown, rapidly changing the topic, and abruptly switching tone. All examples are variations on expressions of "*That's off limits, don't go there,*" that is a boundary. Many, if not most, if not all of us have had experiences where our boundaries haven't been respected, seen, or acknowledged, and we all have suffered the consequences of those experiences in terms of our own felt sense of safety and trust within ourselves, our relationships, and the world around us. And yet, there are times in sex therapy when boundaries need to be looked at, and our motivation for setting them approached and gently questioned, not because they shouldn't be there, but because it is important to understand what we're guarding and why; to understand when and how our boundaries are truly protecting us and when and how they might be locking away harm, effectively walling off our wounding instead.

Where do we go when body, behavior, and emotion are directing us towards areas in need of healing, of deeper exploration and processing, and the mind says "No"? How can we even identify when this is happening?

Ariel is a 30-year-old, cis/het, white female living in the city. She is independent, driven, and has a great job in design and marketing but which she frequently feels overwhelmed and stressed by, but ultimately loves. She has been with Paul (34-year-old, nonbinary, Asian-American) for the past three years. They met through friends, and she loved their sense of humor and free-spirited nature. She instantly wished she "had more of what they've got" in terms of the ease with which they seem to move through the world and their ability to not take life so seriously.

Their sexual relationship has always felt a little off, and they both agree. Paul enjoys penetrative sex, which Ariel states she enjoys as well, but reports always feeling a bit self-conscious and uncomfortable during the experience. She also describes having a great deal of trouble reaching orgasm, something that feels very frustrating to her both in the moment and out. She initiates individual therapy to "learn how to orgasm," after also having worked with a pelvic floor specialist and having had multiple evaluations from reputable obgyn practices in her area. She feels like she has "done everything" and is losing hope.

Therapist: *If I were to ask you what instantly comes to mind when you think about sex, just even in general, what would you say?*
Ariel: *Gross, dirty, uncomfortable …*
Therapist: *Are you able to tie those feelings to specific elements? What about sex is gross, dirty, uncomfortable?*
Ariel: *I don't know … I guess I'd say I think the hygiene part is pretty gross. I just think vaginas are like, leaky and can smell funny and look weird. They like, produce fluid that can just come out of you whenever, which eeks me out. I don't like to touch it and I really don't like my partner giving me oral or anything.*

Therapist: How would you say you've noticed the impact of these feelings on your goal? The challenges you've had with orgasm?

Ariel: I don't know if they really do that much. It's not like I'm thinking those thoughts when I'm having sex. I just try to focus on other things.

Therapist: It feels important to pause here and consider that perhaps one reason you find yourself thinking about other things is because those feelings are very much in the room with you. Your mind is moving you away from engaging in the discomfort they bring, but they come alive in your body nonetheless, having a very real impact on your ability to enjoy sensation, to have a rewarding experience at all!

Ariel: I've always felt this way, I don't really think talking about how vaginas are "natural" or something is going to change that [boundary]. I'd rather focus on techniques I can use to learn how to orgasm.

Therapist: How in-the-loop do you keep your partner with these challenges? Do they know how you feel about sex?

Ariel: They don't need to know this stuff! How weird would it be for me to tell them I don't like my vagina? What would be the point? I would feel stupid sharing that, it's personal.

Therapist: What do you notice in your body as we talk about this?

Ariel: What do you mean?

Therapist: Well, can you name or describe any tension, warmth, looseness, constriction, racing heart, tightness, pressure? If you check-in with your body now, what do you feel?

Ariel: I don't know, I just feel frustrated. That's it.

Starting from the top, what is Ariel communicating to the body with even just the few ideas and feelings mentioned towards and regarding sex and sexuality? How are they shaping her sexual interactions and experiences (because they are)? Let's zoom in on some hypothetical consequences.

- *Vaginas (vulvas) are gross, smell funny, and look weird*: No to touching my vulva, looking at my vulva, getting close to my vulva.
- *They produce fluid that can come out of you whenever*: No getting aroused (arousal comes with lubrication), that is no allowing my body to really enjoy the experience.
- *Sex is "dirty" or indecent*: No to the experience as a whole, it's not for people like me – I'm not indecent or obscene.
- *Sex is uncomfortable*: "No" is with me even as I approach sex – I predict my physical and emotional discomfort in advance. The stories I've attached to the experience are hard for me to navigate.

- *They (my partner) don't need to know this stuff – I would feel stupid, it's personal.* No to vulnerability, sharing, expression of feeling – rejection of the essence of what sex is and asks of us.

All of these separate parts and their hypothetical consequences involve resistance, of which anxiety is a key ingredient. The no's are boundaries, and in this case, like barbed wire protecting the most crucial sources of her sexual discomfort and anxiety, locking away the challenging feelings, values, and thoughts that are directly at odds with her goal, her healing. The therapist must find a way of illuminating how the boundary set (*I've always felt this way, I don't really think talking about how vaginas are "natural" or something is going to change that. I'd rather focus on techniques I can use to learn how to orgasm*) is keeping Ariel back from any forward momentum she would like to see toward her goal. No amount of technique or sexual positions will change that.

We cannot have it both ways: relaying nos to the body alongside shoulds (nos) and having a free, unencumbered sex life, full of easy orgasms. We don't have to consciously relay these nos, they live within us, speaking to our bodies without us having to ourselves. This is different from the important boundaries or "nos" we set with our partners about our experience, comfort, and specific behaviors that are off limits, the boundaries that protect our relational safety. One experience is about distancing ourselves from ourselves, creating restriction. The other is about understanding the parameters necessary to set ourselves free.

The good news? The work she's engaged in thus far is useful! Her time with a pelvic floor therapist helped her come into greater contact with her body, her vulva, the tension she holds and therefore can release in her pelvic floor muscles. The information gleaned from her visits with the obgyn are important for her evolving understanding of her body and sexual anatomy. The critical final piece of the puzzle, the element that rounds out her healing, means addressing the unbypassable psychological and relational factors that inhibit release. We cannot circumvent our own brains, of both what lives on the surface, and what hides behind the curtain. When the mind is at ease, the body will follow. The inverse can also be true, something we can actively exert some control over: when the body is at ease the mind will follow. Between her medical providers and pelvic floor physical therapists, Ariel is in a great position to take on this iteration of the work, her psychological and emotional healing.

Checking in with yourself, what ideas do you hold about sex that could be sneaking into your sexual life, manifesting as physical blocks or struggle? Are there any you can identify from childhood that have an impact still today, despite how much your ideas around sex may have changed and evolved? How are you inadvertently attempting to have it both ways?

What Is the Body Communicating? Common Sexual Challenges Elaborated

The list below offers a brief, condensed insight (beyond what we visited with the pelvic floor) into some of the more frequently identified psychological and emotional causes of common sexual struggles. The list is far from complete and will not include the very real medical, physical, and/or hormonal causes associated to varying degrees as well as sensory processing challenges or variation in experience related to our neurodiversity. All of the above are important, if not primary elements to consider if applicable.

With any sexual struggle, it can be meaningful to understand how our body might be reacting to our relationship with a multitude of factors, as an expression of who we are, our history, and how we feel. The sexual difficulty is the manifestation of larger themes or struggles, very often unrelated to sex entirely.

Pre- or Post-Orgasm Aggravation, Irritation, Sadness, or Shut Down (Postcoital Dysphoria)

> We've been dating a month or so and finally had sex last week. She was so gentle and attentive. I had the most amazing orgasm, and then broke into sobs immediately after.

Postcoital dysphoria is a newbie on the scene, and generally thought of as sudden feelings of sadness, weepiness, and/or agitation/anger/irritability during or most often following what is otherwise an enjoyable, rewarding, or even neutral sexual experience. This commonly shows up directly before or post-orgasm, but it can occur whether orgasm happens or not, and really at any point in the sexual experience. So what gives? One primary factor to consider has to do with vulnerability, and our relationship to it. It is an important player that holds a role in all sexual challenges and the anxiety they kick up. The kind of closeness and sharing inherent in sexual experiences can be exceptional or infrequent in the life of the person, and when we step into vulnerability, we don't get to choose what it brings with it, which is often stored emotion. Most of us work to keep our vulnerability at bay in our day-to-day lives, with differences in degree existing person to person and also dependent upon gender, socioeconomic status, identity (race, sexual orientation, gender expression – i.e. privilege and the felt sense of safety in a relationship to others/the world), and cultural norms. Whatever we are trying to keep back when it comes to vulnerability can come spilling out when we step into it sexually. If orgasm is part of the mix, it's important to consider what orgasm is, namely catharsis: an emotional, physical, psychological, and (for many) spiritual release. Releasing tension, fear, our inhibitions can be tremendously emotional, and also incredibly healing. It can represent one of the few times in life that we've felt safe enough to go there with someone, something that the body can recognize and feel the enormity of even when our consciousness cannot name it. The feelings we feel when this effect takes hold have great wisdom to them, and the less we resist them, the more we welcome them in, the more profoundly they diminish over time as we are doing the healing work of moving them out, which can be its own version of pleasure.

What we're asking for: pleasure, connection, intimacy, play, and so on. What the body is doing: reacting to our own vulnerability, moving through release.

Delayed Ejaculation

Delayed ejaculation (DE) is the inability to control when ejaculation happens and, specifically, the experience of ejaculation (or orgasm for our purposes) being illusive or hard to reach. DE is often confused with edging, which is defined by the experience of taking one's self to the edge of orgasm, just to the brink of ejaculatory inevitability, and then backing off, *intentionally* delaying orgasm. One is involuntary, a reflection of a lack of arousal attunement and control, and is experienced as challenging, the other is very voluntary, a reflection of profound arousal attunement and control, and fun. Delayed ejaculation is often characterized by fast, hard strokes of the penis for a prolonged period of time, which can be challenging to replicate with an anus, mouth, or vagina. This technique can also decrease sensitivity in the penis as any amount of vigorous rubbing on any part of the body will decrease sensation in that part as you continue without varying your stroke, pace, or the quality of pressure applied.

DE, like all struggles, often comes with an anxiety component as the person begins to "work" at ejaculating before their body is ready, striving rather than allowing arousal to unfold in its own time. When we approach the point of ejaculatory inevitability, speeding up our rhythm and tightening our grip can help encourage us over the edge in terms of ejaculation. When we begin this "speeding up" process too early, attempting to encourage ourselves over the edge when our arousal hasn't been able to properly build and the body isn't ready, tension gets introduced and the "work" aspect of the experience gets initiated. That combined with the decrease in sensitivity that comes with rubbing, combined with the decrease in sensitivity that accompanies lack of blood flow to the skin when we are in our stress response, creates the perfect breeding ground for DE. A mistake people often make in the midst of this particular struggle is believing that the inability to ejaculate has to do with the content of the porn they're watching or that the experience they're having must not be stimulating enough.

I must need edgier porn, a more adventurous partner, and so on, which ultimately leads to more striving, working harder, more struggle. DE can also happen as a result of the fear of ejaculating too early! At its most severe, DE can lead to chafing of the penis and other surface level injuries to the skin. At its core, DE is asking us to identify tension, pressure, goal orientation in order to free up sensation and uninterrupted movement through the arousal cycle. It asks us to switch up sensation, pressure, rhythm, slow down, and savor.

Non-situational DE might ask us to take a closer look at our relationship to ourselves, including but not limited to our own sexual desires, preferences, habits, and any shame that may be connected.

What we're asking for: pleasure and orgasm/release. What we're doing: striving/working.

Vaginismus

Vaginismus is the involuntary constriction of the walls of the vaginal canal, or of the musculature of the vagina, which occurs at the prospect of penetration, preventing it from happening. This can be experienced solely with specific objects, like a penis or speculum at the obgyn, or it can occur at the prospect of penetration by any object whatsoever: fingers, a tampon, a Q-Tip, and so on. The body is responding with alarm bells to the idea of or the experience of penetration, as if protecting the person from danger or threat, a sort of panic response. This effect can be the result of sexual trauma and through learning in a real way that this experience is dangerous; it can also be the result of socialization (i.e. messages like "good girls don't"), religious values around sex and abstinence before marriage, an over-controlled personality, inexperience with self-touching and masturbation, deep fears concerning one's own genitals, closeness, or loss of control, tension, involuntary clenching of the pelvic floor.

What we're asking for: ease with penetration. What is happening in the body: panic, tension, involuntary clenching of the pelvic floor.

Erectile Dysfunction (ED)

ED describes the inability to gain or maintain an erection for the amount of time desired during the course of a sexual experience, solo or partnered or both. This can happen for biological or medical reasons (ED can be the canary in the coal mine for heart disease and other cardiovascular abnormalities, circulatory issues, etc.), but given that a significant percentage of ED cases are primarily anxiety-based, it is helpful to think of ED as being less about the loss or absence of erection, and more about our reaction to it. Panic, worry, and concern at the prospect or partial or full loss of an erection moves us into sympathetic nervous system activation, nearly guaranteeing the full loss alongside the inability to regain an erection until the parasympathetic nervous system has come back online (i.e. those emotions have passed). ED, like all sexual challenges, can be highly relational, occurring with greater frequency in the presence of a partner or partners. It is often mistaken for a lack of caring, attraction, or desire. While it *can* be a reflection of these feelings, it is much more often connected to the opposing end of the spectrum: profound attraction, deep caring, and investment that translates into performance fears and anxiety.

> For an erection to be triggered, the smooth muscle at the base of the penis (PC muscle group) has to be relaxed … Erection is a function of the parasympathetic nervous system. If your sympathetic nervous system is activated (in other words, you are anxious), it floods your bloodstream with adrenaline and inhibits erection.
>
> (Keesling, 2006, pp. 65 & 70)

Non-situational ED might ask us to take a closer look at our relationship to ourselves, including but not limited to our own sexual desires, preferences, habits, and any shame that may be connected.

What we're asking for: enduring erections and arousal. What is happening in the body: tension and fear.

Low/No Desire

First and foremost, low desire or lack of desire for sexual experience is only problematic if its absence is missed or feels troubling in terms of connection or intimacy for those involved. Like most things connected to sex, there is no prescribed amount of desire we should feel in order to "do" our individual or shared sexual life "right." This is also a highly subjective area of our sexuality that culture attempts to make prescriptions around:

- We should desire sex with our partners if we love them.
- If we identify as male, desire should be ever-present.
- We should desire sex regularly, at least ____ times a day/week/month to be a "healthy" sexual person and/or in a "healthy" sexual relationship.
- If we're in a relationship, we should only desire our partner.

Whatever feels best for us in terms of our relationship to desire is great! We will all have a unique and specific relationship to desire that will move and shift with our day, week, month, quality of relationship to self and/or others along the way. If we are troubled by the absence of feelings of desire, we can begin to explore what might be getting in the way of it emerging.

Have I felt disconnected from myself lately? Is there tension in the relationship? Am I bogged down with work, kids, stress?

Low or lack of desire can be a consequence of the "shoulds" we hold around what desire should be *for* or in connection with; for example *I should desire an orgasm, or to give oral sex because my partner loves it, or I should desire an explicitly erotic experience.* Low or lack of desire can also be a reaction to trauma, difficult associations, or the consequence of challenging experiences we've had around sex, or discomfort with intimacy and vulnerability, that is anxiety we experience when faced with the prospect of sexual activity with others or self. It can hide in superficial things: *I have low desire because you need to shower more,* or *because our bedroom is a mess.* The superficial causes our brain latches onto very frequently hide the larger issues that have everything to do with us or larger themes in the relationship, such as *I'm feeling insecure about my body, I'm touched out and want to have my body for myself,* or *I haven't felt the desire to come close in any of the realms of intimacy (emotional, sexual, physical, spiritual) since the affair – I don't want to share myself yet.*

Low desire can be a reaction to sexual challenges or "dysfunction," as we're not going to seek out experiences that make us feel uncomfortable, ashamed, or worried. In general, we will not seek out experiences associated with challenging feelings as reward-seeking creatures!

What we're (sometimes) asking for: increased desire. What's happening in the body: emotional and psychological block and/or disinterest.

Note: low or lack of desire can frequently be a consequence of medications we use to treat depression and/or anxiety. In fact, many medications we utilize for mental and physical health and wellbeing can have an influence on desire, sensation, and orgasm. If this is something you've noticed, working with your provider may alleviate some of the symptoms over time.

Anorgasmia

Very rarely is anorgasmia, or the inability to reach or achieve palpable orgasm, due to the inability of the body to understand or provide sensation (i.e. entirely biologically based), although it can be! Most of what we're looking at is inexperience with self-touch, lack of exploration, and importantly difficulty letting go into sensation, emotion, fantasy, and/or connection sufficiently to allow these elements to build and then spill over (which can often be influenced by the presence of pain). Challenges releasing into catharsis (i.e. orgasm) are accompanied by tension in the body or pelvic floor. This tipping point can be scary for some, and parallel to the fear or hesitation we experience when allowing our emotions to reach their fulness in our everyday lives. Some can identify a build of arousal and sensation and then back off, determining it's taking too long or feels too intense. Could we be backing off prematurely, or even intuitively, just as we're nearing that point? Fearing or intimidated by what the spillover may bring? Like many of the other struggles, anorgasmia can be life-long or situational, giving us hints about where anxiety might emerge and what it's made of. It can also be misdiagnosed due to our inability to understand the variability in how orgasms might present! It can feel like a huge catharsis, full-body contractions, or more genitally focused. It can also feel like a tiny burst, a tingly sensation, a relief. There can be great variability in the type of stimulation needed and intensity required to reach orgasm for people with vulvas.

When situational, it is commonly found to occur in partnered sex, where the individual affected doesn't note it happening in their self-touch or solo sexual life. This can be due to: performance anxiety; trauma; intimacy fears or lack of trust (in self and/or other); insecurities and spectatoring; or "watching" ourselves during sex rather than being present and in our bodies; and/or lack of knowledge and misinformation about vaginal versus clitoral orgasms (all orgasms are clitoral, even the vaginal ones that are far more rare – most people with vulvas require clitoral stimulation of some degree for orgasm). This issue seems to disproportionately affect cisgender women who have sex with cisgender men, due in part to the rigid script heterosexual couples are given about what sex looks like, each person's part in it, and the role orgasm plays (often a "must have" = pressure).

What we're asking for: orgasms. What's happening in the body: resistance, holding back, tension, bearing down.

Note: anorgasmia for transwomen who have recently undergone genital reconstructive surgery can be connected to the common causes named above, but it can also be one of the times when sensation and physiology can play a significant role. Post-op bodies are healing, sensation is different, and our brains (and hearts) need time to acclimate and process these evolving differences (because healing takes time). The residual presence of gender dysphoria post-op is common as well (because it becomes something many are intimately familiar with, and therefore often will not simply vanish when and how we want it to), which can cause confusion and impact the relationship we hold to our changing bodies, which in turn impacts the ability to release into them, take a curious approach to sensation, learn, and play. Continued exploration and conversation with medical and sex therapy providers as healing progresses can support ongoing evolution and learning and/or help illuminate vital information around any potential challenges physically and beyond that may require attending to. We all deserve supportive care at all stages in our journeys toward self-actualization.

Rapid, Early, or "Premature" Ejaculation (PE)

A tricky challenge to name (because what constitutes "premature"? How do we know what "early" means for each person uniquely? 1 minute? 5 minutes? 30 seconds?). What we're ultimately working with is the lack of "voluntary, conscious control, or the ability to choose in most encounters, when to ejaculate" (Metz & McCarthy, 2003, p. 1). PE can be a consequence of nervousness, perceived or real inexperience, scarcity mindset (novelty of the experience and/or frequency/infrequency of sexual interaction), shame about erotic preferences/desires, or performance pressure/anxiety. With situational or relational PE, Metz and McCarthy describe the tendency to focus on highly erotic cues or stimuli very early in the sexual interaction with partners to skyrocket arousal. If we take that and combine it with nervousness/anxiety (tension in the pelvic floor) and scarcity mindset (*oh my goodness, this is my chance! This is so hot, I can't mess this up!*), we've got the perfect formula for lack of ejaculatory control.

> Most men [or people with penises] gain a rudimentary sense of ejaculation awareness in adolescence or young adulthood based on their experience with masturbation. They learn to back off the stimulation slightly to last longer and to speed it up to ejaculate more quickly. This trial-and-error learning process usually carries over when they start having intercourse with women [or penetrative sex with partners]. However, for some, it's a learning process that doesn't happen.
>
> (Keesling, 2006, p. 82)

As with all developmental processes, this learning can: get interrupted; be limited by values, shame, and moral code; be thwarted due to lack of privacy, especially under the profound influence of shame and anxiety. Ejaculatory awareness alongside arousal awareness is something we can begin to cultivate today. As with all sexual struggles, we can deepen our development now, correcting course in the present with time and patience.

What we're asking for: ejaculatory control. What's happening in the body: tension in the pelvic floor, fear, often coupled with excitement.

What Else Is There?

Most sexual struggles will visit us at some point in our lifetimes, if not multiple times over, much like sexually transmitted infections (let's be real). Our lives, experiences, feelings about ourselves and our partners, and our relationship to power (within personal and romantic relationships and within larger systems) do not stop at the bedroom door: all elements follow us in, moving through and being expressed in our sexual experiences if we allow them to. This list offers a snapshot into some of the reasons why they surface, how we attempt to cope with them, and how we might conceptualize them differently. Your complexity will add its own details to the snapshots above as they by no means cover everything these challenges are made of or represent.

6 Emotion, Prediction, and Association

What does your anxiety forecast when you approach sexual interaction? What does your brain predict will happen, and how might it tell us this via our emotions? So far, we have named anxiety as the major culprit, at the very least as an important player behind most sexual struggles, elaborating on the emotional concept and breaking it down to understand how to identify and work with it when it steps forward, giving it definition and bringing it to life so it can no longer hide and haunt in the shadows. But anxiety is only one emotion commonly paired with our conversation around sex, as an inherently emotional experience and a profound form of expression. How we understand *what* emotions we're interacting with throughout the experience can determine our relationship with our sexuality, shift our physiological response, and effect our desire for sex at large.

So how are emotions made and how do they inform our associations with sex? Can we unmake them, and influence the body, with the help of our mind? We will turn to the work of Dr. Lisa Feldman Barrett, Psychology Professor at Northeastern University and author of *How Emotions Are Made: The Secret Life of the Brain*, to answer these questions. Her research will give us a window into the emotion–sensation connection and how our brain understands our sex.

The Fabric of Emotion

Ari is in a loving relationship with her partner of a year, Taylor. They engage with each other sexually every Tuesday night and Sunday morning, almost like clockwork. It's a ritual in their relationship.

Lately when Ari and Taylor are sexual, Ari notices clenching in her body. Her heart pounds and palms sweat. As arousal mounts, Ari observes what she identifies as tension beginning to surface as they move through their sexual routine, that then evolves into tears. They hold each other for a few minutes, then go to sleep.

DOI: 10.4324/9781003369080-8

How might these recent experiences shape the description of the couple that we began with? Depending on Ari's lived experience, her past, it might look like:

Description (A): *Ari is in a loving relationship with her partner of a year, Taylor. They engage with each other sexually every Tuesday night and Sunday morning, a challenging routine for Ari. Sex has become complicated, characterized by intense, intrusive, and uncomfortable feelings that she can't comprehend. What she can identify is feeling upset that sex is no longer easy, something Taylor hopes they can get back to, together. Ari worries it's a sign their sexual connection is lost.*

OR

Description (B): *Ari is in a loving relationship with her partner of a year, Taylor. They engage with each other sexually every Tuesday night and Sunday morning, almost like clockwork. Lately, sex has become complicated, but Ari understands this complexity to be healing. With each experience she is releasing fear, sadness, and hard memories connected to intimacy from her past. They build alongside the arousal and are then released in the context of their connection, something they both cherish concerning the safety they've co-created.*

How is it that the same physiological information, identical sensory data at baseline, might lead to a completely different experience, with some similar but also some distinctly disparate emotional characteristics?

To break this down:

- Our brains register raw sensory information from the body ("arousal" + heart pounds, palms sweat, tension) and promptly begin formulating a meaningful guess about the cause to understand how to proceed.
- This guess is informed by:
  - Information from our external world or context (sex/sharing and closeness with long-term partner);
  - Guess work and reference to similar experiences and body states from the past:
    - Description (A):
      - Past experience could include snapshots of sex consisting of fun and exciting interactions with casual hook-ups, but with insecurity and stiffness with long-term partners, including similar physiological symptoms in the body (racing heart and sweaty palms).

- Past experience could also draw from memories of sweaty palms, racing heart, and tension being associated with challenging experiences: auditions, not knowing a lot of the answers to a test, bumbling and not knowing what to say on a date.
  - Past experience could grab inspiration from experiences of not doing something "right," which for Ari has meant she was "wrong" or a failure.

- The culmination of information triggers our emotional concepts, like upset or worry, from those we were taught in similar situations as children.

  - The upset and worry then inspire more upsetting and worrying thoughts and predictions about what will unfold next, building on sensation, culminating in tears for Ari.

Emotions are your brain's best guesses of what your bodily sensations mean, guided by your past experience. Your brain constructs these guesses in the blink of an eye – so rapidly, in fact, that emotions feel like uncontrollable reactions that happen to you, when emotions are actually made by you.

(Feldman Barrett, 2021)

Predictions

Predictions *are* the business of the brain, the way it operates. They are the foundation of our experience, of our behavior, of the big and small actions that fill our day; all of them. The brain is in a stream of constant chatter with itself trying to understand what will happen next from what has happened in similar situations and physiological states before. This process constructs our experience, our present reality being *a* contributor or one factor in our experience rather than an objective element we are in present connection with, and in reaction to. In other words, my experience with a chair (pulling it out, having a seat, settling in) is entirely shaped by my experience with all other chairs before: I am interacting with their imprint and that imprint is the guiding force behind any internal sense of trust I have in the chair's ability to hold my weight, how comfortable or uncomfortable I anticipate it being, and how I maneuver my body as I place myself in position. Despite how imperfect this mechanism may be, full of plenty of room for error, predictions help us understand the world with efficiency. Our brain needs to predict when we're going to stand up from that chair so it can alter our blood pressure accordingly, protecting us from fainting, and it needs to do it quickly.

If predictions weave together every moment of our day, anxiety is what happens when our predictions spiral due to limited and/or negative previous experience to reference. This isn't unique to anxiety, though: all emotions are predictions. Why is this necessary to understand? Because (i) emotions *are* physical, they begin with basic, paired down sensory information in the body, and (ii) if emotions are constructed and made *by* us rather than happening *to* us, we can interact with them differently, potentially changing our experience; we can feel less "out of control" in the face of our emotional activation. We can feel less hijacked in our sex.

Turning Inward

To understand what this "raw sensory data" looks like, we turn to "interception," or the feeling of the sensations that come from the movements inside our bodies. Interception is our "internal eye," the mechanism that senses the status of all our internal systems, communicating this information to the brain, whose primary function is to regulate all of the systems in the body with surgical precision. What does it communicate? It simplifies, condensing our experience down to *pleasantness, unpleasantness, calm, arousal.* Our brain is receiving this feedback ceaselessly throughout the day, paired down to allow us to offer our attention to our external world. Once received, the brain uses the past to construct theories around the cause. From there concepts emerge, memories and past experiences making sense of incoming sensory input, shaping the raw data into emotional concepts. "*Sister knocked your tower down, it looks like you're angry! Anger is a big feeling, isn't it?*" These concepts are introduced to us, learned, modeled, and rehearsed. Emotional concepts sculpt the raw sensations from interoception (*pleasant, unpleasant, arousal, calm*) into the emotions we experience. Absent these concepts, we wouldn't have any of the emotions commonly thought of as "hardwired," the fear, anger, sadness, disgust, contempt, and surprise said to be built in to our design.

> Your brain recreates the past from memory by asking itself, *The last time I encountered a similar situation, when my body was in a similar state and was preparing an action similar to this one, what did I see next? What did I feel next?* The answer becomes your experience. In other words, your brain combines information from outside and inside your head to produce everything you see, hear, smell, taste, and feel.
>
> (Feldman Barrett, 2021)

How might we behave differently, react differently, if we understood that the physical movements and sensations in the body that we associate with distinct emotions have no intrinsic meaning, emotionally or otherwise, that they are simply sensations? In other words, when our brains understand "unpleasant," in a sexual situation, staving off our sexual response, we may have the opportunity to understand that sensation in a completely new way by practicing new responses to it in the moment. I may feel "anxiety," *and* decide to name it as anticipatory energy, helping propel me to take a different step, leading to a new outcome, shaping and creating a new prediction for tomorrow.

Emotional Trade-Off?

Can we control our emotions? Our brains make meaning of the raw data being communicated to the brain in a split second, but then we pick up the ball, participating in the ongoing manifestation of that feeling as we continue to add to the story off and very consciously online, feeding the emotional concept with more evidence for its existence, and proof of its validity. Our emotions *are* our physiology, they exist as sensation interpretation, as forecasting and prediction based on past experience, associations, and memory. Is the raw data being interpreted by the brain under our conscious control? No. What meaning is given to it, the emotional concepts assigned to it, can be influenced. In this way we are confronted, yet again, with the notion that all experiences are constructed. Emotional experience is not an indication of something objective about an event. If we make concepts, we can introduce others, or invite others in with intention. If you change the ingredients that your brain uses to make emotion, then you can transform your emotional and therefore sexual life – shifting our choices today teaches the brain how to *predict* differently tomorrow.

If sex is inherently emotional, what does that mean, given what we now know about what emotions are? What they are made of?

- Remember when we defined sex versus intimacy? Sex being a series of behaviors that we move through that kick up a physiological response in the body, culminating in pleasure, release, and/or orgasm (or not)? Sex is a physiological event, an experience and exploration of sensation, by definition. Sensation is the foundation of our emotional concepts.
- Intimacy takes up the sharing space, an experience characterized by risk as we reveal private aspects of who we are to ourselves or another person or people. Stepping into our vulnerability holds complex memories from which the brain draws information. It is a colorful mixed bag for everyone.
- If we add these two ingredients together, we have the perfect breeding ground for: (i) interacting with and interpreting raw sensory data in the body (*this warmth in my chest feels good, I'm so happy. This tightness in*

my chest feels uncomfortable, tightness in the chest just happened a week ago when I was just about to crash my bike, maybe I'm doing something wrong which will end in disaster [prediction], I'm feeling anxious), kicking up emotional concepts and the memories that inspired them; and (ii) prediction built from complex memory and past experience around an abstract, vulnerable, and misunderstood part of our humanity.

Our emotions are not natural functions, the raw sensory data in the body, on the other hand, is. We can take a conscious part in the ongoing construction of our emotional experience for ourselves, with ourselves. What implications does this have for our sex and our sexual struggles?

Escaping the Past

We can choose which ideas, thoughts, and (now) emotions are reflections of us and our experience, and what might need to be let go of, reframed, recontextualized, or allowed to exist as sensory information on its own, free from story (a practice in itself!). This will not eliminate our relationship with some of our most frequent visitors on the emotion list, but it can help.

Does the sensation I'm interpreting to mean _____ or _____ match what is happening right now (current context) and, if not, can I understand this sensation differently? Can I release my body, my musculature, to invite more sensation in? Can I name this feeling differently as a result?

Associations and Desire

An alternative version of a prediction is an association, which is equally as influential over our sexual experience. An association is a connection, an emotional imprint, a link, as opposed to an estimation of the consequence of something. Our concept of sex can be connected to a constellation of characteristics, these feelings, ideas, and/or images often becoming part of the definition of the word itself, influencing our style when we approach it (playful, jokey, aggressive, tender, performative, verbal or nonverbal, etc.), what we approach sex for (pleasure, connection, release, escape, obligation, etc.), our behavior early on or throughout the duration of the experience (stiff, tense, free, absorbed, attuned, distracted), and ultimately if we follow through with the approach whatsoever (on any particular occasion, or chronically, i.e. avoidance). Despite not knowing what will happen situation by situation, the feelings, ideas, and images linked to our concepts begin in the body before the reality of the concept has begun, sometimes for better (so yay, hooray, go for it!) or for worse (ugh, oh-no, avoid). It is a split-second experience-to-feeling reaction, a merging of a concept to an emotional state or idea or both. What wins out when it comes to our behavior, our literal definition of sex, or the feelings in the body that surface when we think about it? This is the business of associations and the power that they wield in and out of the bedroom, and it isn't new!

Remember Ivan Pavlov, the Russian psychologist who first introduced the world to the art of the learned response via classical conditioning? Most of us have had at bare minimum an introduction to the theory in high school or beyond; but how compelling was the information at the time? How meaningful was the concept of learning through association(s) in terms of our own lives and understanding of ourselves? Let's review these ideas further and take a deeper look at the implications of this theory now (extremely basically, as that's all we need for our intents and purposes), because when it comes to your sexuality, I think you'll see that Pavlov and his dog can tell us a great deal about the associations you've created and why.

Pavlov's experiment breaks down as:

1 When Pavlov's dog (let's call him Spot) is presented with food, he salivates (which was measured via a tiny test tube that was inserted in the cheek of the dog).
2 Pavlov begins ringing a bell before presenting the food.
3 Once practiced several times, Spot begins salivating at the sound of the bell, even in the absence of food. What is happening here?
4 An association has been formed. Spot has begun to associate the sound of the bell with the imminent presentation of food, and as a result an emotional and physiological response was activated in the body.

The formation and strengthening of associations happen continuously throughout our day, week, month, year. We are endlessly in the process of creating or reinforcing associations with experiences, people, places, ideas, and so on. For example, "*I associate sex with shame,*" or "*I associate intimacy with anxiety.*" Unpacking the last one, if every time we approach or think about sex it is tied with the idea of inauthenticity (performance), pleasing the other (performance), accomplishing a goal (performance), being a certain way (performance), how are we going to *feel* about sex? Anxious! From there, can we expect that we would want to do it?

As most of us have noticed about life, and sex is no different, the feelings that surface, that suggest safety or lack thereof, can be actively and subconsciously perpetuated by us. We reinforce the narrative (the felt sense and/or the fully articulated idea), and not-so-suddenly event A gets paired with feeling B in a way that we reinforce over time as our brain continues to collect information that supports the link with each event moving forward. A seed gets planted and grows behind the curtain. Similarly, we can encounter feelings in an experience once, or again and again, which effectively become our "training" around what the experience is, means, and represents. Event A gets paired with feeling B in a way that is reinforced over time because the feelings from our past are so powerful that they completely color the experiences of a similar nature moving forward, therefore reinforcing the association(s). We can live in our associations even as our reality offers the possibility for another experience to arise, arrested by the strength of the connection.

Our desire is governed by these associations. Like our sexual functioning, we were taught that desire exists in its own separate sphere, immune to the impact of life and challenging sexual experiences, ready to be activated, and very easily so, at any moment. In actuality, desire is made and shaped and influenced. We will not seek out experiences that are associated with challenging feelings, threatening or unsafe thoughts, memories, or interactions (even when there is no "logical" reason to feel unsafe in our current context). *If my sexual experiences are characterized by insecurity and embarrassment, I'm simply not going to want to approach them anymore. If every time I ejaculate earlier than I want to, humiliation surfaces, followed by worry that my partner will leave me; sex will be something to be avoided at all costs.* It's that simple. Our desire attempts to work in our favor, showing up and pointing us in the direction of all things awesome and rewarding when the reward is there, but going underground and swapping spots with avoidance and anxiety to protect us from emotional, psychological, or perhaps even physical harm or pain when reward is absent or worse.

Creating and reinforcing new associations is the work of sexual healing; it is what you are actively doing in this moment just by exposing yourself to new content and ideas, and it is what we will continue to do as we move on. Associations will be affected or created by the information shared and the various ways you challenge yourself in relationship to it. Remember how ineffective "the talk" was with parents, caregivers, or maybe even teachers? One of a million reasons why it missed the mark has to do with the fact that for most of us it was a one-off. Sex deserves an ongoing conversation, ongoing thought, questioning and consideration. With learning and information comes a greater sense of connection, and with an increasingly strong connection, there's less room there for anxiety to thrive. The more we interact with sexual content and information, and the more we interact with our own sexuality experientially with new insights in mind, the more we reinforce the kind of associations that make sex rewarding. That can only mean good news for our desire, a feeling born from robust association partnered with fantasy.

In the meantime, what are some associations you can identify that you carry in relationship to sex? What does your brain predict sex will mean?

Activity opportunity: Think about the following words and tune in to the very first feelings, sensations, thoughts, and/or memories that surface. The words may inspire challenging or traumatic associations for some. Proceed slowly, give yourself a minute or two with each word, and stop or pause when needed (listening to and honoring your own boundaries) or skip entirely:

- Masturbation;
- Dating;
- Hook-up culture;
- Oral sex;
- Romance;
- Monogamy;
- Kink.

Do the associations change if you deliberately place yourself next to some of the words?

- Myself masturbating;
- My body;
- Myself hooking up with a stranger;
- Self-love;
- Letting go;
- Being vulnerable with another person.

Now that you've pinned down a few associations that some of these behaviors and experiences carry, return to the list and consider what associations you'd like to carve out and reinforce moving forward, adding some of your own words as you go (e.g. sex *is* sanctuary, my body *is* home). What feelings, attitudes, ideas would you like to embody with these words in a general sense and as they connect to you? It is important to keep in mind that the associations we keep in relation to our own sexual self-concepts exert the most powerful influence over the experience and how it unfolds. Start generally, and then connect with the concepts personally in order to:

1 Begin to conceptualize what associations and ideas we wish to incorporate into our embodiment practice in Part III – associations that resonate with our sexual values and perspective now, free from the "shoulds" we've been beholden to.

2 Bring awareness to the associations that are no longer invited into our lives so that we can begin to put a halt to their ongoing reinforcement. With this awareness in mind, we can begin to ask ourselves what it might take, what even just a first step might look like toward those ends.

If our associations are created and reinforced, will our memory, our bodies, let them go? Not unless we carve out and reinforce new ones, with repetition, patience, and practice (and likely some fumbling around as we do so). If our behavior today directly influences our brain's predictions for tomorrow, our feelings today connect themselves to our experiences, influencing our felt understanding of their definition tomorrow. We've got some really important work to do, always.

7   Putting It All Together
A Word About Pleasure

There was a time in the not-so-distant past when the message we received was that orgasm was the goal of sex. Consequently, if orgasm didn't happen, it represented a failure: either on the part of the individual interacting with themselves, or the partner who was "responsible" for the other person's orgasms, pleasure, or having a good time. So, we ditched that idea and shifted instead to centering pleasure as the goal of sex: "pleasure is the measure!" Yet if we stick around long enough in a sexual relationship with ourselves or other people, what sex will reveal to us is our complexity, as an expression of our complexity as humans. When we let go into what is an inherently vulnerable experience, we cannot control what surfaces, be it grief, joy, sorrow, elation, our trauma – we make profound contact with ourselves in this surrender space. *But if pleasure is the goal of sex and I found myself crying, does that mean I did that wrong? Did I just have bad sex?*

To take this further (and this part is important), if our sexual functions are governed by the parasympathetic nervous system, whose primary responsibility is to help us regain homeostasis, that is to come back to center after a stressful event or even just the events of the day (i.e. sleep), could the main function of sex, at least where our sexual functions are concerned, be to help us regain homeostasis, moving through what gets in the way of our sense of balance, harmony, re-calibration – physiologically, emotionally, psychologically? When we expect this to be the situation, when we understand that our complexity will surface if we truly let go in sex, the process of moving through stored emotion from last week, the tension from the spat with your partner this morning, the anxiety from your presentation at work this afternoon, can feel supremely freeing, relieving, transcendent (forms of pleasure). If we expect sex to be "fun" and about "pleasurable sensation" every time, this experience can feel like an intrusion, pathological even.

In life when we say we want to be happy, what we really mean is: I want to visit more moments of happiness because I understand that constant

DOI: 10.4324/9781003369080-9

happy feelings aren't possible. Sex is the same. We have to make room for pleasure to emerge, make room for happy moments, which means interacting with and experiencing the calm ones, the tense ones, the sad ones, the hard ones. Our physiology is in favor of our homeostasis. Can we join its mission? Do we dare show ourselves or others what that process looks like? Really get "naked?"

For the record, when referencing "pleasure" in this context, we are referring to how society treats pleasure when it comes to sex: as pleasurable sensation, happy feelings, a fun time. How sex therapy treats pleasure is as an umbrella term, something that can include all colors and textures of experience. For example, comfort can be pleasurable, as can connection, closeness, learning, witnessing, catharsis. If we all treated pleasure in this way, sex would always offer something in the way of reward. And yet, can other elements be important, valuable, meaningful too? Pleasure is one color on the color wheel that sex has to offer. Can we invite in all of its rich complexity and, consequently, save sex?

What might happen if we stop making sex our New Year's Eve, an experience from which we expect to receive the fantasy Disney epic party, and are discouraged when it gives us *life* instead? Gives us reality? When we stop trying to force sex to deliver constant pleasure and total satisfaction *"ugh, gotta be a fun time*!!!!" counterintuitively more pleasure shows up. It's no different than placing orgasm as the goal: we're still having goal-oriented, strive-mindset style sex. When we stop trying to force it to be anything other than what it *is* that day, in that moment, in that experience, it reveals itself to us. It offers reward in spades; it is reprieve, sanctuary.

Part II

What Is My Anxiety Trying to Teach Me?

If we lower our anxiety shield, what exists underneath? What is with us as we approach a sexual encounter just by being us, being our age, race, gender, socio-economic status, ethnicity, religion, from a particular family, part of the world or country, with our unique educational experiences, abilities and disabilities, responding to and working with our specific traumas? In this part of the book we will explore some common sources of anxiety that stick to our sexuality simply by being human in a confused world. This is not by any means meant to cover all the bases, there are simply too many to count! But by beginning an exploration into some basic yet major themes, we can and will encounter others that are meaningful to us as individuals. The exploration becomes expansive on its own and gives us practice at attuning to the funky stories, lessons, and ideas that have gone unchecked and unchallenged and therefore live with us and manifest in and through our sexuality.

Is awareness alone enough? It depends! Sometimes awareness of what is with us, what is at the wheel when it comes to our sexual choices and feelings, can be game changing and allow for different choices, a new perspective and way of interacting with ourselves and others, unhooked from guilt, shame, or fear, therefore resolving our struggles! Other times awareness alone falls short, failing to offer us a clear vision for how to move forward, to shift the feelings that surface, or to teach us how to adopt new behaviors. Even when this rings true, awareness takes us a step closer. The more intimately we know ourselves, the more we understand our feelings and choices, the more we trust ourselves, the easier it is to let go.

We will be in conversation with other therapists and experts in the field who will offer us windows into specific cultures, subcultures, experiences, and identities to bring these ideas to life in a greater way. These are tiny windows into a sample of human variety and diversity of experience, identity, and process – each of which deserves an entire book of its own.

DOI: 10.4324/9781003369080-10

Anxiety and sex do not take on an overt presence in many of the areas we'll explore together. That is because these themes are what build our anxiety, construct our relationship to our sexuality. These are the elements "under the hood" when it comes to our sexual makeup. Armed with greater self-knowledge, and a truer sense of how you think about the forces that effect the sense you hold of yourself as a sexual being, we will come into the body in a more experiential way, which we will build on further in Part III, where we deal directly with our sex and anxiety. In the meantime, as the saying goes, *"Everything is about sex but sex."* Let's discover why this is true for you.

8   Arrested Development

Today in Health Class, we're talking about sex! Students file in cracking jokes and laughing nervously about what's to come, anxiety mounting in anticipation of how it might feel to learn about a hush-hush topic in the presence of their peers and teachers. Amanda, a 15-year-old, cisgender, Brazilian, bisexual female in her sophomore year of high school takes her seat. Raised in a strict Catholic family with three younger siblings, sex is a non-subject, which is exceptional even within her church. The absence of this conversation has been anything but lost on her. She began menstruating at 12 years old, had her first kiss at 13, and recognized glimmers of attraction to both same and opposite sex peers around the same time. She finds herself interested in exploring her sexual orientation, and potentially dating, intimacy, and various forms of ethical non-monogamy.

Will I be learning about any of these things today?

The class starts and Mr. Whitley with his flat-affect and tense demeanor does his best to get through some basics around anatomy and how to properly secure a condom on a banana. The lights then switch off as the PowerPoint portion of the day begins. The students spend the bulk of the rest of their class learning about common sexually transmitted infections while being shown nightmarish photographs of the most extreme manifestations. Before she knows it, the day is done. That's it. Pleasure, consent, boundaries, safe sex, gender, communication, kink, polyamory, dating ... a familiar radio silence.

Why do I feel even more anxious now than when I walked in? Why is sex so off limits? Why does it all seem so ... scary?

If it's safe to go there, what are your first memories of your sexuality? Can you bring to mind some of your primary experiences with pleasure, feelings of attraction or longing for closeness, discovering your own body, awareness of your gender, learning about the sexual lives of others – maybe even your parents (whoops!)? What surrounded these experiences for you? How did you make sense of them? Perhaps some were fun, some confusing, scary, or upsetting. Who did you turn to so as to make sense of what

DOI: 10.4324/9781003369080-11

happened? Who was talking you through what they meant and didn't mean about who you are and what you like and/or dislike and how to move forward? Who helped you contextualize it all, assisting you in shaping your sense of self as a sexual being, including exploration of identity, boundaries, and expectations for and from intimacy. For most of us, the answer that comes up is: no one. The reality is, *you* were your primary teacher. Imagine that.

Proper development in any arena of human life requires education, ongoing conversation, support, and guidance. When these requirements go unmet, children, adolescents, and teens are left to fill in the blanks and do the meaning-making for themselves with the brain and life experience they're equipped with at the time. They're left to interpret the silence, the absence or lack of support and guidance on their own, with peers, or online. And finally, they're left to navigate experiences in this realm with no guardrails or real understanding about what to expect or ask for, or where to begin in how they might take care of themselves as they explore. Such a disastrous set-up comes with equally problematic consequences. Even those fortunate enough to be raised in a home where sex wasn't treated as the big bad secret, must contend with the consequences of living in a larger context, a society where sex is taboo, full of contradictions, only for certain "kinds" of people (i.e. able-bodied, cisgender, straight, from designated racial groups, and young), and ultimately an area of deep confusion and shame. They must make sense of this discrepancy within themselves (*Here's where my family stands, here's what I'm gathering from the world around me, now where do I sit?*), intuiting their way through the contradictory ideas and messaging.

Fantasy

A primary way we work to understand ourselves (including our likes, dislikes, desires, dreams, and goals) is through fantasy. We begin practicing fantasizing/imagining at a very young age with non-erotic content that then evolves and spreads into all arenas of human life, becoming increasingly sophisticated and connected to arousal and often orgasm with expanded awareness in adolescence. Fantasy is imagination play-space and adolescence is characterized by it as we understand love and intimacy in more nuanced ways and begin to crave deep connection with people outside of our parents. Though this is established early on, the role our fantasies play remains the same throughout the lifespan, and so just like their adult counterparts, children and teens engage with fantasy in order to: approach the unapproachable; escape; practice; work out longing, lust, unrequited feelings; try on different or new ideas, identities, scenarios, and situations; understand sexual urges and put them in context; go to the places they shouldn't or can't or don't want to experience in their lived reality. It is the place we get to know ourselves in an ongoing way: our sexual thoughts, behaviors, feelings, and how they interplay. It can both serve as an incredibly important offline processing, meaning-making, and self-evolving tool, and also a completely abstract, complex, dream-like space that is entirely about play without any implication whatsoever for who we are and what we want in our lives. This is where we get tripped up, especially as young people. Determining what is OK to think about (which, by the way, is everything), and what our thoughts mean about who we are is one of the great struggles of being human. Anxiety loves it when we believe every thought that passes through our mind, when we decide that random fantasy about sleeping with my teacher or best friend's crush must mean that I've cheated on some level, or betrayed my best friend, or that I must be deeply dissatisfied in my relationship despite all evidence to the contrary. Children, adolescents, and teens are particularly susceptible to drawing conclusions about who they are based on the content of their fantasies, and even simply their thoughts. Distinguishing between a thought that resonates with who we are and how we truly feel and want to move through the world, versus a thought that is not and therefore something to let go of, is challenging even in adulthood. Deep shame begins here.

How quick have you been to draw conclusions about yourself based on thought content alone? Can you recall funky thoughts you wrestled with as a child or adolescent that reflected your confusion around sex? Around your sexuality? How did you attempt to cope?

Children and Porn

If elementary school is a time when we meet and enjoy friendships based on similar interests, middle school is a time when we must adopt whatever interests define a particular group and wear them with precision to fit in, to spare ourselves bullying and ostracization. The middle school years (typically sixth to eighth grade) seem to represent a turning point in the life of the child whereby in-group identity and "shoulds" reign. If you're going to be popular, you have to "do" popular right; if you're going to be "weird," there are rules for that; if you're going to be queer you have to be queer enough; and if you're going to be a jock (athletic) or a skater (skateboarder) you must act the part or else you're a "poser" or worse. Middle school also happens to be a time when children are approaching or going through puberty, when sexuality and sexual exploration explode. With social status and the quest to fit in as paramount, how we "do" our sexuality becomes critical as well. Our reputation is on the line. Where do children go to understand what they "should" be doing when it comes to sex?

These days, the internet, and specifically porn, plain and simple. Consequently, sexual development as it relates to explicit media can be conceptualized as moving along as follows:

- Hyper-awareness of sexuality/sexual feelings/desires around puberty/adolescence + no **conversation or guidance around it** = turn to the only option available to learn, explore, understand intellectually, *and* in an embodied way (porn or erotic media).
- Hyper-awareness of sexuality/sexual feelings/desires around puberty/adolescence + no **conversation or guidance around it** + shame messaging around porn = hidden solo sexual life and ongoing relationship to erotic media in adulthood; a place where I can engage in my sexual feelings, fantasies, and curiosities shame-free.

Children and adolescents long for information, they desire answers and understanding in the same way their adult counterparts do. They understand when information is being withheld, which only adds fuel to the fire. Does an eight-year-old watching porn make him (for example) disturbed? Perverse somehow? More likely to act out sexually when he's older? No. It makes him confused, an emotion we all seek to remedy with answers, with understanding. If that eight-year-old then shows his friend the porn he discovered, does that change our responses to any of the questions above? No, we are still working with confusion and not wanting to feel alone in that experience. Now let's say that these two boys attempt to "play out" some of the media they're watching together. Have the answers changed now? Still no. We are *still* interacting with confused little boys looking to understand the sensations they're experiencing in their bodies, the behaviors that are being modeled or demonstrated to them in the video, grappling with the inevitable question below it all (*"Is this what 'men' do? Is this what my dad is doing? Is this what I should be doing too?"*) – all with the brain and emotional intelligence that eight-year-old children are equipped with. What are we likely to do at any age to understand something more fully? Revisit it. What are we likely to do at any age if there's any amount of thrill involved, even when that thrill is coupled with confusion or shame? Revisit it. What are children likely to do when they (i) see a boundary or rule, and (ii) don't understand why it's there? Break it, especially when emboldened by the presence of another person. Especially when we have a team.

Fear Factor

Circling back to class, how many of us share aspects of Amanda's story? How many of us remember our sex education courses and their "take-aways"? For most, our first real conversations around sex centered on fear: fear of pregnancy, fear of unwanted touch or sexual assault, fear of sexually transmitted infections (STIs), and/or fear of painful sex ("popping the cherry" or breaking the hymen). That fear becomes part of the foundation of our understanding of what sex is, what to expect from it, and therefore an active player in the experience itself.

Fear of contracting an STI on it's own impacts the freedom we experience when moving toward touch with a partner. The knowledge that many STIs are spread via skin-to-skin contact makes even using condoms scary as they cover a limited area of the body. *Letting go, surrender, trust, play, communication, expression, vulnerability* – the STI worry alone impacts (to lesser or greater degrees depending on the person) our ease in stepping into at least several of these elements, and we haven't even considered the others. Is this rational? No. STIs are a normal part of being sexual and most are preventable, treatable, or manageable with proper education, care, and instruction. Tragically, sex education is not about facts and is not an open, honest sharing of accurate and current information, at least not traditionally. In most parts of the USA, sex education has been, and still is, organized around morality, purity culture, and once again fear. Hello, anxiety!

Sexual Imprints

We don't just jump into our sexuality in adolescence; we are sexual, or more accurately sensual beings *in utero*, understanding and often playing with pleasurable sensation (yes, that means exploring fun feelings in our genitals) from the time we discover we can use our hands to touch. For some, genital exploration/play is obvious after the first six months of life and becomes increasingly sophisticated with increased coordination and bodily awareness. For others, purposeful self-stimulation can emerge as young as three to five years of age, and seemingly out of nowhere. This can look like rubbing up against or humping pillows, climbing the pole repeatedly at school and hovering at the top to "see how long you can stay up there" (yes, there were a lot of us), playing with the water pressure in the bath – children are creative and find a plethora of ways to experience pleasure and explore their bodies.

What *is* masturbation for children? Connecting and getting to know sensation in the body, in our genitals, understanding our own physiology, attending to thoughts and watching them pass, encountering the fantasy/story realm of the brain, making contact with emotion and emotional and physical release. It *is* mindfulness, it *is* mindful embodiment practice. What are the implications of interrupting this ongoing practice and exploration? How might we all live and feel differently in our bodies if this wasn't taken away or connected to shame by the outer world? The ongoing effects amount to a thousand paper cuts, it is shame that has been handed down generation to generation, living in the bodies of our parents and theirs, creating a legacy of disembodiment that seeps into daily interactions, into how we relate and care for our little ones.

One example for some can be found in how our parents handle our growing bodies and sexual behavior (and most do the very best they know how with what they were given), directly influencing our understanding of our genitals, our body, our sexuality. When what is heard is *"Don't touch that,"* *"That's yucky, stop that!"* or even just moving the child's hand away repeatedly without an acknowledgment of why, we come to understand that our genitals and exploration of our "private parts" is not allowed at best, and is shameful and disgusting at worst. How were your body parts talked about and treated? How do you think that influenced your relationship to your genitals? What is it like to think about the reality that those reactions were informed by discomfort that didn't originate with your parents, that the feelings were conveyed to them or interpreted from another source or experience, likely internalized by a younger version of themselves who similarly lacked development and education. They were handed down and reinforced. Arrested development is generational.

Play Is Understanding

Our primary route to learning in childhood is play! Like fantasy, play is how children process and make sense of the world around them. Playing house, for example, helps children understand the roles people inhabit, how gender is performed, how negotiation of daily tasks is navigated, how love, respect, and affection are exchanged in an experiential way. Sex is no exception! Children will play out sexual scenarios with one another in order to make sense of what sex means, of what it is. This happens regardless of whether comprehensive, thorough sex education was happening or not; but we can understand the vital importance of play for children when sex education is entirely absent or lacking. We all likely either participated in or knew of children who "played doctor," exploring each other's bodies, maybe even showing each other their "private parts." We are taught that childhood sex play, that normative exploration, curiosity, and touch, falls under the umbrella of trauma, which is not only false but harmful. It is very common for children to walk away from playing doctor, for example, with feelings of confusion and/or guilt and/or excitement. They have simultaneously bumped into an invisible "no" (i.e. private parts are off-limits) and also learned hard-to-access information (What do they look like on other people?), which is the developmental task of childhood: to learn. And let's be clear, children can and do cross the line; not all behavior is benign, much like play in general. "No means no" is a black-and-white concept that children can grasp as young as when in kindergarten, some even earlier. But determining what we can hold them accountable for when it comes to consent and sexual behavior is simply less clear than when considering their adult counterparts. Children do not have the neurological capacity to understand the repercussions of their behavior long term, especially around something as abstract and complex as sex, nor do they possess the wherewithal to get ahead of feelings and desires and act/react from a logical place. The prefrontal cortex, the part of the brain responsible for weighing out the consequences of our behavior in a linear way, is not fully developed until our 20s, hence why even teens can be challenging to work with when it comes to impulsive, risky behavior. The question of accountability becomes clearer when comparing a 14-year-old with a 6-year-old, versus a 6-year-old with a 7 or even 9-year-old, although there are still more considerations when looking at that teen's behavior versus his or her or their adult sibling. All this in mind, what does it even mean to be "sexual" as a kid? Is a seven-year-old engaging in self-touch with a pillow being "sexual" or are they simply having a sensory experience, or self-soothing (sensory experience and self-soothing are indistinguishable when it comes to self-touch: they are actually one-and-the-same)?

What did you do in order to understand sex in childhood? How did it show up between you and your friends? Whatever you did was normal. You may look back on it today and not like what you did or feel uncomfortable about how the others involved may feel about it now, but understand: *you did not know what you were doing*. Period. Anxiety and shame about our childhood sexual play follows us into adulthood and can present a huge barrier to our ease in welcoming in intimacy – to truly *sharing* ourselves with another. If that discomfort is present for you, try to imagine a step you can take to release yourself, and therefore that child, from any misplaced or disproportionate blame and shame. How can you put their behavior in context now? How does their behavior make sense (because, once again, it *always* does). They are not you now, they were a child. Can you find any compassion for their confusion?

~

Everything All at Once

The transition from elementary to middle school, from "child to adolescent," is a rocky path, an infamously challenging time that most of us are happy to have in our rearview. There's a ton happening developmentally: trying on and playing with different identities; getting to know our neurodivergence and its impact (if applicable), exploring gender (it's happening whether we identify with our gender or not); learning about and working to understand our constantly changing bodies, sexual sensations, and feelings; trying to find our place within and amongst our peers and social hierarchy; learning how to navigate romantic and sexual relationships; and attempting to separate and differentiate from our families of origin. All this and more with a brain that is characteristically black and white or concrete in terms of how it conceptualizes the world and the day to day.

Jon Kabat-Zinn, mindfulness instructor and author, talks about how we tend to move through life perpetually and subconsciously labeling aspects of our experience as "good, bad, or neutral." Adolescents, it seems, move through without a "neutral" option. They are either failing miserably or winning, bouncing between the two all day long. This combination of incredible internal chatter and an abundance of self-consciousness and self-focus (*Will I see so-and-so tonight? What should I say to them? Maybe I should just ignore them and play it cool? What should I wear? Did I look dumb in that outfit I just bought? I don't usually wear that color*) creates the very real impression that everything is only ever happening to them, which is why this age classically requires more self-disclosure from therapists. "*Please tell me I'm not alone in this thing I'm going through. Please reassure me I'm not a freak or worse for these thoughts, feelings, struggles.*" The narcissism is real, important, and a part of what it means to be navigating so much change at once; but it's a lonely game, despite appearances.

LGBTQ Sexual Development

Lance is a 16-year-old, cis (but exploring), gay boy from an Irish family at a large high school in the suburbs of New Hampshire. This school, like so many others, has very few queer peers for Lance to connect with, his friends are mostly cis girls who love his sense of humor, quick wit, and big heart. Lance came out reluctantly to his family when he was 11 years old. Both parents are extremely supportive and do their best to provide Lance with ample experiences (camps for queer youth, online groups, visits into the city for drag shows – an interest of his) to bolster his understanding of himself in an ongoing way. In the midst of homework, extracurricular activities, friends, and work at a part-time job, Lance is lonely. He turns to the internet and gets caught chatting and "sexting" with older men, sharing personal information about his life and location. This happens repeatedly, despite getting his technology taken away time after time, and often for long periods. He understands the danger logically, and yet continues to revisit these chats. His parents are baffled and overcome with worry. "Why does he continue to put himself and our family at risk like this? These are grown men, predators online! Why can't we get through to him? What are we doing wrong?!"

With obvious secondary sex characteristics making themselves, well ... obvious around the home, adolescence is the time when parents typically begin to pull away in terms of physical affection and touch. Combined with the pronounced presence of sexual feelings and curiosity, a draw toward intimacy and connection emerges with gusto and adolescents begin playing with romantic and erotic chemistry at school and with peers, learning about what their sexuality looks like relationally via eye glances across the room, texting (or back in the day, note-passing), flirting or "charged" conversation, making out behind the school, anxiously asking someone to dance at homecoming, and gossiping with friends about what it all means. Straight, cisgender adolescents get access to this kind of learning and exploration, this kind of both straightforward and nuanced experiential growth and discovery, on a much more frequent basis and potentially with much, much greater abundance. They get to play with the assumption of their peers' straightness alongside the invaluable advantage of not having to contend with that particular "other" barrier, an aspect of identity often met with hostility, discomfort, and/or distance by those who lack understanding or are confused about themselves for themselves.

Ongoing exposure to sexual and relational information, even when it's subtle, is something that is taken for granted by those of us who went through it. The ability to navigate those waters with others our age is immensely useful in helping to form our understanding of different kinds of relational chemistry, what they mean for connection (platonic versus romantic versus sexual), and what we are interested in experiencing or learning more about. It is painful, frequently characterized by moments of embarrassment, rejection, longing, and anxiety; but it is the consequence of risk in the presence of options (even when they're limited), from engaging with the possibilities or potentials in our orbit. It is the result of "putting ourselves out there," in overt or covert ways, with the hopes of something more. It is the discomfort inherent in growth as opposed to the pain that comes from isolation and the lack of opportunity for all of the above.

Desperation and Risk

Our basic need for intimacy, connection, and understanding, for a sense of belonging, is a desire more powerful than logic. We suffer without it, we "fail to thrive" even as we grow older, and therefore will go to the greatest lengths to find it. For teens, and particularly for trans or queer youth like Lance, this may mean placing themselves in dangerous situations to access exploration, to reach connection (online chat rooms, apps, anonymous or not-so-anonymous pic sharing and text exchanges with strangers). It can be porn and beyond, even potentially with older adults who are both easier to access sexually online and who demonstrate what we're looking to learn. A sexual mentor.

- Hyper-awareness of sexuality/sexual feelings/desires/"otherness" around puberty/adolescence + little to no **conversation, support, or guidance around it** + familial, religious, cultural, societal prejudice and bigotry = turn to the only option available to learn, explore, and understand sexuality and sexual feelings intellectually in an embodied way + often the only place to see examples of others/reflections of self (i.e, porn, chat rooms, social media).

We have all experienced the degenerative quality of chronic feelings of "aloneness" of any kind at some point in our lives (if not collectively during the COVID-19 pandemic). Helping our adolescents and teens find community is preventative and lessens the sense of deep desperation for understanding and connection, the felt sense of necessity that overrides logic and inspires dangerous risk-taking behavior. Helping ourselves find community in adulthood dampens, if not completely eradicates, the anxiety we feel about who we are and what our desires are made of. The far-reaching consequences that we are only beginning to understand come along with social media and the online universe, which has made community (virtual camps, support groups, classes, clubs, even shows) possible, even from a distance. We can discover others that reflect back who we are and how we love outside of the performative example porn provides.

Where did you find yourself searching for understanding? In what ways did you risk in order to obtain it?

Socialization and Sex

In terms of our working definition, "socialization" refers to the ideas, values, beliefs, and rules that are all rolled up in the scripts we inherit as we grow up in and move through the world. It is an extremely powerful aspect of our "training," providing us with the framework for "how to human" correctly, or at least according to the ideals, values, and influence of those in power throughout the generations, passed down, manifest and perpetuated by family, culture (with distinct particularities within social and cultural groups), and at large in society. Regardless of our gender now, whether you identify as female, male, nonbinary, agender, and/or trans (among others); regardless of our sexual orientation now and the scripts associated with being straight, gay, asexual, pansexual, and so on, nearly all of us are socialized according to scripts constructed around and associated with our genitals and with heteronormativity in mind, namely straight, cisgender, male, or female. Our socialization is terribly challenging to separate ourselves from, as the messaging is not always apparent but (and also *because*) it is deeply engrained.

As teenagers, we simultaneously challenge everything and nothing at all. The rules and "norms" that are not rebelled against are often treated in overly concrete or literal ways as a reflection of the concrete thinking characteristic of this time in our development. For example:

> *You're not supposed to have sex until you fall in love, which probably happens at around seven or eight months of being together, so we're really close.*
>
> *I'm a virgin and am planning to wait until marriage to have sex, so my boyfriend and I just have anal sex instead.*

Teens find creative ways around limiting ideas, rebel against them, or stick to them like glue, making the confusing and often harmful messaging received particularly problematic. If a behavior or set of behaviors is a "norm" within a friend group, there is the additional pressure to conform simply to maintain relationships and status amongst peers. When not rebelling against ideas and values, teens will "perform" more extreme versions of the gendered messaging that is being taught to them in order to convey that they get it, they're mature, confident, and much closer to their adult counterparts both physically and mentally (and therefore sexually – sex being associated with adulthood) than to the child they were in the not-so-distant past, despite how problematic that can be. This in mind, in terms of our sexuality, our socialization happens in relation to family, culture, religion, society, and (importantly) our peer groups.

Exploration Opportunity

Let's scratch the surface in terms of the messages we received around what it means to be sexual as "male" or "female," interacting with who is presumed to be opposite sex partners. Add to this list in an ongoing way as it will be influenced by a multitude of factors, including (but not limited to) past and present community, faith, race, and socio-economic status to bring awareness to the anxiety and pressure that follows you uniquely into the bedroom and plays itself out at baseline, simply for having the genitalia you have or had. As you move through, consider not only the thoughts that come up, but the feelings that surface, and the experience you have in your body. Our thinking mind may tell us we no longer have a relationship to a particular idea, while our bodies are relaying a different message. By uncovering what still lives within us and how it manifests, we are able to adopt and live (practice) new or more resonant ideas and values that align with who we are and how we want to love and "do" sex, with our authenticity and personal, current ideals fully at the wheel. It provides us with the ability to start to chip away at the anxiety that lives underneath and is woven into our own more personalized, unique, and specific challenges regarding sex.

Socialized male (people with penises):

- Sex as performance;
- Sex is goal oriented;
- Desire is ever-present;
- Must provide orgasms;
- Must take on more dominant role in sexual interactions;
- Penis must be "ready to go" at all times;
- Sexual prowess and performance as indicators of manhood ("real men score");
- Penis is central to good sex (if it doesn't do "its job" the experience is a failure);
- Rock hard erections only;
- Penis must stay hard long enough but not too long;
- Penis must look the part;
- Must ejaculate inside partner;
- Sexual experiences are win/lose, good or bad.

Socialized female (people with vulvas):

- Sex is about the other;
- Good girls don't;
- Must please the other: do not disappoint or risk upsetting the other (even if it's to our own detriment);
- Look "sexy" and achieve the perfect body to attract and arouse the male;
- Must be submissive;
- Should not deny sex to romantic partners;
- Must be giving;
- Too sexual = slut, not sexual enough = prude;
- Do sex to get love;
- Must have an orgasm to satisfy other's ego;
- Vagina must be "tight";
- Sex as performance;
- "No" has relational consequences (hurt feelings, agitation, anger, and beyond).

The ideas in the lists above create anxiety precisely because they are harmful. Our body is giving us a warning that we've strayed from what sex can be and into territory that at best causes disappointment, and at worse enables sexual violence. Our relationship to these messages deserves our attention; *we* deserve better in our intimacy. Our comfort with sex requires it.

How we were raised, how the topics of sex, intimacy, and relationships were demonstrated or discussed, how we navigated those areas for ourselves we did so with little to no support from our world, having been exposed to conflicting and confusing ideas about what to expect and what it all means. We have more control now, more of a sense of where to look and how to learn to further our development along, to undo what has been done to our intimacy and sexual sharing.

You were your primary teacher, and you were not equipped for the job. Yet look at what you were able to understand and work through. Look at your ability to connect, share, and cultivate intimacy with friends, colleagues, family, and/or romantic and/or sexual partners (even if it's not easy) despite it all. Keep that with you as you continue to explore, both in this book and beyond: remember your teacher.

9 Family Matters

We're in Sex Therapy, Why Are You Talking about my Dad?!

We move through life managing emotional closeness and distance with others. Ever find yourself picking a fight with a partner for no reason? Yeah, that. The intimacy we cultivate is guided by blueprints that we play out, with more-or-less ease depending on the nature of the relationship. Where and when and how we allow others in is not a coincidence, not random, nor is it due to the exceptional magic of the person (not to say magic isn't involved). These blueprints are modeled to us, demonstrated with us, and therefore normalized in childhood. They are our training in what it means to be intimate, close, vulnerable, and open, just as they are also our guide for the roles we inhabit and what our worth is relative to others. They are complex, deeply engrained, and we are either living them out or reacting to them (instinctually or intentionally choosing other ways of living and loving) as we move through each day. For better or for worse, or complex, or neutral, they are processes that were passed down by our parents or caregivers, who were given to them by theirs, and so on. We embody them in our own unique way, informed by our own unique lens, and add to the evolution of these blueprints in ways that offer new possibilities for growth and healing, for ourselves and our children if we have them. Our comfort with, desire for, and what we actually require so as to feel steady within ourselves and in relationships in terms of closeness, connection, and intimacy, is influenced by these blueprints and, even at times, powerfully governed by them. With this in mind, what does our family have to do with our sex lives? Everything. Can we exert more authority over the continued life and presence of our "training" in our sex and relationships? Absolutely.

Rhea

Rhea (29-year-old, cis/het, Black female) jokes about how controlling she has always been. As a child, she would attend to her siblings (one younger,

DOI: 10.4324/9781003369080-12

one developmentally disabled older) after school and when mom and dad ran late at work (a regular thing). She balanced homework and social obligations alongside extracurricular activities, sports, and church. She was meticulous with her dress so as to appear studious (her dad was a professor, someone she admired) and in order not to attract the attention of the group of white boys that would catcall her on her walk home from school (from elementary through high school), one of whom lived next door. She planned her outfits and accessories for the week every Sunday evening (a routine she still participates in). When her parents would have friends over, she would sit by, watching and counting the number of alcoholic beverages her parents would consume, since intoxicated people made her uneasy, and was the "designated driver" in high school. She can trace the anxiety that has been with her as far back as her memories will allow, and the desire to control the environment, including the people in it, that has accompanied it.

Flash forward and Rhea finds herself in relationship after relationship with men who drink or get high excessively. Big partiers, she doesn't find herself with people who do these things 24/7, but when they do they take it to an extreme – blacking out or getting sloppy, incoherent, inaccessible. This makes some sense to her, as a socially anxious person she enjoys drinking to calm herself and make it easier to "be herself," so she is often meeting these partners in party settings. Yet, she is baffled by her pattern and resentful of all the caretaking she gets herself into.

The dynamic is far from sexy. Inevitably as she moves into a caretaking role, she loses attraction for her partners and her desire to be close sexually falls off. To add to this, she finds intimacy is hard. Sex feels awkward, but she'll go through the motions in order to get to the love, the commitment. She enjoys masturbating on her own, but when with partners finds it challenging to relax, to feel any kind of comfort or ease in her body.

She comes to therapy wanting to learn how to orgasm with her partner, how to feel more aroused during sex. Where might we begin? With arousal and orgasm?

This example clearly demonstrates a common sticky spot in therapy: naming and having to debunk the very understandable notion that sex, our bodies, our sexual functioning is to blame for struggles whose roots go much deeper. Is this issue even about sex at all? Let's break this down:

- Her history of anxiety and its coping partner, control: When we are as familiar with anxiety as Rhea has been, when it has felt like an organizing principle in one's childhood, we become incredibly familiar with control: seeking it out, struggling in its absence, engaging in behaviors, rituals, and processes that allow us to access the illusion of stability it seems to give us momentarily. Existing outside of this system becomes challenging and can feel foreign. Where and when can she let her hair down? When does she feel free?

- Rhea's relationship to alcohol: Despite associating alcohol with anxiety, Rhea drinks herself. What gives? We often think of substances that alter our experience as mechanisms that move us out of our inclination to control, as a way into an "out-of-control" state. The counterintuitive element that lives at the core of this experience is that the feelings that come with inebriation, even the experience of being "out-of-control" itself, is an exercise *in* control. Rhea understands what alcohol gives her, or more importantly what it moves out of the way in order for her to feel more at ease and able to connect. Alcohol and substances for all of us become a way of accessing a different constellation of experience, in a way we can anticipate, and therefore another way to control or try to shape our reality. Needing to drink to feel comfortable places her in a set-up where she is likely to meet other folx who do the same, some of whom do it in a way that is more extreme or problematic (which feels tough to determine or define) than her. Meeting potential partners who are not as connected to substance use requires learning to be with her anxiety, letting it accompany her as she puts herself out there as sober, risking living out and stepping into the challenging feelings and fears that come with that version of reality, whatever that may look like.

- Caretaking: Rhea took on the responsibility of attending to her siblings when mom and dad weren't available, stepping into a parental role at a young age and navigating the learning and specific developmental needs of each child whilst being a child herself. Watching, diligently counting her parent's drinks, scanning for differences in their behavior – what happens to Rhea's sense of being a "child" when attempting to monitor and manage the adults in her environment? Even if only in these particular settings and situations, she is also practicing moving into a caretaking role relative to her parents. Without conscious recognition, the felt experience even for a child is one of being in control while the adults around are not. Anxiety mounts as children sense their adult is not accessible in the same way, not as predictably "them."

- Racial and gender identity: Earlier in the book we referenced our unique experience of safety in the world, which directly influences our felt sense and understanding of anxiety and relationship to it. It is important to consider how racial and gender identity (i.e. what it means to move through her world as a black female) and how she's seen, "understood," and treated by her white counterparts plays into her inclination for control and how it manifests. The white boys in the neighborhood were the source of unwanted and challenging attention that had a powerful impact on her relationship to her body, safety, and sexuality. What was her understanding about why *her*? What was the composition of black versus white families in her neighborhood? What did she perceive white people saw when they saw her? Her family? Who could she turn to for protection? For understanding?

- Treatment plan:

  - Making contact with "little Rhea" and her relationship with control that began in childhood: Getting to know the version of Rhea that first learned to cope with anxiety by leaning into control will assist her in understanding what that little girl needed then, and therefore what she can provide herself now.
  - Creating a context for and then learning to let go in a routine way, building familiarity with the experience and sensations involved in release, and learning to trust that she can do just that and still be safe.
  - Relationship to herself: Looking at the intersection of race, gender, and sexuality as it relates to the management of distance versus closeness she exercises in romantic partnerships and beyond. Identifying the insecurities at the heart of her personal relationship to alcohol and what it helps her cope with and distance from. If Rhea struggles to allow vulnerability in (i.e. relinquishing control), and to feel comfortable with who she is, that discomfort will impact her ability to trust herself and to release fully into the experience in the bedroom (sensation, emotion, arousal, etc.). Who is Rhea outside of her anxiety and control? What can she learn about herself as she learns to step beyond it?
  - Alcohol within the couple: Working with their shared relationship to alcohol confronts the caretaker–child dynamic they have created and that directly disrupts desire. It will be crucial for Rhea to understand that control and caretaking are fundamental parts of her "training," parts that we can work to separate from via the active relinquishing of control on her part alongside the stepping up of her partner (requiring a reworking of drinking habits or quitting altogether).

Sex therapy symptoms are not only manifestations of larger themes and challenges: they come with a level of connection to our family and upbringing (i.e. to primary lessons in intimacy, closeness, trust). To begin by working with arousal and orgasm might effectively tap into, or scratch the surface around, the forces at play that are preventing their ability to unfold in the first place (lack of trust, need to control, tension in the body, discomfort with own sexuality, difficulty with vulnerability and closeness), but more than likely starting there would be like trying to help someone stop crying without addressing their sadness. We would then miss the larger forces toward progress, the stuff that makes for freedom from anxiety and our sexual inhibitions, the heart of true, lasting change.

Holding Accountability and Love in the Same Place

We can feel a lot of resistance to taking a meaningful inventory of our childhood, our "training," and more specifically the things our parent(s) or caregiver(s) weren't able to provide. Navigating complex feelings as they relate to these figures, the people from whom we learned the most profound lessons in life, is tricky and requires holding seemingly contradictory emotional experience in the same place, for example love *and* disappointment, or accountability, or anger (to varying degrees – it can also feel like overwhelming grief and anger in the absence of love). It means understanding that, even under the best-case scenario with truly engaged and loving parents, they are human and incapable of understanding all our unique needs. They simply don't have access to all the parts of who we are growing up (we don't even have access to all parts of ourselves), and therefore are doing their best at making informed guesses around what might be best in handling what they do see, the sliver they are able to access all while interacting with and attempting to cope with their own traumas, wounding, challenges, and stresses of the day to day. For example:

> *If Andy's parents value "success," placing tremendous pressure on him to win or get the A's or excel above all else, then Andy is likely to approach sex as another thing to accomplish, something his ego needs to tackle as an indicator of his worth. With that much on the line, sex will be stressful. Who is he outside of his accomplishments? Does he even know how to let go and enjoy just for enjoyment's sake? Do his parents? What drives this strong desire in them? A history of poverty? Of wealth? The values handed down to them by their own parents? How is the overwhelming quest for "success" or accomplishment a reaction to their own lived experience?*

It is common to feel protective of our parents as we delve into what our blueprints are made of. That feeling is a reflection of the goodness that existed and remains within the connection and memories made. Those things are real and can live and breathe right alongside our understanding of where they inevitably missed important information about what we needed, missed an important choice on our behalf, or weren't able to provide the sense of safety and connection we longed for to the degree we needed it in a general way, or at different points in life. We can love them and come to understand where we needed more "training" or where we would've liked the lessons learned to be different, or simply edited. Adulthood is the place where we get to look back with the information we have as the people who lived those childhoods, the people who actually experienced our experience, and identify where we can fill those needs and edit the learning in our adult lives. We pick up the ball from our parents, and that's where our reparenting comes in. It's on us now.

Reparenting Our Littles

Why is it helpful to conceptualize some of our distancing strategies, anxieties, and fears that feel unrelated and unwelcome in the now as our "little" or "younger" selves, rather than simply originating from them? Because it creates that sense of space, of welcome distance and detachment, from identifying with the experience *as* us, as just part of who we are. It is the difference between:

- Thought #1: *I'm anxious during sex and have to work to manage my anxiety* and
- Thought #2: *A part of me gets anxious during sex, thinking I need to look and be perfect – ideas that were engrained in me as a pageant kid. I can hold that part with compassion now, and trust and let go into the beautiful complexity and messiness of my sensuality.*

Both identify the feeling, but Thought #2 gives us a way of interacting with it and ourselves in a way that actually addresses why it's there, or a meaningful aspect of its origin story. We can interact with and talk to that "part" as if talking to the pageant child, tenderly inviting ourselves back into the present, our bodies, our sensuality, and ultimately a new and healing message and experience. It recognizes the influence of our training and gives us a frame for our brain's predictions in the moment.

Memories as Gateways

Is there a vivid memory from your childhood that visits you from time to time, or maybe even regularly, that feels important? Like a particularly detailed moment or experience? Can you think of an approachable memory that feels connected to your primary relationships or sexuality? Why do you think this memory feels so vibrant, still, after all these years? Why might it visit you? What message do you think it has for you as it relates to your life now and the choices you make for yourself?

Our most accessible memories carry the most profound messages. They maintain their poignancy because they represent significant moments of learning and growth, stand out moments for better or worse, in complex ways and without exception. They can also represent moments in time where we get stuck, or frozen around a particular developmental theme or idea, leaving this theme or idea to be played out, replicated, or left to be attended to in a similar way as we grow older, as we saw with Rhea. We don't exclusively replicate behavior, however; we also very frequently step into the emotional, psychological, and cognitive frame and perspective of the version of ourselves who lived through it. We can take on and inhabit qualities of that younger person as they're brought to the surface in the face of similar experiences. Let's look at another example:

> *Darren (nonbinary, 36-year-old, pansexual, Vietnamese-American person) and Jenni (43-year-old, cis/pansexual, Vietnamese-American female) have been together for six years. Darren is in graphic design and Jenni owns her own clothing retail business. They seek therapy because they've stopped having sex. Both describe not feeling particularly desirous in the context of their relationship. Darren, however, has cheated on Jenni multiple times in the past two years. They describe three of the incidents transpiring with strangers, and one time with their mutual friend. All of the occurrences were disclosed to Jenni nearly immediately following. Darren's drinking and partying are excessive, and are part of what Jenni looks to when attempting to assign blame and make sense of Darren's acting out. Darren has recently even gotten in trouble at work for chronic tardiness and missing deadlines. They have attempted to set boundaries and create agreements to allow Jenni to feel more respected and met in the relationship, but Darren struggles (or refuses?) to follow through.*
>
> *When talking with the couple, the therapist notices Darren rolling their eyes, slouching on the couch, and mocking Jenni. Darren feels like a 15-year-old child in the room. Why is this version here?*

As the therapist delves into their family of origin story, Darren recalls a memory at 14 when they were in the backseat as their parents got into a huge fight in the car. Dad took Darren and their mom back to the house, dropped them off, and before he drove away looked back and said, "*I'm done with you all.*" This memory brings Darren to tears as it's recounted, and the therapist can feel them completely immersed in every detail of the story.

1 *What might Darren have internalized about themself as a result of this experience as a 14-year-old?*

    That they were not only not worth sticking around for, but that they were so disliked by their own dad that he wished to never see them again.

- Even though we understand this to be much more complicated from an adult lens, that is not what we're interacting with. The message is internalized and felt from the perspective of the little boy (Darren references this version of themselves as "he"), who thinks in extremely black-and-white terms, and will assume (as children often do) that their dad's behavior is their fault.

2 *What might Darren have desperately craved from their dad that was lost?*

Love, acceptance, to fight for him and their connection even whilst the marriage was falling apart. To prove to Darren that he is lovable and deserving of love not only from others, but from him.

3 *What might have been the takeaway lesson as it relates to intimacy and closeness?*

That it is untrustworthy, unreliable, dangerous.

4 *How does Darren's behavior make sense given this context?*

Being at the place in their relationship where the attachment has become more familial, less lust-based, their vulnerability and attachment wounding is surfacing. Darren *is* that 14-year-old boy, stuck in a cycle of testing and intentionally breaking boundaries and agreements, waiting for Jenni to leave like dad, waiting to prove the lesson correct yet again. "*Will you stick around if I cheat, even with one of your friends? What if I'm frequently reckless and irresponsible? How far can I push before you'll leave too?*"

5 *What does this have to do with sex (i.e. why does this have everything to do with sex?)?*

- The boy is scared of getting too close, the boy is fearful of intimacy. He would rather act out and have the leaving be connected to behavior rather than who they are, sex being an expression of who we are. Ideas that may be at work behind the curtain for Darren:

    1 *What might Jenni understand about me as I let her in, allow her to see and interact with who I am in ways I can't control?*
    2 *With that degree of closeness involved, what might she discover about me that my dad did, that made me someone he was capable of abandoning?*

- Jenni, on the other hand, is reacting to the childlike persona of her partner, and the loss of respect that comes with reckless, immature, and inconsiderate behavior. Where has my partner gone? Why am I suddenly feeling like I'm parenting and trying to manage this fully grown, capable, adult?

- Therapeutic considerations: How did Darren understand what makes someone valuable growing up? How did they feel valued? Where else does the theme of rejection reveal itself in their history? Have they felt rejected by others or community for who they are? What has their journey with acceptance looked like as they've navigated their gender identity, racial and ethnic identity, and coming out process? How has this relationship with Jenny furthered them along in their healing, influencing the daily impact or shadow of the memory (because it has)?

Revisiting Sex's Asks

When it comes to our unique training in the categories below, challenge yourself to think expansively about the answers; they need not be loud or blatant, sometimes our most powerful experiences are found in subtilty (a wink of an eye, a comforting smile, an expression that we understand to mean one thing even though it appears to be something else on the surface). If parents or caregivers are tricky, think about other influential people in your upbringing, others whom you felt close to. Their presence may have been just as influential, if not more so, than that of your nuclear or adoptive family.

When moving through the questions below, try to hold the frame of "How was this present and how can I continue to elaborate on and strengthen my relationship to what I already know in this area?" rather than allowing your focus to zero in on the absence of. Even the smallest examples, the tiny bits we can find to work with, represent the presence of these skills in our lives and within who we are. They are real, tangible elements of our learning or "training" that are always available for expansion and editing.

- **Vulnerability:** Can you think of an example of someone being emotionally brave with you? Letting down their pride in favor of the relationship, sharing an apology/forgiveness? What impression did it leave? How vulnerable do you allow yourself to be today? How much will you allow yourself to risk emotionally?
- **Expression:** Can you recall a memory where love and care was expressed to you in a way that you could receive? This could be by a family member, friend, or first romantic partner. What did it look like? Was it overt and verbal, or via hugs/affection, attention, protection, or gifts? How do you express yourself to those you love or care for?
- **Letting go:** What did it look like when people let their hair down in your house? Who seemed the most at ease? Where do you let go today?
- **Self-acceptance:** What part of you when growing up felt the most embraced by parent(s), teachers, peers, or extended family? How did it feel to have that part reflected back favorably? Where do you find the most self-acceptance and positive self-regard today? Professionally? As a friend? Partner?

- **Sharing:** What person in your journey so far has kept you "in the loop" of their life in the most meaningful way? Do they reveal their struggles, triumphs, day-to-day experience? Conversely, can you think of something another person shared or revealed to you that felt important or significant to them? How did it feel to be trusted in both scenarios? Whom do you trust to share your life and challenges with, in an ongoing way or on occasion?

- **Exercising and respecting boundaries:** Where were loving, or respectful, or containing boundaries the most present in your home when growing up? Where were they the most clearly articulated and spoken to? Who demonstrated the most respect for your likes/dislikes/yes's/no's? How did that relationship feel to you as a result? How do you honor your boundaries today?

- **Play:** What were some shared and solo activities and experiences that represent "play" in your life? What are the feelings associated as you reflect? How do you incorporate play in your life presently?

- **Communication:** Who in your family or friend group growing up seemed to be the most heard or understood? How do you think they accomplished that? Was their communication verbal, non-verbal, behavioral, respectful, loud? What did you learn from that person in terms of your own communication style? How articulate are you about your wants, needs, feelings, and what do you have an "eye" on in terms of your approach (because we all need work here)?

- **Embodiment:** What was one message or value you can identify from family, health class, or peers that centered connection or care for the body? In what ways are we granted permission to be in connection with our physicality in ways that are celebrated (athleticism, "gut-instincts," etc.)? Where do you give yourself permission to come into loving or caring or even neutral contact with your body today?

Understanding what we're working with, the important and also challenging impressions, lessons, and ways we've taken on and lived out elements from our past, our training from the people and communities who loved, cared for, or were responsible for us, creates the space required to understand what was important and to continue our learning in a way we choose while also giving us examples of the experiences and ways we practice what sex asks of us currently to draw from – as a starting place. It is both disconnecting (from unconscious processes that are no longer invited) and connecting (in terms of real ways the elements above are alive and present within us, reflecting our very real ability to be in relationship with them). It also helps us get clear on what sex means to us today, and how we want to understand and experience love and connection in our lives and relationships, free from the confusion of previous generations, unbeholden to the past.

We can edit our own blueprints.

10 Your Relationships

Just as we are different versions of ourselves in the various chapters we move through in life, we are also different versions of ourselves in different relationships, which means we will often want or yearn for different things from and within them, sexually and otherwise. If you look back on your relationship history, can you make sense of why you chose certain people at specific times? Why *that* person then? We learn about ourselves through our relationships, which moves us along in our development, our healing, our understanding of what it is we ultimately want to invest in. We "try on" partners or dating experiences like we "try on" identities as adolescents or young adults. We react to our previous partners with the next partner (and yes, we're doing it right now). It's a constant, ongoing exercise in self-understanding and exploration, and if we stick around in relationships long enough, all roads lead to sexual challenges. All roads. It's our sexuality's way of attempting to continue that development in all realms, to evolve and even deepen our capacity for intimacy and connection. To what end? Let's talk about it.

- When sex got perfunctory what did I need?
- When I no longer was interested in X, what might that have meant?
- When sex became illusive, what needed to be asked?
- When sex felt one-sided, what needed to be said?
- When I felt insecure sexually, what was my insecurity showing me?
- When sex was no longer fun, what needed to change?

When reading through these questions, did any answers reveal themselves with ease as you sifted through the memories? Did they stir up anything interesting or surprising to get curious about? Or were they all kind of browsed and moved past? It can feel futile or like a waste of time to reflect on our sexual struggles from the past, but rewinding the tape is the business of therapy as we can learn a great deal about ourselves from the snags we've experienced throughout our lives. If we can't or don't bother to try

DOI: 10.4324/9781003369080-13

and answer questions like the ones above, we miss out on the important learning that leads to more comfort, more opportunities to put to practice what we've learned, and therefore more embodied and connective experiences.

Can you go back to these questions once more and really sink your teeth into them with this in mind? Anything we unearth is connecting us to ourselves in a way that chips away at the anxiety we can encounter as a result of distance, hyper-focus on the other, and performance narratives. In other words, the more connected we are to our sexual self-knowledge, the less disconnected the sex (hello!).

Comfort Is Complex

Clearing the way for comfort and ease in partnered sex requires nurtured relationships, or the cultivation of relational environments that enable us to expand ourselves, take risks, and grow. This means making an effort to bring our best selves to the table in an ongoing way (as we did when dating – bolstering our "relational self-esteem"), actively advocating for and discussing our wants and needs, showing up for conflict (and learning how to do it) rather than brushing challenges under the rug, and creating space and time to connect and appreciate intimacy of all brands. This does not mean we have to spend every second together. Nurturing our relationships means accounting for distance and the importance of time apart. Why? Because we will discover significantly more ease when stepping into vulnerability, sharing, revealing, playing, connecting, expressing ourselves, and letting go if we feel good about how we're showing up (being content with our behavior in a relationship), our partner, and the context we've created together (not a hostile, resentful, or overly parental or sibling-esque system). An added bonus, when healthy distance is fostered, we up the odds of showing up eager to learn and connect, much as we did when learning and connecting were intoxicating, all-consuming forces in the beginning (i.e. new relationship energy).

What kind of comfort are we referring to? Comfort in terms of *verbalizing my feelings and boundaries, sharing my evolving sense of self with my partner (including my ever-changing body, sexuality, emotions), my feelings about who I am and my value in this relationship, and connection with my partner.*

What crosses the line? A sense of comfort born from trusting our stories and our ideas about the other so completely that it obfuscates the respect and reverence for the separateness of the other almost completely. It's comfort and a sense of "knowing" that manifests as taking advantage, taking for granted, feeling entitled, or even assuming what the partner must want.

And here's the deal: we all bring our worst into our closest partnerships as well. It is inevitable that the mask will slip, the facade fades, and routine and predictability conjure up a sense of comfort that *will* lead us to cross that line. We have built-in emotional distance when we begin dating someone new. We feel that great space in-between, and it breeds curiosity, a desire and enthusiasm to know more, and that desire motivates us to do and be our best to get there. Once that new relationship energy begins to evolve into the kind of attachment to the other that feels much more familial (which can happen at any point and is very specific to the relationship itself but is often found at points that represent further merging, e.g. moving in, engagement, getting married, having children, in no particular order), our familial "stuff" begins to surface. In other words, as the intimacy we cultivate with our partner(s) takes on the quality and feelings familiar from and to our family of origin, our wounding surfaces. Our first lessons in love, trust, and acceptance surface, including what was modeled to us by our parents, what we were on the receiving end of in terms of our own treatment, and the role we took on in the family (nurturer, peacemaker, parent, black sheep, etc.). Our "training" when it comes to what it means to truly get close kicks in, and the strategies we'd acquired to keep ourselves safe emotionally and psychologically – strategies that helped us adapt and cope with not getting specific needs met, with challenging or traumatic situations in the family, with abandonment (emotionally or otherwise) from a parent or both, with the processes unfolding in front of us or directly to us (communication patterns, our parent's relationship to expression, communication, connection, closeness and how that manifests) – embed themselves in the dynamics of the partnership. As such, as adults in relationships, our connection moves from being driven by lust and/or longing to resolve the mystery and be as close as possible, to being driven by the deep intuitive need for individual healing in the context of connection, where all wounding originates. Couples therapists call this "finding the 'I' in the 'We,'" and embarking on this path allows couples or relationships to move toward the center and experience the kind of connection that is both close and intimate, and yet holds plenty of space for us to thrive and continue to learn about ourselves as individuals. It's the relationship sweet spot.

Differentiation

In high school I dated an "older man," meaning I was 17 when I met him, and he was 21. If dating a "college guy" wasn't sexy enough, he also happened to be in a fairly well-known punk band in our area and played bass. We dated for nearly two years and despite the ups-and-downs, I never tired of walking into the concert venue to see my guy on the stage doing his thing. I loved watching all the eyes on him, especially the other girls. After each show, I felt a revived sense of lust and longing for him, an expanded sense of appreciation for our relationship, and just so, so much pride. That's what I want in my marriage now.

(Janice)

Yes, this is a sexy set-up, but why? What common thread weaves the following together?

1 Older college guy;
2 Punk band;
3 Others' desirous gaze;
4 Witnessing of talent.

The common thread is differentiation, something we simultaneously love in terms of desire and attraction and find threatening in terms of our experience of safety in relationships. What is differentiation? The felt experience of definition in terms of the identities and emotional and psychological experience and presence of the individual parties in a relationship. It is our ability to hold onto ourselves and recognize the "other" while in connection. All of the elements above describe aspects of the boyfriend that made him "him," that allowed him to have a distinct presence and identity within the relationship, and that allowed Janice to experience him as separate, with his own talents, unique qualities, and things that she could witness others appreciate in him as well. When enough distance is created for us to recognize the things we appreciate in the uniqueness of the other, we call that pride, and pride would not, could not, exist without differentiation. It is born from it. Can you recall a moment when you felt proud of a current partner or a partner in the past? That sense of awe, admiration, and respect (subtle or profound) *is* differentiation, and as author and therapist Esther Perel explains in her book, *Mating in Captivity: Reconciling the Erotic and the Domestic* (2006), it starves and struggles to survive under the weight and consequences of our own anxiety as closeness moves in, meaningful attachment forms, and our desire for emotional safety reigns.

Anxiety likes to take the healthy space that exists between self and partner(s), the space that illuminates difference and ignites desire, and frame it as threat. Taking sexuality as an example, feeling like we lack understanding, exist outside of the ins and outs of our partner's erotic life, including desires, fantasies, curiosities, edges, and transgressions, is part of what makes the experience of coming together sexually so thrilling when dating. There is the unspoken understanding that we are being let in on something that is very much theirs, and not only that, but assumed not to be readily and openly shared with others. That is the intoxicating nature of intimacy. Yet when we enter into long-term partnerships, what was once a thrilling adventure in learning, exploration, and discovery becomes something we need to understand fully, something we need to control even, in order to quell our own insecurities. *I need to understand everything about your inner sexual world to not feel like your desires, fantasies, curiosities, and edges will take you away from me.*

Counter-intuitively, differences create closeness, a gap to bridge, open space for curiosity. A focus on similarities stifles intimacy, creating the illusion that there isn't anything meaningful to learn, bringing forward a sense of "knowing" that results in the illusion of safety, leading to the kind of comfort that *means* taking advantage, taking for granted, ultimately fanning the flames of disinterest. Sexual struggles can be an indication that this effect has taken hold, an alert to back up and find a sense of ourselves as separate in order to feel open and receptive to relational and sexual sharing.

Relationship Myth-Busting (or, Saying Goodbye to Disney's Love Story)

We all eventually find ourselves face to face with disappointment in relationships. We all come to understand that the fairytale isn't real and that relationships are immensely challenging. This is tough, but this is the beginning. Once the shiny veneer has fallen off, we can begin to look at relationships for what they are, what they can realistically offer, and where they challenge us to grow. Therapy has to center the reality of both being human and taking on the extraordinary task of healing and also revisiting our trauma alongside another person or persons on a loop for as long as we occupy the containers our relationships create. Moving unhelpful stories and ideas from the world out of the way is one step in the healing direction, one step away from the anxiety that comes with not living up to the fantasy (which we simply can't accomplish anyway), and one step towards finding and executing realistic goals and agreements with partners moving forward.

What the fairytale sold us versus reality:

- *We meet and find "the one."* We can find meaningful connection with many people throughout the course of our lives. There are many exciting, challenging, and powerfully intimate relationships out there for us. The world is big! A scarcity mindset can backfire and cause us to miss the important cues that let us know someone might be a good match in our anxious attempts to seek out perfection (because if there's only one, they had better be perfect).
- *Our partner(s) should meet all our needs: sexual, emotional, spiritual, intellectual, etc.* Unfortunately, this idea pervades modern relationships, and we suffer for it. In our monogamous relationships in particular, we tend to strap our personal aim to accomplish fulfillment, comfort, pleasure (sexual and otherwise), and sense of stability onto our partners, and onto our relationships to inherently provide, otherwise they're "broken." We are responsible for our own happiness, for co-creating the relational space we desire with the other or others (which means work, accountability, and bravery). This also means attending to the

other forms of connection and the other ways we get our needs and wants met throughout life: e.g. community, friendships, hobbies, professional connections; taking the impossible burden of being "everything" off an imperfect but alive and evolving relational system that offers so much but can't possibly be what we're meant to find in the world and other forms of relationships around us.

- *Healthy, "good" relationships should be easy (i.e. void of or very little conflict).* Partners need to know how to argue and how to do it with skill. We need to care enough about ourselves, care enough about the relationship as a whole (caring about ourselves *is* caring about the relationship), to show up when things get hard and give voice to our struggles. Challenge is a key ingredient in healthy relationships: it lets us know that we're changing and that we care about the changes that are happening and how they get incorporated into our lives. "Easy" in long-term partnerships can alert us towards "avoidance," when there is nothing more worthy of our time, attention, and, yes, struggle, to co-create something that protects what our connection is made of today. We uphold the status quo, which can push us out over time, or we push up against it in favor of change so we can stay. It's the most meaningful hard work there is.

- *There are no secrets (i.e. no private life).* Secrecy and privacy are two very different concepts, and it is important to make the distinction in relationships, otherwise big assumptions get made that can lead to trouble. To feel that separateness we continue to reference, we need to feel our own sense of autonomy, of individuality, including a relationship to our own private world that is just ours. We do not become boundaryless in relationships, which is an extremely problematic dynamic that is at odds with desire. So, what makes a secret a secret? Information that is being withheld or concealed in the knowledge that it violates an agreement (which is precisely why ongoing understanding and discussion of agreements is so vital – our relationships are an ongoing constellation of them) or an overt understanding that the thing or behavior being concealed would cause harm. Outside of those parameters, our private life, including fantasies, desires, and past experiences, are ours to own and ours to occupy. If framed as "secret," we carry around millions or more every second of our day.

- *No more attraction or feelings of lust for other people: "I only have eyes for you."* We choose a person or several while continuing to stumble into or cultivate chemistry with and finding feelings of attraction to and for other people. We cannot shut off admiration for other bodies, curiosity about other people and experiences, and interpersonal chemistry and connection with others. They are part of being human. Part of an active and alive sense of wonder, a fantasy landscape of possibility. We work to create romantic partnerships that are vital and dynamic and rewarding so that we continue to make our choice, to return to something that makes the doors we close worthwhile.

- *No solo sexual life (or very minimal – but what does that look like?).*
  With everything our sexuality provides us, with all that is built into our design, the notion that we would abandon our individual experience with and relationship to it when we partner with another is not only unrealistic, but also places undue shame on our shoulders when many of us inevitably fail at this mission. Why? Because our solo sexual life and relationship has been with us since we were children and is deeply woven into who we are, manifest in ways both big and small. It can be fantasy escape, a way of navigating and coping with our feelings, a way to feel alive and connected to ourselves, a break in our day. Many (though not all) of us *do* have a solo sexual life, we simply miss the many ways it reveals itself to us: celebrity crushes, feelings of longing for a character in a book, flirtatious back-and-forth with a co-worker or bartender. It doesn't always look like masturbating or watching porn, although it certainly can.

Relationships, Anxiety, and Sexual Dysfunctions

The bedroom can seem like the most unlikely place to bump into versions of the harmful relationship myths spelled out above, but they are frequently found to be at the heart of why and how we get sex wrong. *Does my partner shame me when I struggle sexually? What expectation does that illuminate? Is there a huge power discrepancy in the relationship? What do I perceive my role to be in romantic or sexual partnerships? Do I feel a responsibility for my partner's arousal and orgasms? What other responsibilities do I assume in my relationship that are hard to live up to? Is my relationship on the line when it comes to our sexual life?*

When it comes to sexual challenges, whether they originated in the dynamic or followed one participant in, the relationship inadvertently organizes itself in a way that either eliminates or reinforces the struggle. When it's the latter, all partners participate in the active maintenance of the issue, despite intentions. This can be due to a plethora of complex reasons, but commonly spotted dynamics include (keep an eye out for our "myth" items):

- Power dynamics in the couple:

  - When one partner feels intimidated by or inferior to the partner in a general sense and/or sexually;

- When one partner feels like the other has one foot out the door and has to work hard or stifle their own needs to keep them in (i.e. pressure to please);
- When one partner is being actively ridiculed or shamed for a sexual issue;
- When one person feels entitled to sex or places responsibility for their sexual pleasure on the other who they perceive to be failing or insufficient;
- Sexual inexperience relative to the partner.

- Misinformed ideas about why the challenge exists (some of which may be, but often are not, true), which directly impact behavior around the issue:

  - They must not be attracted to me;
  - They must want to cheat or are cheating;
  - They are intentionally withholding.

- Upset (on the part of the partner or self) and/or "show stopping moments" when the challenge occurs:

  - How the couple treats the issue, and each other around the issue, in and out of the moment, can either pave the way towards healing and even resolution of the challenge, or it can actively maintain and strengthen its power. One tactic that absolutely never works is bullying, shaming, or aggression of any kind. Bullying or pushing our partners to have sex more frequently, to get over their insecurities, to enjoy the same things sexually that they enjoy, and/or to stop having that sexual "dysfunction" are coercive, first off, and also a great way to assure our partner's lack of desire for sex, and particularly for sex with us, in an ongoing way. We have just effectively strengthened a sex = discomfort and pressure association, therefore adding to the difficulty long term.
  - When something happens in the bedroom that feels "off script": someone experiences pain, gets triggered, ejaculates earlier than they'd like to – couples will often halt the action completely which can then turn into a display of frustration and embarrassment and/or a cryptic conversation about the future of the relationship at large. These "record-scratch" or "show-stopping" moments leave a residue, depleting our motivation to re-approach, communicating a lack of versatility, resiliency, and creativity connected to our sexual life, placing an enormous amount of pressure on the sexual relationship to be perfect, or else.

- Difficulty being open and honest about the issue with the partner/
  partners:

  - Openness and honesty are – vulnerable and intimate experiences,
    precisely what sex *is*. Practice in the realm of communication and
    sharing paves the way for greater ease when sharing ourselves sexu-
    ally, communicating during the experience itself, and in learning how
    to negotiate a pivot (which is required for a satisfying sexual life).
    Keeping our experience, our concerns, our wants, boundaries, or
    challenges to ourselves when they have important implications for
    the interaction, for the relationship, distances. It requires mental
    effort to "hide" how we're feeling and what we need. We move into
    "power-through" mentality.

Alex (cis/het, 29-year-old, white female):	*It's angering that we're here. It's taken him so long to do anything about this. It's been seven years! Seven! And he still can't fuck me or make me cum. Like, I've done so much for this relationship and have sacrificed a lot to be with him and he doesn't even care enough about me to try to figure this out all this time. It's infuriating, I can't tell you how resentful I am. I feel like he's robbed me of my sexuality.*
Therapist:	*Can you talk more about what sexual strug-gles you both are dealing with? Actually, Max can I ask you to answer before I jump back over to Alex? Alex is that OK?* (Alex nods head yes, eyes to the floor.)
Max (cis/het, 32-year-old male, Indian-American, identifies as having autism spectrum disorder (ASD)):	*Well, yeah I mean she pretty much said it. We haven't had, like, I guess intercourse or what-ever because I lose my erections every time before we can even get there.*
Alex:	*And he can't make me cum, like with his fingers, his mouth, anything. He's plenty happy to receive all the blow jobs from me, though! My last partner was so much more giving, I had an orgasm nearly every time we had sex.*

Max: I don't understand what she wants me to do here. I don't feel like she's explaining herself clearly other than telling me how angry and disappointed she is in me. How much of a failure I am to her. We'll be making out or something and then suddenly she's furious and it comes out of nowhere. I literally don't know what I've done wrong most of the time, or what she'd like me to do so she's happy. If she'd just tell me how to touch her...

Alex: I shouldn't have to explain how to have sex to a fully grown man. I AM disappointed. Who waits this long to get help learning how to fuck their partner, who is this negligent?!

Therapist: Max, is this what all of the conversations about sex are like between the two of you?

Max: Yeah, they're all pretty tough on both of us.

Therapist: OK. I appreciate both of your honesty ... and I'm going to try and be very clear here. This issue is twofold: Max, we will attend to your erectile dysfunction and the anxiety, insecurity, and longing for direction and instruction that fuels it. Alex: we will address your desperation and the hostility being directed towards Max around something deeply personal and intimate both individually and between the two of you. They are completely and inextricably interwoven. Alex, I want to understand what your anger is made of, not because I don't believe it's valid, there are real beliefs and ideas that inform its magnitude, but because we must hear it, understand it, take any meaningful information away from it, and then determine if it can be let go of. It has to be for our work to proceed. I will not ask him to risk coming close to you sexually while it's here. It's not safe for either one of you. Right now, the anger and intimidation IS the erectile dysfunction and avoidance, they're one and the same.

The therapist will need to immediately address and seek to understand Max's experience of his ASD (of which he is the expert), bringing Alex up to speed and in touch with both how best to convey her experience and how to conceptualize and more properly address her frustration. Like any couple, both partners need to understand where accountability can live and where we are simply bumping into how the brain, or ASD, works. Therapy would also require looking closely at the cultural differences between the two, including religious influences if applicable, how sex was treated by both families, what gender norms were taught, and how closeness and love were demonstrated.

Infidelity and Shattered Stories

How could you do this to me?
It's like our whole relationship has been a lie!
You never really loved me!
I don't know who you are anymore!

We will be in a perpetual state of information gathering, of working to understand just like we saw with Alex and Max, because the fact is we will never really "know" our partner(s). We will never have full access to all of their parts (just like our parents with us), to all of the things that make them "them." We are influenced and shaped by forces, experiences, and people we can't acknowledge or even access in memory, despite their ongoing impression and influence, forever sitting in the presence of a great mystery with ourselves and our other or others, only ever working with a sliver of the whole. This is pretty incredible – and scary! So how did we or do we find ourselves concluding *"I know you better than you know yourself"*? Or, *"I know what they're thinking just by looking at them"*? Or, when it comes to infidelity, *"I don't think I ever really knew you."*?

When information enters our orbit that counters the stories we've created about who people are, what their inner lives look like, who we are to them, the things they do and (more importantly) would never do – this disrupts our sense of safety in those relationships. Our stories are, by their very nature, designed to provide a sense of control, of consistency, of security. Yet injury-free, devastation-proof intimacy is not possible in relationships that are characterized by change, by shifting and evolving needs, by the constant unfolding of different iterations of ourselves. When we are met with this reality, it not only rewrites our ideas about safety, it irreparably transforms our relationship to trust, but often in ways that are more connected to reality (a blessing and a curse). To summarize a few hard truths and their realities that make themselves known with infidelity:

- *Complete safety is an illusion.* Romantic partnerships are inherently risky and conditional. We can and do and sometimes *need* to fall out of love if the relationship has run its course, if we're no longer compatible, or if we're on the receiving end of chronic neglect, abuse, or mistreatment.
- *Trust is not and was never black and white (despite our best efforts).* We move around on a scale throughout our day/week/month/year. Many people understand what it feels like to exist in partnership by trusting at around 50–70% on good days. We simply determine that living with that discomfort is worth what we gain.
- *We are enough as people (fully whole and complete as we are) but cannot be "enough" to meet all the needs and wants of our partners in relationships, sexually and beyond.* We make sacrifices in order to have "close enough" or "good enough," and the rest is on us to attend to, manage, cope with, or fight for if the sacrifice becomes too great.
- *We can always find reasons to cheat in long-term relationships.* Justification will always exist because relationships are an ongoing

cycle of, as Terry Real (2008) puts it, "harmony, disharmony, and repair." We have a collection of war stories and grievances at our disposal at any given moment. This is an inevitability with time. Looking at these elements in isolation takes too narrow a view, neglecting all of the other important pieces, relationally and individually, to consider within the complexity of infidelity (relationship to self, desire to escape "realness" of adult life, desire to connect back to fantasy version of ourselves, deep need to access parts of ourselves left out of our current relationship, etc.).

All these hard truths crack open a new level of anxiety, of fear, of uncertainty about ourselves, our partner(s), and our place in their life. In order to alleviate some of the discomfort this anxiety carries, we frantically reach for control in the form of an endless stream of information gathering or the inclination to collect as many details about the affair as possible: *Who were they? How old? Where did you meet them? Where did the two of you go out? How often? What were they like? What did you two do sexually?* And so on. This mission is futile, as no amount of information gathering is going to undo the hard lessons learned. It will not restore the illusion of safety, of comfortable and complete trust. As such, it routinely fails to satisfy and ultimately leads to more pain, despite anxiety's message of "*just keep searching for clues, ask another question, you'll feel better if this detail is understood.*" No amount of digging will alleviate our brain's inclination to make this about our worth, a theme that brings us back to childhood. We will not find "closure" or comfort behind door Z. One question answered leads to a collection of others. Once we accept our new understanding, we can move into working with it in favor of stronger connection, of greater intimacy, of a new frontier of emotional and relational understanding.

Tina (cis/lesbian, 30-year-old, woman):	*We've been sleeping in separate rooms for the past year and a half. It's been this way since I discovered the cheating.*
Therapist:	*A year and a half is quite a while! Have you been intimate with one another in that time?*
Lexa (trans/lesbian, 32-year-old, woman):	*A few times, but at this point it's been nearly six months. The longest we've ever gone by far. I get it, but I also don't at the same time. I'm just trying to be as understanding as I can.*
Therapist:	*Understanding of?*

Lexa:	*Of her feelings and where she's at after everything that went down. I was in the wrong and I know I caused a lot of pain. So, I get that I need to try my best to win back the trust that was lost and to prove myself, I just wish I felt like we were making progress.*
Tina:	*That's not true, it's just hard. I think we've made some strides! I'm just not ready to go back to the way we were before. I know you're trying, and I'm trying too. I'm just not there.*
Therapist:	*What does "there" look like for you? Where are you hoping to land?*
Tina:	*I'm just so anxious constantly. It's exhausting. Whenever she leaves the house, goes out with friends, is late getting home after work ... my mind goes wild! I desperately want to trust her again, but I just don't think I'll ever understand why it happened. I can't make sense of it, even after all of the talking we've done. I just need more time, I think. And I need her to take all of this seriously.*
Therapist:	*"All of this"?*
Tina:	*Our lives! I need her to come home after work and not f__ around! I need her to consider my feelings and maybe text a few times when she's out with friends. It's hard for me every single day, I just need her to care about that and be a little more responsible for a while.*
Therapist:	*Predictability in behavior over time is one way we cultivate trust. It's important that our agreements are treated as sacred during this time, which is why we want to make sure we're comfortable with them before making them. Lexa, part of repair means responsibility to the relationship, attending to it as you would a wounded pet: checking in on it, making plans with it in mind, nurturing it back to health. And Tina, it's important to understand that, despite Lexa's best efforts, a sense of complete comfort and security is unlikely to show up, especially while your shield is up. Distance begets distance and can become enormous over time. Let's talk about how you'll know you're ready to risk again, how you can better understand your fear and anxiety, so it doesn't trick you into believing it's safer to stay behind your shield than to let it down, opening your heart again.*

Despite how very uncomfortable it feels in one way, being in the position of wearing the armor (which represents safety), witnessing our partners express desperation to have us back alongside behaviors and "showing up" in ways we've always craved, is powerful. We are unlikely to remove ourselves from that position, to make ourselves vulnerable again without a nudge, or an internal and loving shove from ourselves, if return to the relationship, to connection, is what we want. If we wish to move on.

Why do so many people cheat?

- *When someone has a crush on me, I feel _____.*
- *When someone is excited and curious about me, I feel_____.*
- *When someone expresses attraction towards me, I feel_____.*
- *When someone is flirting with me, I feel_____.*
- *When I can feel another's desire for me (from someone I like), I feel_____.*
- *When I feel genuinely wanted, I feel_____.*

(Answers to the questions above will vary from person to person. There is no one-size-fits-all when it comes to sexuality, attraction, and interpersonal chemistry.)

New relationship energy will be compelling for many of us at different points in our lives; this is normal and not necessarily an indication that the relationship is in crisis (i.e. no reason to panic). Settling into long-term relationships means allowing someone to get to know us, *really* get to know us, beyond the idea or image we want to convey when dating. As they get to know, they form a relationship to our wounding, our trauma, our flaws and imperfections, and to our darker or more challenging qualities and sides. We are in the palpable presence of that ourselves as well, both in relationship to our own "realness," our bumps and bruises, but also to our partners. That realness lives in our homes, comes to our dinners, is right next to us as we drive to the grocery store or stroll through the park, and it is simultaneously beautiful and real, or beautiful *because* it's real. There is something fantastic, profoundly healing, to be at the place in partnership when we experience that kind of intimacy, the experience of *"I see your complexity, I experience it, AND I love you. I choose to be here."* We can and do take it for granted, allowing the significance of it to slip past us as life becomes perfunctory and our jobs, our routines, wear us down.

Many of us never stop wanting to feel wanted. The desire to be close and have others seek out closeness with us is what it means to be social creatures. Many, if not all, of us crave escape from our reality, from the realness we are in the presence of in our day-to-day, from our own inner complexity. New relationship energy, another person or experience, can represent that escape. It can represent the place where the shiny, sparkly veneer reveals itself again, not just for the other person, but for us. It is the place where we get to visit the fantasy version of ourselves. Can we do this in other ways that leave the integrity of our agreements intact? Yes. Do some people struggle to understand how? Yes.

People cheat for a large variety of complex reasons, all in need of investigating, all requiring understanding and learning. Relationships can emerge stronger on the back of this process, armed with new processes for moving forward, new ways of relating and understanding. A first chapter in the sequel begins, an entirely new relationship between the same people is sometimes called for. Sometimes infidelity lets us know when it's time for an end, and sometimes it is the unfortunate break in our reality that is required to allow us to see the beautiful realness right in front of us.

Attraction

- What first drew you in? *Their eyes.*
- What did you make up about their eyes? *They looked kind.*
- Then what? *Their humor.*
- What did the humor mean to you? *They're fun and don't take life too seriously.*
- Then what? *Their attentiveness.*
- Why attentiveness? *It feels like care.*
- Then what? *Their body.*
- What did their body communicate to you? *That they're strong but not too strong, not intimidating but protective.*
- Then what? *Their talent.*
- What does their talent represent to you? *Passion, focus, dedication, all qualities that I think are important in trying to build a stable life with someone.*

When asked what you find attractive in a partner (or specifically, *your* partner if applicable), how do you respond? Can you imagine those qualities now? How many of those characteristics are physical in nature? How many have to do with personality traits? How many with accomplishments, occupation, or hobbies? What does this say about the nature of how your attraction works and what creates a "pull" or "draw" towards other people?

- Have you ever been physically attracted to someone only to get to know them and have that attraction completely melt away?
- Have you ever felt zero physical attraction to someone initially only to get to know them and have attraction grow?

In the "rules" of dating and finding a partner or partners, physical desirability has traditionally been treated as of primary importance. Dating apps lead with pictures that we get to scroll through, judge according to our own subjective criteria, and factor into the equation that determines whether we want to strike up a conversation and take things further. Some people begin with the pictures, then move onto the actual content of the profile once the person is experienced as attractive enough; others begin with the content of the profile and visit the pictures with more or less importance. Either way, the predominant cultural narrative places physical attraction as critical when dating, something that *must* be there or else your relationship is doomed to fail. Why? Likely because we've linked physical attraction to sexual attraction (which can be, but isn't always, linked), and we've placed sex as of primary importance in lasting relationships (which it can be for some, but not everyone). On the flip side, we've also determined that, once in a relationship, we should see beyond the other as an object; and that it is selfish, cruel, superficial, and wrong for us to struggle with the physical desirability of our partners, and that we need not worry about what or how our partner's feel about our own. Beyond the confusing and contradictory messaging, we find that attraction is so much more than meets the eye. It is layered, and multi-dimensional as the opening questions suggest. What can we assume, then, about how attraction gets dismantled and what that may or may not mean for our relationships? When do we need to worry that grief (regarding one form of attraction or the relationship as a whole) is on the horizon?

When couples present and one is breaking the often very painful-to-hear news that they are no longer physically attracted to the other, it is a starting point. What were you attracted to originally? What drew you toward your partner? What was your attraction made of? Often many of the qualities named are still there. What have they been overshadowed by? What has entered the relationship since, eroding the appeal those qualities possess? Resentment, for example, can steal away the desirability behind even the most appealing characteristics, making what was once experienced as charisma look like desperate performance. Working to eliminate or minimize the presence of unsavory relational characters (animosity, resentment, disrespect) can clear the way to begin shifting focus to the qualities we've lost sight of, or any new ones that have emerged. Noticing both old and new can require intention, part of the work of long-term attraction, of the art of keeping it alive.

What is anxiety trying to tell us when it comes to attraction? What does it really mean or point us towards in terms of implications for the relationship? How shape-shifty can we count on it being?

One important element to consider is how much worth we derive as individuals from how our partners present to the world. How much do appearances matter across the board? In other words, *if you don't look the part, it reflects poorly on me; if you do look the part (some sort of fantasy person or ideal that's been created), I've somehow proven myself to my peers, or my family, or (arguable mostly) to myself.* Our past can get involved as well, in terms of the associations we form in relationship to different qualities, sizes, changes that occur over time, or even our own struggles.

> *I was a scrawny kid growing up. I was relentlessly bullied for it, so in high school I started working out and everything changed. Suddenly I was popular, started actually dating, and was able to leave that scrawny, puny little guy behind. Since my partner of six years got a new job that occupies all his time, we don't work out together. In fact, he no longer works out at all. His physique has totally changed and I can't help but see that weak kid when I see him. I've lost all attraction entirely.*
>
> (Jason)

Lack of attraction can direct us towards places *we're* stuck, or that require further healing and guidance. It can have nothing to do whatsoever with the person in front of us, as illustrated above. We can react to aspects of our past, our conditioning, our messaging and misattribute the cause. It is important that we check in with this when loss or lack of attraction surfaces: it could be an opportunity for greater expansion, more learning to help us stay in relationships that we value, to help us continue to love who we love without contradictory messaging, "phobias," or internalized shame getting in the way.

Sometimes attraction is lost because the person we fell for is no longer there, the ingredients of attraction have left with the changing of the person, and which signifies a need for an end. Other times, it's buried under complexity and is calling for our attention.

The Dimensions of Desire

"I want my partner to want me, to desire me." What can we expect from "wanting" after the felt sense of "knowing" has arrived? What new discovery can be had from seeing our partner's naked body? We've seen it. What new discovery can be had from having sex? We've had it. What is there to want? It's all here. Returning to Esther Perel's work (2006), can we want what we already have? The answer is yes, but the wanting *can* (and often does) feel different.

As discussed, a sense of separateness and autonomy is one crucial variable for the maintenance of desire. It allows for distinction, the sense of definition between partners required for curiosity to emerge, for the kind of "Who are you today?" to create a "come find out" that both partners can grab a hold of. It makes space for us to see our partners with fresh eyes, noticing the things that make them "them," enabling visibility of their unique qualities. Will that create the butterflies we first experienced in our dating days, though? Will it reignite *that* passion?

Let's say we arrive home one day and there's a beautiful chocolate cupcake on the counter: the cake is moist and buoyant, the icing perfectly placed, with a shiny chocolate covered cherry on top. You haven't had a chocolate cupcake in years, so you begin to imagine how good it's going to taste when you bite into it. You approach and it's just as delicious as you'd imagined, so good in fact that you leave a bit for the next day. In the subsequent few days, you notice the details of how delicious this cupcake is: the moistness of the cake, the deep chocolatey flavor, the perfect little crunch of the tiny sprinkles on top, and the bitter/sweet combination of that chocolate covered cherry. So, you acquire the recipe, and then you're making chocolate cupcakes whenever you like. Is it as exciting as it was that first day? Does the cupcake taste as mind-blowingly delicious? Do you crave it, looking forward to getting home to it each day after that week or so of constant cupcake eating? Maybe not, because these cupcakes are available to you now. And even though you aren't running home to them every day, longing desperately for one more bite, now you return to the cupcakes because the feeling of the icing on your tongue is still nice, the chocolatey flavor reminds you of home, and the ritual of baking and eating something you once couldn't go without is now comforting.

This is what we're working with in the vast majority of long-term relationships, the ways in which the wanting changes. Will it look the same as it did when we were dating? When we couldn't get enough of exploring each other's textures, flavors, and beauty? Likely no, but just like the tradeoff we make with new and long-term relationship energy, we can swap desire and wanting made from "hit-you-over-the-head" novelty for the kind of desire and wanting made from more subtle ongoing learning, from the deep love we feel and the "pull" it carries. It is wanting born from the ongoing fantasy we hold of our partners, the stories, qualities, and attachment that survives the test of time, expansion, and growth. And if we zoom out enough, we can catch a glimpse of *those* eyes (because they're still there).

11 Disconnection

Sex *is* connection. It connects us to sensation, our subconscious, erotic imagination, play, emotion, each other, vitality, our physiology, spirituality, our learning. It is part of what it means to be human, an animal, a part of the earth, the earth itself. Our sexuality is an expression of this story, reminding us of who we are and where we came from, as primal beings underneath rules and roles and expectations. As modern life continues to create the perception of distance between ourselves and the earth we are a part of and inhabit, we risk betraying and abandoning the very ingredients that make sex what it is.

Sex as Life Force

When sex is discussed as "life force" or "life force energy," it can take us to a fairly "woo-woo" place, a potential roadblock for those less spiritual. One way of conceptualizing this understanding in a more operational way is by considering sex's "asks" that we've reviewed as themes at the core of what it means to be human. Vulnerability, play, connection, revealing, sharing, letting go, expressing, communicating – in order to grow, in order to move through and process our emotions and experiences, in order to find intimacy with self and others we *need* access to ongoing experiences within these elements. So, if sex is a place that encapsulates and provides access to ourselves, the "I" underneath our conditioning, our homeostasis, sex becomes something far more than meets the eye. It becomes healing, it *is* intimacy, our way beyond our own armor in order to experience the "home" within ourselves. It is a visit back to our childlike, unarmed, fully present, and bare selves. Like sleeping is to waking, it is the counterpoint to the pressure and grind of what it means to be human in modern times.

So, if sex represents our vitality at its core, then it is no wonder we endure such profound consequences when it is harmed or even descended upon by our own egos. It makes sense, then, that we avoid approaching

DOI: 10.4324/9781003369080-14

sex in order to avoid the grief we feel in our struggle to reconnect or access its power, the access it grants us to another realm of experience (like dreaming). When sex is not allowed to be the force that it is, the magic that it is, the transcendent and healing space that it is, it becomes precisely what we've created with and of our humanity in general: an anxious attempt to distance ourselves from our primal nature, and "perform" being an idea or a concept rather than ourselves.

Disconnection permeates nearly every challenge we face with our sexuality, and it doesn't stop there. Our relational struggles nearly all originate with or become fueled by the feelings we encounter when experiencing both fleeting moments or deep periods of disconnection, and everything in-between within our relationships and within ourselves. Disconnection can be found at the heart of our shame, depression, insecurity, anger, and rage, all feelings that lead to behaviors relationally that perpetuate it, resulting in: trauma, body and gender dysphoria, racism, bigotry, sexism, misogyny, addiction, violence, and ableism, among a plethora of others.

Taking gender dysphoria as an example, Jordon Anderson, a transgender-identified clinical social worker and certified sex therapist, gives us a window into the complexity of disconnection, even in our conceptualization:

> The language of gender dysphoria comes from 19th century sexology. It is outdated and historically has been about cissexuals naming transgender experiences. The language of gender dysphoria is part of the problem; it is inherently about distancing self from body, both for trans people and for cissexuals, and thus results in experiences of disconnection. It posits a negative experience, rather than an embodied or curious one. As therapists, we ask people, "tell me who you are," we do not ask, "tell me who you are not." When we center dysphoria, we ask individuals to engage in mental gymnastics. When we recenter gender-pleasure, gender-play, gender-curiosity, as Lucie Fielding argues, we then can ask better embodied questions of not only trans and gender non-conforming folxs, but of cissexuals as well.
>
> In addition to encouraging a disconnection between self and body, the centering of gender dysphoria also disconnects us from the historical reality that throughout the whole of human history and across cultures, there have been natural varieties of gender expression, and that not all those who are gender-**expansive** are transgender. Many cultures and languages have a variety of identifiers and names for themselves. The gender binary and thus the language of gender dysphoria are products of white-settler colonialism; we must connect with old wisdom and deep-knowing that gender is **expansive**. Dysphoria is not a prerequisite for breaking or expanding beyond binaries. Western-practicing therapists must resist trying to classify people and groups as one thing or

another. This requires respecting indigenous wisdom and history, recentering these indigenous narratives, and dismantling the hegemony of gender dysphoria.

(Anderson, 2024)

What is your experience of connection like today? How might you describe the quality of the connections you hold with your family, peers, community, colleagues? Or your body, your gender, your sex? Is there a particular brand of connection you seek out? Or avoid? Or are fearful of or challenged by?

Sex asks us to shed our human scripts and prescriptions, and connect back to something organic, unbound, and ultimately primal. The more disconnected we find ourselves in relationship to our animal body, the more we fear and want to distance ourselves from it, the more tense and cerebral sex becomes. It is wet, sticky, rich with smells, tastes, noises; it is unkempt and wild (even when it's slow and tender). In our attempts to distance ourselves from our fellow animal species, we've effectively denied, rejected, and labeled elements of our nature as gross or repellant, elements that can and often do come to life in sex if we're letting go enough to allow them.

Can we make peace with (or even fully embrace) the fact that:

- We secrete fluids, including vaginal fluids;
- We ejaculate (and pre-ejaculate) fluids;
- We emit smells from our bodies and armpits;
- We pass air through our bodies (we fart, we queef, etc.);
- We sweat;
- We have scars and cellulite;
- We have soft bodies, large bodies, thin bodies, fat bodies, wrinkly bodies, disabled bodies;
- We have bodies with stretch marks, folds, and dimples;
- We make noises;
- We have circumcised and uncircumcised penises that are straight or angled, of all sizes;
- We have big, small, thin, long, wide, deflated breasts;
- We have long, flat, wide, puffy nipples;
- We have different sized labia, both inner and outer;
- We have breath that can smell and taste of the food we ate that day;
- The landscape of our own skin contains different colors and textures.

Which of the items on the list can you identify as being challenging for you, either now or in the past or both? Are there any you can add? Can you identify some that you've already embraced, perhaps even eroticized, perhaps even celebrated?

This list is not meant to suggest that we should completely disregard our social conditioning entirely, tossing out what we understand to be "norms" of human hygiene, social rules, and care (unless both parties are into it), but can we lessen our hold, our deep desire to control, slightly? Can we care a little less about being doll-like versions of ourselves, squeaky clean, imperfection-free, smelling of roses?

This list is to remind us that, although we are human beings operating within systems that dictate social rules and norms, we also live in bodies that are messy, organic, performing functions outside of the control and management of the conscious mind, and made from the same parts as our mammalian counterparts. We are not robotic, despite where our evolution seems to be steering us, and sex that feels as such is lacking a central ingredient: liberation.

Serina Payan Hazelwood: "What Did My Ancestors Hope for Me?" Coming Back to Ourselves, to Earth's Body

Serina Payan Hazelwood (S) (she/her) is a queer, Indigenous-Chicana, scholar, author, educator, and community gatherer. She is a certified holistic sexuality educator and yoga teacher dedicated to liberatory praxis through Indigenous knowledges. Her work is rooted in the cosmologies of the land. Reclamation, ritual, and renewal are the guiding value systems that inform the human experience of her work.

Paula
Leech (P):   Humans have moved further and further away from the kind of intimate relationship, both spiritually and physically, that some of our great ancestors had to the earth, the land, and the animals that inhabit it. How would you say that evolution has had an impact on our relationship to ourselves, our bodies, sensuality, sexuality?

S: I will say the first thing that I felt in my body was the word "evolution," and the distinction that would make more sense to me would be the evolution of colonialism, and specifically capitalism and supremacy. With each generation through my line, we have become more and more disconnected because of the systems of colonialism. First we have the removal of the lands, someone coming in, taking the lands, and then saying "OK, you can come back to these lands but now you gotta work them and whatever is produced from those lands that you used to 'own,' ('cause there wasn't really ownership)," and so it becomes this extraction of not only the land and producing, now it's no longer a part of ourselves, now we're also the product, now we're the laborers. And as capitalism and supremacy have strengthened, the more disconnected we became, right? So maybe my ancestors were in hiding with their ways of knowing, but still connected. Or maybe half of it was hiding and half was outward. And then as these systems strengthened and there's more violence, there's more of a necessity to assimilate, to be safe. So, with what was required in order to be outwardly safe, inwardly those rituals and those ways of being connected to the earth slowly diminished over time and suddenly "Here I am, so disconnected from my food sources, and from nature."

P: Just to be clear, how do you conceptualize what colonialism is? What are we speaking of specifically?

S: It's such a big word! Without delving too deeply, it's when a group comes in to dominate (and we're talking more settler – there're different kinds of colonialism but I'm speaking more to the USA, Mexico). Europeans in these cases, but also the Spaniards by way of Mexico, and they seek to remove the people from the land and all that is connected to the land. We remove the people and then they use those resources to profit, to build wealth. It's a violent act, colonialism is violence. I also want to say to decolonize is also violent, a violent act. And colonialism isn't an event, it's a structure, it's a system, so to say "Oh, this happened between these years and these years and then it was done" is not true, it's actually ongoing, it's an ongoing structure.

P: That we're still involved in.

S: That we're still involved in! We've created this country from removing the people from the land and then enslaving stolen people and using bodies, immigrant bodies, to build wealth and um ... always makes me sad talking about it, right? And of the many systems that feed into this big machine are things like our educational system, our political system, our financial system. And we're now here, you and me, in this very well-oiled machine, and for so many of us, and I'll speak for myself, I can't completely remove myself from it. So how can I still feed myself and have a home and have joy and these ways of taking care of myself and my body and also reconnect with that which was systematically removed from me?

P: Does the system, the machine in and of itself and everyone involved, which is everybody – does it represent disconnection for everybody?

S: Yes, I believe so. I believe that so many of us don't even know that we're disconnected, until like in *The Matrix* when you take the pill, the blue pill or the red pill and you wake up to the fact that you were not just randomly disconnected from it but you were, all of us were, *removed* from it, including the settler. The settler had to be removed from the land and their connection to the land to do the acts that they did.

P: I'm almost hearing you describe like a severance from the root that has happened for us. And how that has translated into how we experience our bodies, sensuality, our sexuality, what we contend with as a result of that profound disconnection feels like … trauma.

S: Yeah! Sever to me would be like [she makes a breaking motion] severed, and when I think about it, it's more dormant, or maybe like some or most of that root has died and when we pull out a plant sometimes we think it's dead, but it's not – there's a little piece of it showing you something else and you're like "Oh, this little piece is still alive, let me just plant this in there and see what happens." That piece is your vitality, that is your life force. And what is our sexuality? It's our life force, right? They are one and the same. So for me, to separate the topic of sexuality from everything else, it's not possible, it's connected because *that is* our life force, that is how we get the vitality that we feel, this drive for life, enjoying the pleasures, as well as experiencing pain. I believe, the more we do the work to reconnect to earth's body in a meaningful way, it also helps us to grow that root, to make that root come alive where it becomes this plant and it's full and rich and healthy even when it has these insects eating at the plant. If you have a strong plant, its resistant! It's like "Oh, yeah this little bug that's eating me, I'm resistant to it, I'm strong enough for this."

P: Right, because so much of what sex therapy *is* is undoing narrative. We walk into a room with another person and we're confronted with a multitude of scripts about how we should be doing sex, and ultimately these are stories about how who we are and how we express and receive love just isn't enough. So, a great deal of the task of sex therapy is to look at how we get underneath all of this so that people can access what feels transcendent about sex, and in that transcendent place we're tapping into our primal being, who we are outside of these systems, their narratives and the consequences, and surrendering to *that*. And that to me feels like what you're describing in a larger way with how we connect back to the earth and to who we are underneath all the training that we've received. You know? Sex is one path.

S: Yes, to who we are!

What I return to is, "What did my ancestors hope for me?" And what do I hope for my descendants, whether that's from my line or descendants in my family, my community – what do I hope for them? It's actually the same thing, right? And it doesn't involve things that have to do with capitalism, that's for sure. It's more like joy and harmony and pleasure. I find that also learning about history, the things that we were not taught, is essential. Because sometimes we must tell our stories, we have to go back and think about or reflect upon our stories in therapy to get to where we're at or where we want to go. I also believe that to be true when we're talking about earth's body because it's important to understand *why* we were disconnected and how that connects with our sexuality: how we are to "perform," and have gender roles, and marriage, and the question of who owns our bodies and so on. It's learning about colonialism and how it affected us and our families, even if we don't have their stories. Healing can also come from understanding or reflecting on the whys: "Why am I here at this place and I'm disconnected from my body?" Well, there's a reason. It's on purpose.

P: Right! Which presents challenges for all of us in terms of getting back into the body, finding reconnection, or even understanding a way. And what I'm hearing you talk about is the ripple effect of reconnection to earth's body and how that translates on this foundational level to reconnection to ourselves and our own sensuality and ability to connect with other people ... how it's all part of the same thing.

So, from your perspective if you had to boil it down ...what has colonialism, what has capitalism done to sex? In a general sense what is this disconnection made of, what has it moved us towards?

S: OK, so here's how I see how capitalism effects our sexuality or vitality or life force. So, there's the extraction process, the violent extraction, then there's a consumption of those things that were extracted, a metabolizing of those things, and then it spits it out into this other thing, it's processed, right? And I think that capitalism has really done that damage to us in telling us what our sexuality is supposed to be and what it means to be sexual beings. From the extraction to the repackaging of it. And if you think about the essence of who we are, and you even said it, like this primal ... natural, our bodies are wise but we have been told by these systems that our bodies are not wise, that we need to listen to this authority on what it is, and how we should be, and what we should know, and how we should know it. For generations we've believed that, and we've even taught it to our own descendants because that's what we were told but also that's what kept us safe. To act any other way would mean we would receive violence, we would be harmed. Capitalism, supremacy, and colonialism have produced compliance to the scripts instead of trusting ourselves. Sometimes I think the anxiety comes from the not-trusting because we have this larger narrative telling us what this performance should be (*What does capitalism tell me I should be?*), but we can feel another way internally, intuitively that conflicts with those messages, and therein lies this internal struggle.

P: As you're talking, I'm thinking about how the production part of it requires so many rules, right? You have to "do" things, life, a certain way. And I think there are lots of reasons why people have decided sexuality is threatening, but I think that in the experience of sex itself, you are not completely in reality space, you're interacting with and deeply into fantasy territory, immersed in an experience, in sensation, in story which may be why this is such a struggle for folx, because consciousness, our conditioning, comes online and reminds us that "there are rules for how I'm supposed to fantasize," "there are rules about what I should be fantasizing about or even if I should be in that space at all," "there are rules about how I engage with my body," there're just so many things in the production that seem to completely eradicate intimacy. The stuff at the heart of sex.

S: What comes to me when you're talking about that is the binary. It's such a binary, right? Thinking about the fantasy piece, it's like, "Oh here's how to fantasize by this movie, this is how fantasy is supposed to be, don't come up with it on your own, if you do that you're weird." Yet when I think about the earth's body and all the things connected to it, it's so non-binary. There's no right or wrong, there's no one way, it's flexible. Capitalism, supremism doesn't want us to have the qualities that exist within the non-binary, it makes those things inaccessible to us.

P: It's also reminding me of how in adulthood many of us have had a collection of experiences that awaken the realization of, "Oh, nobody really knows what they're doing, we're all kinda lost!" Despite our best efforts to organize, study, and understand – despite our attempts at boxing life in! Boxing sex in! And like you said, what is the earth? It is wild, ego-less, fluid and moving, and can I trust that? Can I lean into that when it comes to my sensuality, my sexuality, or do I need to continue to listen to what confused people have decided together in their confusion and fear over the centuries?

S: That is so true. And when we even think about psychology and where that came from, who was being studied, who was doing the studying, and who was saying "this is the way you must – here's how to be normal" – the fuck does that even mean? Right?

P: Right. So, what does healing look like from your perspective?

S: It gives me great comfort knowing that there's no final destination. For me, it's a constant process, a constant journey. Just like in the process of working with the earth and gardening and noticing all of the cycles, right? Healing is that process: death, rebirth, death, rebirth, and sometimes old shit comes up again but maybe in a different way. Sometimes we get stuck in cycles longer than we think we're supposed to, sometimes what we need and what we want are two different things.

It also takes work; healing takes intentional work. I do think as humans that we want a "yes" or "no" way of doing something or we want something done, or not done. And so, when we talk about these things related to colonialism, and we talk about these things related to earth, sometimes it's frustrating for even me where I'm just like, "I just want the answer. I want an immediate answer because we feel like we have the right to know everything," which is not true. So sometimes when we're talking about healing, I know it can seem like it's up here [her hand makes wave-like motions in the air]: ethereal and just like air, and sometimes it is! Which is why this conversation, this book, will be balanced with something that is perhaps more binary, like "This is how you do this." We get to learn from and be with both on our way.

12 Insecurity and Confidence
(Your Relationship to You)

We might reference "getting naked" when speaking of "getting real," or candid, or honest. We use "stripping down" in the same way. Why? Because we all understand, without saying it, that revealing ourselves in the ways sex asks means to encounter without our defenses, the ways we hide, conceal, both literally (*I can't hide that part of my body I'm self-conscious about without particular clothes and their placement*) and psychologically/emotionally (*will they "see" my insecurity, my lack of experience, the imposter underneath the persona?*). When thinking about who we are in our sexual experiences, we must consider all of who we are and how we feel about those parts, our many pieces. They are with us in our "realness," our naked, stripped-down, attempts at making contact, real contact, with self and other; the kind of contact that leads to the dream-like experience we all know sex can be as an event that blends and blurs the lines of both fantasy and reality.

What are your pieces made of? What follows you, in ways that are advantageous and in ways that are challenging, into your sex? If you could bring your armor, your defenses, into your sexual experiences with you, what would they protect you from feeling? From noticing? From worrying about? What would they remove from the room? Let's explore.

Deep "Knowing"

- What version of yourself was the wildest?
- What version of yourself was the most held back?
- What version of yourself needed extra care and nurturing?
- What version of yourself do you want to revisit?
- What version of yourself was the most vulnerable?
- What version of yourself is the most present with you today?
- What version of yourself bears the brunt of your anger?
- What version of yourself is grieving?

DOI: 10.4324/9781003369080-15

- What version of yourself could you use more of in your life today?
- What version of yourself do you need to make peace with?

Romantic or invested partnerships demand more and more of and from us over time. We want to feel the emotional presence of our partners in an ongoing way, which requires coming to the table, sharing, communicating, expressing, and advocating (and yes, sometimes even fighting), over and over again. We have so much more control over what gets shared, and the version or versions of ourselves we want to bring to the table in the beginning phases. Over time, that control slips, along with our efforts to "put our best foot forward" as we get comfortable, and the deep complexity of who we are steps forward. The relationship begins to feel and react to how we think about ourselves, our relationship to our history and past versions of ourselves, and the ease with which we navigate our feelings. It may sound strange, but we go through a similar process within ourselves as we work to self-actualize. We can't out run ourselves, we can't out run our feelings, and we can't out run our trauma and our wounding. Significant figures from our childhood are called to the carpet in our adulthood in ways both overt and covert, reflected in the quality of the connection in the present, the ways in which we relate to one another, the memories and hurts we dance around. We attempt to organize our lives accordingly in order to keep the ghosts, the tension, and the irritation at bay; and we try to engage in a similar process with ourselves with much less success.

When we attempt to keep ourselves from ourselves, we suffer tremendously. There is no "good in moderation" when it comes to living within our own skin, although many expend significant effort attempting to fill up or busy our lives in order to try. Moving away from ourselves signals danger to our nervous systems, giving anxiety the green light to thrive, stealing away vital ingredients to intimacy. We are versions of ourselves, unfolding one after the next; behaving in ways that make sense given our context, developmental stage, and understanding of ourselves and the world. It always makes sense; we just have to look close enough to find it. Do we dare? Who might we be, how might we love without the shame we carry from the past?

- How do I feel about how I show up in my relationships with family? Particular family members?
- How do I feel about how I show up in my friendships?
- How do I feel/have I felt about how I've shown up in romantic partnership(s)?
- How do I feel about how I show up in my relationship with myself? How do I feel about how I treat or take care of myself? How much time do I take to care? Where is my relationship to self on the priority list?

Say you worked in an office at your former job, one that required formal business attire. This cost time and money and required effort each morning, attending to every detail: the wrinkles in the clothes, the smell of your skin, the placement of each hair – something that could get tiresome and burdensome day to day. Then you find yourself in a new role having been offered better pay elsewhere, and this job is remote! You roll out of bed, put minimal effort into appearance (*because I don't need to, yay!*), and jump into a few virtual meetings followed by a dozen or so phone calls. Business on the top, pajamas on the bottom. This saves time, money, and hassle and yet it doesn't have the anticipated effect. You walk into the bathroom to glance in the mirror and feel like you don't recognize yourself, don't like what you see. You are confronted with a sense of loss and sadness as you stare at your reflection and then return back to your calls. What happened?

Turns out that the time and energy invested was meaningful time and energy investing in *you*, your identity within your professional role, the presentation of and care for yourself. The attire felt fitting given your worth, your value within the company, as a reflection of your own personal pride. Without that care for and attention to, there's less of a reminder of those qualities in yourself, less of a routine celebration of your inherent worth. You notice this loss and yet continue to go about the same new routine you've adopted, shifting the message to self, neglecting your own feelings and the important message they provide. How does your sex life suffer as a result? How are these things connected?

Chronic experience of grief and sadness related to self + inaction and bypassed opportunities to attend to and problem solve (lack of care and investment in own experience) = decreased feelings of openness and enthusiasm to share self with another (sexually and/or emotionally).

Experiences that we visit and revisit that make us feel bad about ourselves without being attended to or corrected are also bad for our desire and bad for our ability and willingness to connect; it's that simple. It all truly begins and ends with our attention to self and how we respond to our own pain and struggle. *How do I feel about how I showed up in my relationship today? Not awesome, I was more critical than I would've liked to be when discussing our finances this morning. How might I repair tomorrow? What would that look like? I will take accountability for my mood and apologize, let them know I care about how I treated them.* If we rewind the tape daily, considering our behavior and care for ourselves and the relationships we value in our lives, we will inevitably feel more accountable to them, to ourselves, sending the message to our heart and mind that "I" matter and hold an important and powerful place in my life and in the lives of those around me, resulting in meaningful changes that reverberate out. Is this effort? Yes. Are we tired? Yes. And what could be more important? We won't easily find or have access to intimacy, desire, and potentially even sexual functioning (if it's responding to our feelings of anxiety originating from our insecurities) if we neglect it. How else do we keep ourselves stuck in insecurity? Held back from connection?

What's Left Without Feeling?

Attempting to keep back and bottle in expression of feeling has a ripple effect, impacting our physiology and tampering with our ability to connect with sensory input as emotion is built from sensation. Our attempts at keeping emotion and our own vulnerability at bay only serve to amplify the presence of what are deemed more socially acceptable emotions to demonstrate or walk around with, feeling states like anxiety, tension, agitation, anger. These feelings and concepts can follow us into the bedroom and take on a presence as a means of guarding us from the harder stories underneath. This "protection," paradoxically, signals a lack of safety to the body; the body then inhibits sexual response.

Our emotional concepts and sensory data are the wisdom the brain turns to as a means of determining whether the conditions are right to release, turn on, and play. Comfortable? Great. Excited? Sure! Nervous? Maybe later. Scared? Definitely not now. There is no such thing as neutral, we are always reacting to what is happening, may happen, or is very much about to happen to and with us sexually and within the context and what we understand or make up about the other person or persons involved. Even as we grab information from our reality and blend it into our fantasy world (e.g. *I don't know this person well, but they seem kind of feisty, which I like, and kind of look like that person I had a crush on in high school*), we are helping ourselves access and/or move through feelings, associations, and therefore predictions that bring us closer to arousal. Throughout the interaction, our emotional concepts wrap themselves around sensation in the body, amplifying that sensory experience, taking us further into full surrender and immersion in connection, or encouraging us out. Whether we are actively trying to hide our feelings and convey a different persona or are subconsciously protecting ourselves from them, the body will notice that discrepancy. Our hearts know the difference.

Sex can show itself as the counterpoint to how we move through our daily lives. In other words, *in my professional and personal life outside of my sexual experiences, I am a very controlled person, private, and reluctant to express and show my feelings, but in my sexual life all that melts away and I am exceptionally connected to my vulnerability, expressive and free from the control I partner with the majority of my day.* It can also be an extension of our mode of operating in our daily lives, which tends to be the experience for most. If we have an adversarial relationship with vulnerability in general, we can inadvertently work to resist or hold it back sexually (a losing game). This *seems* to work for some when being sexual with strangers or people we aren't terribly connected to or invested in. In fact, for many in these scenarios our sexuality flourishes and we feel the most sexually uninhibited and free. This begs the question: Are we actually being less vulnerable or are we freed up to be fully vulnerable without the fears and insecurities that accompany deep investment in outcome, the person, the relationship? We have greater room to imagine what is being shared, having no or lacking meaningful history, which is connected to fantasy and how we imagine the other person sees and experiences us. Until we are in a relationship where we begin to understand each other's complexity, alongside deep care for the other person, the challenges with vulnerability are less apparent, less problematic. It gets harder to hide, imagine, or story tell as we draw nearer, too powerful to compartmentalize. We *have* to understand the fear at the heart of our inclination to hold back, what our brain is referencing in its prediction of danger at the prospect of sharing, of being seen.

- What version of me learned, really learned, that I'm not good enough to be loved for who I am? What version of me began understanding that it's better to hide and hold back than to reveal and express?
- What message did they need to hear then?
- What do they (this version of me that still and will forever occupy residence and space within my psyche) need to understand from adult me, now?

Depression

When we invite someone to engage with us sexually, we invite them into the story we hold about ourselves. We invite them into the feelings connected to those stories, whether they're consciously felt or not. For all of us, this is complicated, and each of us is more-or-less skillfully able to bypass some of the more challenging elements of our story in order to feel more fully into the parts that open the door for desire, comfort, and connection to emerge. The bypassing requires that we, again, have some comfort within ourselves to work with, an appreciation or even neutrality that can be experienced in a regular way. When what we have to grab for or rest into becomes increasingly elusive, and the challenging aspects of our story seem to take up the most meaningful space, we will distance. Depression is often paired with low desire for this very reason, and it is not our fault. It's simply the nature of the beast. Depression traps us in the challenging stories we have about ourselves and dresses them up as who we are, causing us to lose motivation, isolate, and distance from intimacy. It can even be thought of as serving a function, for example: "*My low desire protects you from my heaviness, my sadness, my shame.*" In a seemingly backwards way, the low desire becomes a version of loving and caring for the partner, in the midst of the great distance, loneliness, and isolation depression creates.

Is there a part of your story of yourself, your understanding of who you are, you can visit that gives you a sense of meaning or purpose, that keeps your energy going when things get stressful, that quiets some of the chatter? Most of us don't think about how we think about ourselves throughout our day, but we should! It's more than just positive self-talk (although that can help): it's concept building, self-worth scaffolding, deep self-tether creating stuff!

Addiction

Our relationship to our feelings/emotions, our past, and our predictions *is* what creates and sustains our addictions. Fueled by enormous complexity below the surface, what we often see manifest is the anxiety pulling us towards our substance of choice. That is we look forward to a drink after work (relief from anxiety and stress/sense of control), a glass of wine or a beer with pals (relief from anxiety and stress and social anxiety, inhibitions – paving the way for "connection"/sense of control), maybe even getting wasted on New Year's (relief/complete escape from anxiety and stress/sense of control). Addiction is a challenging topic to discuss given that our definitions of it are lacking. However, when it comes to sexuality (i.e. the expression of, and release into, feeling), extreme ideas around what it means to have a problematic relationship to substances is not required. Our alcohol consumption, for example, doesn't need to look "excessive" in order to have an impact on our sexuality. We smoke marijuana, drink alcohol, or engage in a variety of other substances to gain a sense of control, to move away from aspects of our experience. In that "moving away" we are distancing ourselves from ourselves, and by virtue of that, distancing ourselves from others. We are also tampering with our physiology and circulation, altering the quality of blood flow to the surface of the skin and to our genitals, and therefore our experience with sensation and pleasure, for better and for worse. It is important to note if sex and substances frequently go together in your life. If so, what parts of yourself do they hide or diminish in order to help bring more comfort forward? What predictions and associations connected to sex are being replaced with predictions and associations connected with inebriation or alcohol?

When considering what is often framed as "true addiction," what comes to mind is someone whose consumption is part of their every day, an organizing principle to their life. When this is the situation, a few things can happen:

1 Aspects of our development get arrested when the addiction becomes an entrenched process in the life of the individual. Relationship to our emotional experience gets altered by the substance or substances, interfering with the constant learning they offer throughout each day. Consequently, it can feel like we are in a regressed place emotionally and psychologically once the substance has been abandoned. In many ways, we pick up where the addiction started. Suddenly we're back at 18, for example, with the relational and emotional skills of that version of ourselves, attempting to learn how to feel and cope, pivotal elements of our development the addiction hijacked, among others. An incredible task.

2 When we give up the substance, and move into sobriety in a meaningful way, the feelings, memories, and challenging lessons that we had concealed with the addiction are there to greet us in addition to challenges we may face navigating those feelings without the coping/distancing mechanism that was once the go to. This experience can be immensely challenging, as we often come face to face with years, possibly decades, worth of accumulated emotion that has been stored underneath the barrier of the substance(s). Stepping into vulnerability can feel like approaching a tidal wave of powerful emotions.

This level of newness, rawness, tenderness can feel overwhelming. Learning how to step into and befriend vulnerability, coming face to face with the powerful reasons underlying the origins of our backing away, is a process that takes some time, experience, and support to acclimate to. The good news is, with this process comes the opportunity to truly take a beginner's mind to our sexuality, something important but also something we are not inclined to do unless cornered. *What does sensation in my body feel like now? What am I learning from it? What feels interesting, good, or neutral today? What am I curious about exploring? How might I check in with my partner (if I have one)?*

With access to this new realm of feeling comes access to joy, passion, and pure, electric pleasure, feelings that are able to emerge following the grief, sadness, shame, and/or guilt we are first met with. Patience, awareness, presence, and our willingness to feel (accompanied by the guidance of a skilled therapist) will get us there.

You Are Not Too Much or Too Little, but Your Behavior Can Be

We talk about "being enough as we are" throughout this book, under-standing that we are worthy of loving and being loved as is. Though this is true, our inherent worth doesn't give us the green light to behave however we'd like, it doesn't mean we need not consider and work hard to be rela-tionally smart and protect others from our challenging parts, our unpro-ductive or harmful coping behaviors, our emotionally assaultive outbursts. What are the ways in which you mishandle conflict? How do you get in your own way in terms of communication, connection, and problem solv-ing? Do you shut down? Get intellectual? Blame and criticize? Dodge responsibility? Are these things "part of our personalities"? Or are they adaptations, methods we've developed that our subconscious understood as the only or the best option for negotiating tough times as children. When we view aspects of ourselves as fixed, we pass the buck onto our partners or those around us to accommodate, change, and tolerate. This may ease anxiety in one sense, *"this is just me, take it or leave it,"* but it ultimately ups the anxiety experienced in our lives as our relationships suffer, and our partners are left to shoulder a degree of change that should be ours to understand and attend to in the evolving relational dynamic. Counter to this, fixed traits can have the effect of stirring up a great deal of anxiety *"I get snarky and sarcastic when I fight. It's such an ugly trait, but it's just me! My dad was like that also. It makes people feel small and I know that. I feel like I ruin really great relationships with this aspect of my personal-ity."* Without any sense of agency, we can feel stuck, doomed, or trapped inside ourselves. Worse, it eats away self-trust. And it doesn't need to be this way.

We are complex beings with equally complex feelings and parts to us that come alive or reveal themselves in different circumstances. None of us are entirely angry, or shameful, or sweet all of the time. We all do things we're not proud of on our quest for comfort and place in the world. What do we do when faced with seemingly "fixed traits"? It is fairly easy to find justification to do nothing via "self-empowerment" posts on social media. Sentiments like "you are not too much, they're just not enough for you" can simultaneously validate our inherent worth, while invalidating others, and inadvertently reinforcing potentially problematic behavior. Behavior that potentially gets in the way of being seen or heard or met in a meaning-ful way. Let's take Jill and Nadia as an example:

Jill:	*We don't communicate. It's our main issue, it's why we've been to multiple therapists at this point. We just can't seem to figure out how to talk to each other.*
Nadia:	*Well, speak for yourself please. I have no problem saying what I need to say to you. You just won't listen, or conveniently*

you'll vanish when you know I have something important to say. (Turning to therapist) *I try to talk, she runs away.*

Therapist: *Jill, can you tell me about what Nadia is calling "running away"? Can you understand why she would perceive that in you?*

Jill: *Well, yeah I understand why she would perceive that. I do run away! She is a very passionate person, something that drew me to her and that I love, except when we have something serious we need to talk about or when one of us is upset. She goes from zero to sixty and I can't handle the yelling and screaming and swearing. I just can't. It's like my whole body reacts to it, I can feel my heart start to race even just thinking about it.*

Nadia: *Well maybe I wouldn't get so upset if you would actually take me seriously and listen. I'm tired of chasing you around, begging and pleading for you to listen. It's not fair and I'm exhausted.*

What needs to happen here? If Nadia were to tell her side of the challenge to her friends over dinner, they might say something like *"Jill is neglectful! You have a right to say what you need to say! If she can't handle it, that's on her! You need someone with more of a backbone, who can appreciate how passionate and direct you are."* If Jill were to confide in her circle, they might come to the table with something along the lines of *"Nadia is abusive and out of control! It's not OK for her to rage and scream at you like that! She needs to figure out how to manage her anger, otherwise you need to leave this relationship."* Is Jill "avoidant" and Nadia "verbally assaultive"? Or is Jill *choosing* to avoid and Nadia *behaving* aggressively? Either way, both partners need to shift their part in the dynamic in order for attention and connection to happen, for conversation to emerge, and for real learning and solutions to take place. What does this mean? Both have to:

- Understand the function their behavior serves:

  J: My parents would yell and scream, I learned to hide in my room and tune out.

  N: I lived in a house with five older siblings, I learned I had to "get big" to get attention.

- See the barrier it creates:

  J: My retreating creates more desperation for connection with those I love, I am making myself inaccessible.

  N: My aggression is a distraction from my message. My partners become overwhelmed and intimidated by the expression of my emotion, preventing them from doing anything other than focusing on and reacting to just that.

- **And learn how to get out ahead of/work with it themselves:**

    J: I can speak to my overwhelm, stay connected by placing my hand gently on Nadia's arm, and ask for what I need to engage.
    N: I can take breaks when I become overwhelmed, attending to my activated part and working to release the adrenaline so that I can return and speak *to* the emotion rather than hurling it at my partner. I can speak clearly and slowly. My vulnerability is something I can step into now.

Caring for ourselves is an antidote to anxiety. Learning to "do" conflict, communication, connection more skillfully is self-trust, self-intimacy, and self-worth building. Our personalities, attributes, and behaviors are made of a million ingredients, and while all of the ingredients are meaningful and what make us "us," none are unshapable in how they get expressed. Some of them require work, others can live in certain contexts but not others, maybe a few have to go entirely. It's our job to know the difference, and to do the hard work required to improve our lives for ourselves and those closest to us. Our complexity is what makes us unique, funny in our own ways, and interesting. It informs the way we see the world and the important choices we've made along the way. And some of it must find its place in the back seat when it threatens our ability to drive safely.

Body Image

When do you recall first noticing how your body looks? How it does or does not fit the definition of "beautiful" or "handsome" or "valuable" at the time? When did you begin imagining what might be different if *you* were different, your physicality more in line with what the world, or more specifically the media, defined as beautiful or sexy? At some point all of us have bumped into the consequences of our training here, our training being the non-stop, daily, if not hourly, barrage of emaciated or artificially muscular (i.e. steroid) bodies being held up as the standard of beauty for decades. The pop culture magazines displayed at physicians' offices, salons, barber shops, and the dentist – all ridiculing celebrities for putting on that 15 lbs and daring to go for a swim on family vacations. Now we contend with different ideals, different definitions of beauty and what makes bodies valuable, worthy of loving, worthy of desiring. It evolves alongside us and is a reflection of our cultural ideals and where we place our physical being, our aesthetics as a reflection of how much value we have as people relative to others. And there's a larger, more insidious, story here.

In her book, *Fearing the Black Body: The Racial Origins of Fat Phobia*, Sabrina Strings (2019) reveals the idealization of slenderness to be a means of "using the body to validate race, class, and gender prejudice." As Hanna Carlan summarizes:

It wasn't until the late seventeenth century that fat became a recourse for racial categorization. The writings of early race scientists like George Cuvier, J. J. Virey, and Georges-Louis Leclerc who linked gluttony, stupidity, and the characteristics of Africans, whose idleness was attributed to their warm climate (a pervasive trope also found in colonial discourse about India). Enlightenment-era rationalism elevated food to the moral plane of asceticism required for intellectual pursuit. Soon, a thin physique had gone from being a sign of sickliness to evidence of the moral and intellectual superiority of Europeans, supported by the writings of anthropologists and naturalists seeking to codify and biologize a racial hierarchy.

(Carlan, 2020)

J. J. Virey's writings, mentioned above, included:

In our white species, the forehead is projecting and the mouth retreating, as if we were rather designed to think than to eat; in the negro species, the forehead is retreating and the mouth projecting, as if he were made to eat rather than think.

(Strings, 2019, p. 86)

Through our history we see how deeply seeded our ideas about race embed themselves, seeping into our Calvin Klein adverts alongside a million other popular brands proudly displaying emaciated bodies to sell clothing in the early 2000s and beyond. How does this brief window into our history shift how you think about *your* body? How does it influence your conceptualization of what weight means or represents, or has meant and represented to you in your experience, or the experience of those who've struggled around you? How can you further your learning in order to continue developing an understanding of weight, "beauty," and value that is less governed by feelings, ideology, and hatred that has traveled through time and through our bodies? Our current cultural shift towards a new rhetoric around body positivity means extricating ourselves from a long, pervasive, and racist history whereby fat was objectified as an indication of racial inferiority. Beauty has been defined by hatred.

Missing the Mark

Our day-to-day struggles with beauty, body, and weight make little room for victory. Despite our best efforts, this beast is never full, never satiated, as an aspect of human existence and experience that is entirely subjective, emotional, and personal at its core. Proof of "body perfection" evasiveness can be found in our modern-day celebrities, as even those who have gained fame and adoration from their bodies and physicality alone continue to engage in plastic surgery, ceaselessly editing and sculping. We may arrive at a place of contentment, but it's often fleeting as our bodies continue to grow and change and slow down and speed up, doing exactly what bodies do, and we work, sometimes making ourselves miserable, trying to keep up. *This follows us into the bedroom!*

Fixation on body and size can be a way of directing attention to an aspect of our lived experience we feel we can control or exert a degree of control around (despite how extremely challenging that control can be). *If I don't like you seeing that part, I can shift my posture. If I don't like that pooch underneath my belly button, I can suck my stomach in and focus on my crunches during workouts.* Yet, the physical appearance of the body itself is not it, as was demonstrated in *Fearing the Black Body*. What ideas we have about ourselves that live in connection to what those "imperfections" mean to us, how they reflect larger themes about ourselves, our lineage, our worth, and our desirability, are what we are reacting to. In this way, body image is self-image, *an understanding of the kind of person I am, based on how my shame links up with my weak chin, my social anxiety links up with my crooked teeth, my feelings of not being good enough link up with my flat chest.*

Flood your social media stream, saturate yourself with images of diverse bodies of different sizes, races, shapes, abilities and disabilities. Begin constructing and determining your definition of beauty for yourself, now, and work to prove it to yourself on repeat. We have decades, no centuries, worth of messaging to overwrite toxic and harmful ideas that were promoted and reinforced, and so we must do the same in the other direction.

Gender Dysphoria

Alongside the package of rules and "shoulds" we are exposed to regarding our bodies comes a complex set of expectations, rules, and "shoulds" for how we express and live out our gender (which is distinctly different from our sex which is solely determined by our genitals at birth, namely "male," "female," or "intersex"). Gender is the *expression* of the characteristics that we have *associated* with what it means to have those genitals, which traditionally has been in relation to what it means to be male or female, masculine or feminine. When our relationship to these characteristics is not clean or when our perception of ourselves does not match what and who we are told we are meant to be, with everything that encompasses, we can experience gender dysphoria: the experience of incongruence or disconnection between the sex you were assigned at birth (vulva = female, penis = male) and how the world determines we are meant to behave, dress, feel, act, and relate simply by possessing those body parts. For example, if you were born with a vulva, the script given around what it means to embody femininity or be a "girl" frequently involves dresses, princesses, pink, dance and gymnastics, being empathic and sensitive, longing for and having crushes on people assumed to have penises, or who possess more "masculine" characteristics (which often translates into being unemotive or lacking emotional expression or range, being a provider, being "handy," athletic, muscular, assertive) and look like "men." Gender is made up, something that humans have created and continue to co-create, including all the norms, rules, and expectations associated with all genders (because we have many).

Not living in accordance with who we feel we are, how we truly feel, and what the expression of that authenticity feels like for us uniquely has profound consequences for our mental and emotional health and wellbeing. Understanding from the world that we are not worth knowing and loving if we fail to live up to expectations and adhere to the script is deeply wounding, depriving us of real intimacy and connection as we "perform" for others' comfort. If we hold, as Jordon Anderson described, a gender expansive lens, resisting the inclination to classify complex, unique, distinctly different people living amongst tremendous variety and complexity, perhaps we will find an entirely new level of intimacy in our peer relationships, in the formation of new friendships, as we rely less on our predictions about who the person is, how they likely behave, and who they likely love based on two rigid and distinct categories.

What Is Confidence, Really?

- If I look confident, then _____.
- If I act confident, then _____.
- If I feel confident … will I *be* confident?

Confidence is held up as the ultimate sought-after attribute. What do we imagine it has to offer? What is inside the "confidence" package that is locked in the glass case far from the reach of most of us?

- Ease socially?
- Bravery professionally?
- Less internal analysis when taking risks?
- Comfort within our skin?
- Feelings of trust in our decisions and instincts?
- A general sense of trust in ourselves?

What does it mean when someone seems confident? That they have managed to wipe away their flaws? Become a genius? That they are emotionally and relationally sophisticated? Healed? How do we understand self-trust and ease in the way confidence seems to promise? Does confidence equal – perfection?

"Fake it till you make it" has withstood the test of time. This is not to say that this strategy cannot work, sometimes we can show ourselves that we can deliver the presentation with charisma by stepping into our performance of the associated qualities, but the idea that we need to pretend to be something or convey something or embody feelings that aren't real for us as a way to demonstrate confidence or competence seems problematic, especially with sex. We not only risk being seen as a fraud (I'm sure we can all think of someone who has essentially "told on themselves" by talking themselves up too much, bragging about their accomplishments, one-upping others), and transparently insecure, but we effectively buy in to the notion that our own humanity is a form of weakness. We subscribe to the idea that there are those who move through the world insecurity free, never at odds with themselves in any way. If you imagine a person who seems "perfect," would you want to be friends with them? What would intimacy look like? How might you learn to lean on or trust someone who cannot relate to what it means to be a fellow human, dealing with our "baggage," the broad spectrum of feelings, working and struggling to perpetually better ourselves, a journey we are all on forever and together. We have conflated cockiness with confidence, grandiosity with "having it all together," not caring with coolness without ever really looking at the implications of these qualities for our intimacy, when oddly enough, most of us understand what cockiness feels like when it enters the room – and it does little to inspire connection.

> It is more about authenticity than it is about outspokenness, because being the loudest voice in the room is really just about volume. The type of confidence I want to see is one where we carry a deep trust in our personal gifts and inherent value – and we extend that same compassion to others.
>
> (Davidson, 2021)

Confidence isn't perfection, if it was no one would have it. Confidence means understanding our humanity, our imperfections, our unique complexity, and owning/embracing it. It means holding that we are fallible, make mistakes, and have a unique and complex past *and* are good and worthy of being in connection, of being valued. Confidence looks like apologizing, taking responsibility, sharing, getting curious, transparency, emotional expression, advocating for ourselves and others, admitting when we don't know, being open to constructive criticism (and being able to filter it); it looks like vulnerability rather than defensiveness.

Who we're trying to be versus who we are: sex shines a light on that discrepancy and asks us to ditch it. It beckons us into acceptance, into open-hearted intimacy with self and other, that touches all of who we are and where we've been. If we take its lead, confidence will follow.

What Else Can We Do?

We can appreciate the ways our humanity has held wisdom throughout time, cultivating understanding between the "me" of today and my former "selves." For example, say we were a bully in junior high, the one doing the tormenting, throwing food at the "weirdos" in the cafeteria, making others feel small. How hard is it to face that version now? What feelings surface as you imagine them within you? Now look at the context they were embedded in, the insecurities they were working with that directly fueled that behavior, the ways they felt small and/or tremendous pressure to secure their place in the social hierarchy at a time when it can feel like its "kill or be killed." Who were they trying to impress and why was that so hugely important (because it was)?

When we can approach our pasts, and the behaviors and experiences they confront us with, armed with curiosity and steady in our present self, it can be challenging to avoid greater understanding and consequently compassion for our other versions (which then can translate to greater comfort within ourselves today) – is that not confidence?

That girl that gave her body to anyone who seemed interested. I want to hold her hand and let her know that she didn't need to give sex to get love.

That person who raged at their partner for years before finally getting help. I want to hug the little version and let them know that I hear them when they learned that no one else would.

We talk a lot about formulas and patterns as predictors of long-term outcomes. Things like "do one thing for you each day to stave off depression," and so on. Although we can't get that specific, the suggestion here is to simply strive in an ongoing way to like yourself more than you take issue with yourself, to feel like, at the end of the day, you're worth sticking around for. It's not perfect and will never be, none of us get to reach 100% because we don't even know what that would mean or look like. But to know deep down that despite that shitty comment you made earlier, the terrible things you did in college, the times you broke the trust in the relationship, you're a good person, worthy of sharing deeply with others, worthy of being appreciated and loved. The presence of that knowledge, felt meaningfully, will keep us open, empowering us to risk and to break our cycles of immobility.

Gay Men and Body Categorization/Celebration: A Conversation with Dr. Israel Martinez

Dr. Israel Martinez (I) (he/him) is a gay man, a sex and relationship therapist, and an author who has been working with the LGBTQ+ community on a professional basis for close to 20 years. This background provides him with unique expertise on issues that tend to be a part of the lesbian, gay, bisexual, transgender, and queer experience.

I: When I think about gay men and body image and sex, what comes to mind, which I think is unique to our community, is the specificity of what a body should look like, which is categorized according to multiple or varied desirable forms or body types relative to the straight world. Essentially, there's one or a few ways that women are supposed to look to be "beautiful" or "attractive" (and I'm thinking of porn or movies) that includes a certain or specific waist size and breast size and hair length. With gay men, we're famous for having these categories which are "hot" or "sought after," from a Twink, or someone who appears skinny, hairless, and youthful; to a Bear being someone who is sort of the opposite of that, regarded as older, a bigger person, with hair all over; and then you have an Otter which is essentially like a skinnier Bear. We have these categories that are considered "sexy," but if you don't fall into one, it can stir up an identity crisis, making it difficult to search out and feel confident about being desirable.

A lot of gay men are looking for partners and sex on the apps and the apps are asking you to put yourself in one of these categories. They're asking you if you identify as a Bear, Otter, Twink, or Jock, etc. ... consequently it can feel shaming if you don't fit into a category easily. If you happen to have an average body or not a ton of hair but some hair, it can create insecurity as you're unable to communicate who you are cleanly to potential prospects who are looking for someone who fits the descriptions the categories provide. While you may think "Oh wow, you can be a heavier person and be hot and sexy" ... yes, but even within that Bear type, you're expected to look a certain way. And with some of my non-binary or even feminine-leaning gay clients, if they don't fit the stereotype of non-binary being, for example, rail thin, if they have curves, or even an average-build body, they can be left feeling like they won't meet expectations, or worse, just avoid having sex altogether to avoid the anticipated rejection.

There're also people who don't want to identify a certain way but feel forced to because of their body type. For example, this idea of a Bear as being dominant or aggressive, maybe someone who is into leather, a bit kinky, and celebrated for their size. Some may physically look like Bears but don't identify with the attributes that typically go with that stereotype.

So, "My community is saying that I am supposed to behave a certain way based on how I look and I don't know that I want to celebrate the things they want me to celebrate – I'm not dominant, or kinky, or assertive." When you have these questions about whether you fit what you're supposed to fit or if you're going to be or live up to the stories people project onto you, it keeps you away from wanting to be naked and vulnerable with somebody else. Despite all this, despite what can feel like rigid categorization, it isn't everything. People *are* able, and often do, step outside of the mold, and still experience themselves as someone that others want to have sex with.

Paula Leech (P):   The straight world has its own rigid ideas around beauty and what makes a body "sexy," and what those qualities mean, but how do you make sense of how or why the gay community continues to lean into these categories so overtly?

I: That's a great question. One potential theory is that gay men can grow up needing more external validation than their straight counterparts, on account of possessing this feeling or understanding that you're bad, sinful, wrong from the inside, right? If you can't validate yourself internally, you'll look for it externally.

Another factor may be connected to internalized homophobia and this idea of masculine versus feminine. Within these extremes, one can imagine that hooking up with a "Twink" might feed into a sort of "I'm more masculine because I'm going to be with someone who is more feminine," idea, right? The Twink being seen as more feminine, as having a more stereotypically "female" body type. And then having the Bear profile represent a sense of masculinity, at least how we think of it in the traditional sense.

P: Right! What I see is that these rigid categories also have stories, like you said, they have characteristics and attributes, so to a degree I'm interacting with a character that I've imagined rather than the real person and their unique qualities. It's interesting to think about that and how that relates to our own vulnerability.

I: Right, yeah! We don't have to be as vulnerable, right? How much are we invested in learning and sharing, or spending the time to dig deeper if the person is just a character we're interacting with where we already know their story, and vice versa, we feel like our story is already told?

P: And what I'm hearing you say too is that a real challenge can exist in having to figure out how to part from these categories if they don't fit, still risk and put yourself out there, all the while grounding yourself in your own internal validation, including your own thoughts about what makes *my* body valuable and beautiful as it is, what are *my* values around this in order to effect my outward lens?

I: Yes, and gay men, it seems, have an oversampling of relationships where you have a fairly significant age discrepancy, so I've seen that naturally the older partner's body is changing more swiftly than the younger person's, resulting in some issues around attraction and sex. I also think the gay male world is famous for prematurely aging our community. For example, there's a "hot, older males" porn site that's for men aged 30+. It's treated as a joke but it reflects a reality that in the gay world when you hit around 35 you're invisible and a dinosaur, right? And part of that is simply your body is not what it was or as easy to maintain or keep looking a certain way, a natural part of aging. And then as you continue to age it can become so much more isolating and you just begin to perceive yourself as ... not valuable.

P: I think a lot of straight women identify with that also, the experience of feeling invisible when they are no longer being noticed for their appearance. We've placed so much of our worth on our youth and desirability, at least within straight cisgender partnerships and amongst gay men.

Circling back to your point about external validation, I think people in general contend with this, but it seems like we can also assume that perhaps there might be a little of the "my partners look a certain way which validates who I am. I can get the hot Twink, or I've still got it because ... look who I surround myself with." You know?

I: From partners to friends to what your apartment looks like to what you drive to where you hang out ... it's often about what does this say about me? I think it makes it more difficult for a man whose aging and body is evolving as bodies do, to be able to see for themselves that they have value and are deserving of great, passionate, stimulating, whatever it is they want to get out of sex. And again, the messaging is there: "You're old, you're invisible, you're not valuable."

P: The external validation piece becomes untenable for us all and then we have to figure out, "Who am I underneath or beyond my appearance, my identity as 'beautiful' or 'sexy' and why is that important?" Some of us wake up to that reality earlier than others, some of us have to be in that reality all along because, for example, "I don't fit the categories and so I have to look at 'who am I? What else do I bring to the table?'" Doing the internal work to feel like "I can be vulnerable enough to really put 'me' out there, not an idea of me," you know?

I: It's tough because our community, our culture, our history, part of our evolution is connected to these labels. While they can be harmful and limiting, they're also a part of us, a part of so many people's identity, so it wouldn't be all or nothing to say "gah, I wish they would go away." I guess I wish they were more voluntary or something that people felt were options to step into but not that they *needed* to fit into. Like, "Great, these are some options that some of our cultural narratives have been around *and* there's so much more than that." To have our community realize that on a broader level. Even just to have a consent component to it: "Don't tell me I'm a Bear, ask." "I'm skinny and don't have hair but maybe I'm a Bear," right? Just to have more fun with it, to have options but for it not to have to look a certain way. That would be nice.

I just encourage my clients to really think about what they want to get out of sex and separate that from what they want to project as their identity.

13 Sexual Prowess and Inexperience

Shouldn't this chapter be an extension of the previous one? Why aren't we talking about sexual inexperience in relationship to insecurity? Because they don't always go hand in hand, and they certainly don't need to! We link experience with confidence, mastery, and skill; and therefore, inexperience must mean insecurity, incompetence, and a bad time. This formula and our awareness of it becomes, in and of itself, a major source of anxiety, perpetuating and solidifying the narrative in the mind of the person carrying it as the anxiety plays itself out in behavior and lack of connection (when with us sexually, anxiety is always our primary partner – three's a crowd). Life doesn't like a binary, neither does our sexuality.

Can there or are there very real advantages to having relational experience (i.e. sex with other people) under your belt sexually? Sure! Experience *can* put us in touch with how our bodies show up relationally that is different from how they operate individually, and therefore how to accommodate and work with those differences. Experience can help us learn how to be connected to others and with ourselves at the same time. We can practice holding multiple focuses of our attention, moving from our own process and exploration to our partner's body and experience. We can practice how to communicate our boundaries while holding the other's in mind as we let go into trust in whatever way it is present. We can elaborate on this list because it is true; experience helps us learn! And yet all of the above are possible, but not always present. Sometimes what we learn is not helpful whatsoever. Sometimes the lessons make sex hard. The real catch here is that all of the benefits mentioned above and more are only available to us if we're in our bodies, in connection, and in our own experience enough to receive them.

The flip side of that coin takes us back to the conversation around the futility inherent in trying to "master" an abstract, moving, breathing, emotionally infused experience that is made and in the presence of wildly different factors and contexts each day. Just like being a therapist, thinking

DOI: 10.4324/9781003369080-16

we "know" how to do sex and therefore can just apply the same formula every time is limiting and problematic. What do we miss by defaulting to the generic blueprint as opposed to the curated experience? To generalized knowledge versus personalized attention? To a self-help book versus your own personal therapist?

Curiosity Is Confidence Is Sexy

How was your date?

It was fine. They were super sexy, which caught me off guard at first. But then they opened their mouth and never closed it. I don't think they asked me one single question about myself.

When falling in love, we often hear people describe the exceptional in a person. *"They really get me," "I feel so seen," "They just understand me in a way no one has before," "When I'm with them, I feel like the only person in the room."* We all seek validation for who we are, and we spend our lives looking for it. When this is showed to us, when we feel heard, seen, and like someone is excited about the things they hear and see, it is the ultimate salve for the "not good enough" story that we all contend with to various degrees throughout our day, week, month, life. In this way, part of the honeymoon phase means falling for ourselves! Feeling the high that comes with another person or persons' desire to continue to uncover more about who we are because they're enjoying or even loving what they've uncovered so far. The same is nearly always true with sex. Who doesn't want an attentive and attuned lover? Someone who is interested in our experience, in understanding how your body works, keen to learn about your pleasure today?

We discussed how depression takes us into ourselves in a way that can prevent us from being emotionally, spiritually, and psychologically available and attuned to other people. We can feel completely consumed in and paralyzed by the enormous heaviness that can come with being who we are, with the stories we carry, the memories we work to reconcile, our sense or lack of identity and connection. Insecurity, which we all possess to varying degrees, is the same. Self-doubt puts us in constant connection with self-analysis, strategizing, and second-guessing – all experiences that take us out of connection with other people. Insecurity makes us anxious, uncertainty about ourselves is anxiety provoking, which holds us back, keeping us from taking necessary risks, the primary ingredient required for building the sense of self-trust that confidence is made of. To be in our insecurity is to be in an isolated place, where the only way out is to risk connecting.

"What do you want?" vs. this is what I think you want.

"Does this kind of pressure feel good to you?" vs. this is what most people tend to like so I'll go with it.

"Want me to go faster?" vs. I'm kind of into doing this a bit longer but I think I'm supposed to start going faster now.

"Show me how you like it" vs. my last partner loved it like this, so this must be how they'll like it too.

To demonstrate curiosity with ease, which requires a strong belief in its value, translates as genuine interest in the other and for the other. It allows the person on the receiving end to feel cared for and attended to while serving the very important function of allowing learning to unfold alongside intimacy. It communicates the knowledge, awareness of, and appreciation for the uniqueness of the person or persons we're interacting with. As such, it is the ultimate expression of desire to know, get close to, and make real contact with the person, their layers, their body. Through curiosity we honor each other's individuality – what could be hotter?

That in mind, what feels more like an expression of confidence: asking about what feels good (with ease), or staying quiet and guessing?

Practice: Say the following few questions one by one out loud to yourself in the mirror and repeat them as many times as it takes to feel comfortable. Say them using the tone, pace, and rhythm you might use with a partner (one example being hushed, slow, matter of fact rather than over the top):

- *How does it feel when I touch your body like this?*
- *Where can I kiss you? Where does it feel really good to be kissed?*
- *Can I put my hand (body, face, tongue, penis) here? I love touching (licking, feeling, pressing up against) you here.*
- *Are you ready to move on or do you want me to stay right here?*
- *What do you want me to do to (with, for) you right now?*

If you're with a partner who is uncomfortable communicating about sex and/or during the experience itself, try introducing the following:

- *I'm going to caress your skin like this. Would you like me to be more firm? Or more soft?*
- *I'm moving toward your breasts (stomach, thighs, _____). Does that feel how you'd like it to feel?*
- *I love touching this part of your _____. Can I stay right here? How do you like to be touched on this part?*
- Practice the "narrating touch" experience with yourself and/or your partner as in Chapter 21.

Do you have lots of experience to draw from? Or little to none? Use curiosity to your advantage with both.

The following are more "advanced" examples with what some might consider to be a more erotic charge. We are inviting in the "no" at the beginning of the experience and/or along the way: "*It's OK if you need to say no.*"

- *Show me how you do it for yourself.*
- *I want to know exactly how you turn yourself on, take me there.*
- *What's that thing you're doing with your hand? Use mine.*
- *Show me what you do when I'm not here.*
- *Tell me what you want.*
- *I love touching this part of your body, does it feel good for you? How can I make it feel even better?*

Practicing in this way can stir up feelings of self-consciousness. Why? Because we feel vulnerable, like we're stepping outside of what is "normal" or "cool" or a demonstration of confidence (e.g. *I shouldn't have to ask, I want them to think I just "know"*). This is part of the problem, an ego barrier to intimacy, and therefore this solo practice also helps us begin to break down inhibitions and "shoulds," stepping outside of what hasn't worked and into a new way of exploring, relating, and learning.

While taking the temperature around consent throughout the interaction plays a key role in the cultivation of safety in some sexual experiences, especially with newer partners (i.e. experiences where we seek to create the sense of safety and trust required to let go, surrender, play, express, communicate, etc.); "front-end" consent and negotiation of boundaries has a meaningful place in the interaction as well. In other words, inviting our partners to set boundaries with us from the start, and conveying the understanding that they're important to the ongoing sexual connection shared, frees us up to check in and practice curiosity as it comes up organically or around specific aspects of the experience, rather than constantly, diligently, and in a way that impedes ease and free movement throughout.

What this might sound like is:

> *Your comfort is important to me. If at any point you want me to stop or do something different, please let me know. I want you to want this, which will only happen if you feel safe with me. I will never be upset with you for saying "no."*

Is it unfortunate this has to be specified? Yes. We should all feel safe enough to say "no" and exercise limits with others. Sadly, the reality for many is one is which sex *is* pressure: to engage, to partake in certain behaviors, to service another, to abandon ourselves for the sake of the other or others. We emphasize this message by checking in periodically and asking when we'd like to explore something specific or that goes beyond what feels like your shared baseline behaviors (which often include things like kissing and caressing), especially with new or newer partners. Implied or "front-end" consent + curiosity/pointed consent check-ins = the scaffolding required to allow us to lean in and let go without fear and learn along the way. Asking for consent with every move = distraction, and requires constant cerebral engagement. Absence of or unclear consent request or giving = uncertainty with the potential to do harm.

When we slip out of curiosity, we begin to make assumptions with blinders on. We limit our view, our story. What might happen if you dared to study your partner's sexuality, their body, for the rest of your life? Knowing that, like most things in life, the more you know, the more you know you don't know, versus deciding you've figured it out?

Masturbation and Inexperience: Masturbation *as* Experience

One major source of learning that we tend to take for granted is our experiences with ourselves. Considering the major presence we have (not to mention the requirement of presence for our own safety and boundary setting) in a sexual experience with another person, this omission from our socialization is particularly harmful. If sex *is* intimacy, how do we understand how to share ourselves sexually if we don't pay attention to what it is that we like, dislike, are curious about, what kinds of touch are welcome, unwelcome, when to speed up, slow down, where to touch and for how long, and so on? This learning is foundational, it allows us to feel at ease within ourselves as someone else embarks on their learning experience of our sexuality, our bodies. We can answer questions, direct (with consent), provide information, set boundaries, help ourselves along!

We learn how to be with our arousal and how to interact with it in different ways when we masturbate mindfully. So don't tune out here! Watch explicit media if that is exciting for you, but also note what is happening in your body and mind. The more information, the better equipped we are to embark on relational sexuality and to be able to navigate and provide a detailed map that makes for a dynamic experience. And guess what? This is real experience that really matters and that we can revisit as much as we like, because it is built in and walking around with us all day long.

Train Like an Olympian

What transpires between the onset of anxiety (and its accompanying thoughts and feelings) and an avoidant reaction? Visualization and storytelling. For example:

She just put her hand on my leg, oh god, I bet she's going to try and cuddle. I bet she expects me to kiss her or initiate something. Why else would she be touching me like that? But oh no, if she expects me to lean in for a kiss I bet I'll be super awkward about it (enter visualization of herself reaching around stiffly, moving her body to face her partner in a very contrived, clinical way, and then kissing her with a pillow's width of distance between their bodies). I bet I won't know what to do next, I'll just stare at her awkwardly. She'll probably be totally weirded out and feel pressure to take over. OK, I'm gonna just pretend I need to go to the bathroom.

We are profoundly proficient at visualizing and mentally moving through worst-case scenarios, getting our sample of the potential feelings they might conjure up, feeling our physical body respond. What we tend *not* to do, however, is visualize or consciously and intentionally predict the best-case scenario, or even just a good-enough experience. What are the consequences? Do our worst-case imaginings set us up for worst-case experiences? Or best-case for optimal ones? It turns out athletes have been intentionally employing visualization techniques as part of their training for this very reason. The benefits are very real.

According to Schmalbruch (2015), the effectiveness and utility of "visualization" has been proven in a research study by Russian scientists who compared the training schedules of four groups of Olympic athletes. Each of these groups practiced a different combination of physical and mental training, broken down as:

- **Group #1** = 100% physical training;
- **Group #2** = 75% physical training, 25% mental training;
- **Group #3** = 50% physical training, 50% mental training;
- **Group #4** = 25% physical training, 75% mental training.

Group #4 outperformed the others at the Olympics, altering how trainers and trainees alike conceptualize their learning and skill-building moving forward. "We stimulate the same brain regions when we visualize an action as we do when we actually perform that same action," writes Srinivasan Pillay (quoted in Schmalbruch, 2015), Harvard M.D. and author of *Your Brain and Business: The Neuroscience of Great Leaders*. In short, when doing the meaningful learning in a way that actively creates a blueprint or map for the body and engaging in a form of advanced practice from the comfort of our own chair, or bedroom, or living rooms.

Oh God, what about that awkward part where I need to put on a condom?

Mentally rehearse an alternative to awkward.

Am I going to freeze up when it's time to get sexual?

Visualize effortlessness, curiosity, and comfort with the other.

I have no clue what to do with my body or face even for that matter, after I put on lingerie.

Picture a scenario that allows you to enjoy the lingerie for yourself, with them.

We may need to look for examples of what we long to demonstrate or feel sexually, and that's OK too! Any effort in favor of building and envisioning an alternate narrative is better than sticking with the anxiety one. Once we have that new narrative solidly in mind, play it and replay it, in excruciating detail, over and over again. Add different elements, edit the story with other possibilities so as to minimize the very real risk of things feeling "scripted" in another form in the bedroom. We are imagining ease, we are imagining what comfort might look and feel like, rather than specific scenarios to duplicate exactly.

Visualization is one way we let our mind and body know what we're looking for, laying out a map, and providing rehearsal for our brain. If we "practice" awkward scenarios and sexual blunders in the theater of our own imagination, we are likely to step into that story in real life: our brain doesn't know the difference. If we "practice" direct communication, eye contact, deep, passionate kisses (if that's what we like), and exploration of a wide variety of sexual play in detail, our audience (i.e. our brain, which is paradoxically also the director) may draw inspiration from the scene to cast its prediction about what the reality will look like as we approach it. It is experience under our belt in another form; our brain understands it as experience, nonetheless.

Pivoting

Next time, or rather every time, you watch a sexy movie, or even porn (as long as we're including some more documentary-style, or less "performative" and preferably ethical or feminist porn selections in there), notice not only the more obvious activities, but the smaller ways they engage: the outward expression of passion or emotion, the places they attend to each other (or others) in different forms, how they linger for moments, where they may apply different kinds of touch, where and how they may include kink or more imaginative play, all the places they kiss or lick or explore each other, the moments of rest and energy. When our experiences don't unfold in the way we anticipate, we need to have a sense for what we can shift to instead, where we can explore next, what we are curious about, or what else on the menu might be interesting today. Without a selection to explore, we risk freezing, our anxiety making it challenging, if not impossible to understand how to proceed when working with limited options. This creates the perfect set-up for a "show-stopping moment," where we inadvertently reinforce our rigidity: *See, when **this** doesn't happen, the whole experience is ruined!*

Create a list (the beginning of one is available in Chapter 18) and then use visualization to imagine what some of the items might look like in real time, in your reality, alternating between roles. Go down the list and give each activity life in your erotic imagination, weaving it into a scene, spending significant time with the details, allowing it to incorporate itself into your sexual blueprint or schema. Every minute given means sexual and erotic expansion, it means dismantling rigidity, it means evicting anxiety from our sexual imagination, predictions, and experience.

Expansion: Growth is Clumsy

Expansion means trying on the new things we uncover and experimenting. This can be clunky or awkward or messy! Just like learning how to drive, we have to orient ourselves, practice, return, and try again in order to achieve ease. So, just because I stepped into role play with my partner and found myself feeling stiff and unsure of what to say, doesn't mean that was "bad" or a failure, or something to avoid or abandon. It means we're expanding and learning! Why would we treat our sexual life any differently than our day to day? Learning requires practice, uncertainty, vulnerability, and feeling around in the dark a bit, or a lot. An adventurous spirit, a sense of humor in the face of our growth, and the ability to take ownership of our clumsiness (i.e. hold it with levity rather than apologize for it) will go a long way and give our partners the permission to do the same (which they *will* experience as their own learning curve if they're interested in expansion, i.e. interested in a sexual life that isn't characterized by boredom, as well).

Expansion is what we hope we do as we age. It is growth, maturity, wisdom, understanding, accountability, creativity, and healing. In this place we find possibilities and doors to new kinds of experiences, different ways of experiencing ourselves and others. Without the mess expansion brings, we stay in one place, sex holds its routine, and the ways in which life feeds us dry up. It is an unavoidable part of our growth. Without learning how to drive the car, we stay home.

14 Sexuality and Aging, Sex and Death, Grief in Sex

Sexuality and Aging

- My sex life looks like this _____
- My orgasms feel like this _____
- Your body works like this _____
- You get turned on by this _____
- My pleasure works like this _____
- Our pleasure looks like this _____
- I can move like this _____
- I can feel like this _____
- My sexuality is this _____

Life unravels the stories we carry, directly challenging our commitment to them, and yet we are so very committed to them. By the time we've reached our 40s, 50s, 60s, we have grieved and grown a million times over, in ways both subtle and even unrecognizable, and in ways that are blatant and profound. All we need to do is pull out photo albums to understand how much we've changed, how hard and important those changes were, and therefore the tremendous price we've had to pay in order to accomplish that changing. We have practiced at this and somehow it doesn't untie our attachments, doesn't lessen grief's grip, doesn't make us more proficient in letting go. Constancy feels like safety, love and pleasure feels nourishing and needed because they are, endlessly; we will always cling to aspects of life that fall into these categories, we will attach and invest, identify with and commit to, often until we're forced to do otherwise. And we will spend a good portion of our lives worrying about when those times will come and what our suffering might consist of. Our worry shows us what we have to lose, a mirror that reflects back how precious it all is. Sex is no different. When our previously full-body orgasms are elusive or don't feel the same, when our erections are less reliable or lack the strength they once had, when skin thins and tears with penetration – the main plot points to

DOI: 10.4324/9781003369080-17

our sexual stories become erased and we struggle to fill in the blanks with new content. Change ushers in our anxiety, stifling access to creativity and possibility, placing a period where a semicolon should be.

Old age is the place in our evolution where growth seems to slow, and loss proliferates. We conceptualize it as exceptional due to the amount of blatant or profound changes that begin to occur with greater frequency, much like they do in puberty and adolescence; but it is rather a continuation. The elder years bring us into greater contact with death, with a more rapid evolution of our bodies, with disability of all forms. How does our sexuality respond? With curiosity. How do *we* often respond? With grief over the loss of our sexuality, full stop.

> "How do we untie the knots that we have so carefully constructed to avoid discussions of sex and sexual identity?"
>
> (Duclos, 2023, p. 10)

To review. In the developmental lifespan of a sexual relationship with a partner, it seems we move through several phases:

- Dating and early life of the couple = sexual exploration, curiosity, enthusiasm towards learning and unveiling the mystery of the other.
- Settling in (which can come with moving in, engagement, and/or marriage but can also simply come with time) = enough sexual likes/dislikes, and understanding has been discovered by both partners to create a "sexual script," becoming the go to way of having sex. The seeking out of, and enthusiasm around, learning slows in favor of the illusion of "knowing" and the power, gratification, safety, and sense of closeness that comes from mutual understanding.
- Maintenance and consistency = *Why not do more of what we know works?* The learning is still there, it always is, it can simply take on a less profound presence relationally as the comfort that comes with consistency steps forward, as we move out of discovery and into doing what we know works, what tends to spark pleasure and fulfill our basic wants, over and over again.

When we settle into processes in our sexual relationships and neglect to invite new information in as each person evolves, they become problematic, much as they do in our relational life in general. These processes then become representative of versions of ourselves that in many ways are no longer here, a sexual life and pattern that no longer fits, despite the comfort it may bring. As we age, we continue to learn about ourselves sexually as individuals. That information makes its way into our psyche simply by moving through the world, by being alive, by having a body and imagination. When we create sexual processes, and sexual relationships without honest, open communication built in, we leave ourselves out of the picture in major ways as we and our bodies evolve, depleting intimacy from the interaction, kicking up tension (even if it's only experienced internally) as we no longer feel satiated and seen sexually. Very early on, many of us begin to think of the sexual relationship as fragile, unable to tolerate new information and desires, and therefore we leave it out even as years upon years go by. This feels like a protective move, but it can isolate both partners over time, increasing our sense of loneliness with one another. And when loneliness is experienced sexually, it frequently blurs the lines and is experienced in a generalized way with sex being so much more than a series of behaviors and therefore capturing so much more for us in terms of our basic need for intimacy, sharing, and connection.

> Whether it's hearing, or vision loss, or arthritis, or pain, or prostate problems, structural change in the relationship and in the sexuality of older partners is warranted. Moving from talking to touch helps. It shortens the distance. It is also an ecological change: there is movement from the past and its discontents to today and its nothings. We have to make room for play by putting aside thoughts of yesterday. Anything that happens more than 24 hours ago need not be discussed. An empty mind is not an anxious one.
>
> (Duclos, 2023, p. 8)

Resistance to change creates tension (a reaction to what our anxiety is telling us about what this change may mean), and that tension inspires avoidance. *I don't know what my body is going to feel like after this surgery, and I'm afraid to find out. Can I accept myself, let alone risk seeing if my partner will as well?* The relationship adapts only as it is given the opportunity to do so; but that can be tricky! Coming to the table with different wants and needs or coming to the table unable to identify what our wants and needs might be in this changing or changed body requires acknowledging and feeling that change is a variable at all. It requires a level of acceptance to help extinguish the avoidance. And what are we avoiding here? Grief. But only once the wall of grief is cleared can we begin exploring new possibilities. We grieve and then we see what's possible on repeat. Because we always have access to possibilities.

We forget, or take for granted, that, like our experience with growth and loss, our relationships (if we're in them long enough) go through significant structural changes many times over, as they grow and shed versions of themselves alongside us. Relationship and family systems fight for sameness, but change pushes up against the practiced status quo and our relationships are busy working to accommodate it. Although not always successful, being with anyone for any significant amount of time (whether that be a year or 30), requires navigating and accomplishing systemic and relational change continually (when we move in together, when there is infidelity, when we have children, when we move, get new jobs, etc.). What would happen if we trusted that more? What does it mean for us when this doesn't feel true? How are we committed to sameness ourselves out of fear for what grief may await us if we risk stepping out of beat?

Anna (cis/het, 67-year-old, first-generation Armenian woman):	*I'm here for my husband.*
Therapist:	*What do you mean by that?*
Anna:	*I just mean that I am fine with our lives just as they are. I don't need sex anymore, I've come to terms with it and there's nothing to do about it. It just is what it is, my desire is gone. I don't believe in trying to resurrect the past. He just can't move on.*
Therapist:	*Davit, your wife has described being here for you. What do you think she thinks you want?*
Davit (cis/het, 65-year-old, second-generation Armenian man):	*I think she thinks I want to have sex like we used to, that I expect we're going to make love for hours and that I can't tolerate anything else. But that's not what I'm saying and it's nothing I've ever said for that matter. She hears what she wants.*
Therapist:	*Davit, can you clarify, then, what it is that you're asking for? What would you like to see happen?*
Davit:	*I just want her to be close with me again. Just to cuddle, or hold her, or for her to let me kiss her again. It feels like overnight we became strangers to each other and it's lonely! It needs to end.*
Therapist:	*Do you feel that way also, Anna? Have things felt more distant between the two of you?*
Anna:	*A little.*
Therapist:	*How do you make sense of that? Davit, you speak of it feeling like it happened over night. I wonder if you might go first in talking about your experience of that.*
Davit:	*I was diagnosed with stage 3 lung cancer seven years ago. It was a very hard time and required a lot from both of us. She took great care of me and*

> *was there for me through the whole thing, right by my side. I would've thought we would be closer than ever after surviving that experience, but it seemed to have the opposite effect. She won't talk to me about it and she's completely pulled away.*

(Anna turns away slightly, tears in her eyes.)

Anna: *Let's not talk about that, please.*

Sex and Death

Death and sex both live in the shadows, both unspeakable or challenging to approach, yet inextricable and fundamental aspects of our humanity and awareness of ourselves. We have traditionally looked to sex for life, but sex represents creation (of connection, love, play, fantasy, adventure, chemistry, power, etc.), even when procreation is not a goal; and with life/creation comes death and endings. Events on opposing ends of the same spectrum, sex is synonymous with connection, death with disconnection. And when death touches us in real time, our capacity and/or longing and/or experience of intimacy is shaped and influenced, impacting the manifestation of our intimate lives: our sexual desires, feelings, and behaviors. We can find ourselves turning to sex to remind us of life, connecting us with life force energy, and maybe even to a sense of ourselves as that energy itself, a comforting link to a sense of spirituality, a connection to all things. Conversely, we might find ourselves turning away, particularly in our meaningful relationships, suddenly reluctant to feel the very connection that has been threatened in the window we were granted into what that absence might feel like, distancing ourselves from intimacy as a means of protecting ourselves from the enormity of the feelings associated with its loss.

Eckhart Tolle, author of *The Power of Now*, says that death is a stripping away of everything that is not you, until you realize that there is no death. Jon Kabat-Zinn, author of *Full Catastrophe Living*, calls this "dying before you die." Sex similarly asks us to strip away our facades, our performance, our people pleasing, our rules and "shoulds," our conditioning, and enter into something else entirely. A nameless, shapeless space that can feel like God to some. It asks us to leave our ego at the door, something many if not most of us have no sense of how to accomplish in a world that is about who we are as a brand and how many followers we have.

For those of us particularly connected to ego, sex *is* threatening. To be invited to take down our facades, our performance, means risking confronting what led us to cling so strongly to these elements to begin with. *If I'm not this person I've created, this character, then who am I?* Sex *is* death from this lens as we are forced to abandon strategy, intentionality, control, and let go into everything that lives underneath it, including the insecurities and fear at the heart of its origin story.

Anna had to face the prospect of losing her husband, Davit. Death entered into their lives, home, and relationship as an ominous and threatening third party, and still is to a certain extent, as is inevitable on the back of battling cancer. How might Anna come close after facing the fear of his absence? Of the obliteration of her whole life as she knows it, and with it her sense of herself, an inevitability after decades shared. How does their culture, their shared heritage, interact with death? What does death mean for their understanding of life?

> But this association doesn't make sex something fearful … at least, not so fearful as to dissuade people from participation. To the contrary, it makes sex more intimate, more exciting, more important and meaningful. The connection with death is what makes sex powerful.
>
> (Robertson, 2019)

Grief in Our Sex

Grief affects all parts of who we are, living and seemingly embedding itself in our psyche, our memory, our muscles, and, yes, our sex. This can make the experience of letting go into our own vulnerability, into catharsis and parasympathetic response, appealing or frightening depending on the day, our emotional state (as touch is the great amplifier of emotion), and our developmental trajectories with grief. Though grief can often be experienced as leaving a "bruise," or a hurt that we simply carry with us and relate to in different ways throughout time, at a certain point our day-to-day experience can seem to reflect having "gotten through" it's enormity, as it no longer feels as though it's sitting right below the chest or throat as we attend to routine obligations or tasks. But when we go to engage the body, or our sexuality at large, we are visiting different perspectives or embodied experience of the pain, therefore bringing that source of grief and its current iteration to the surface. This is how the enormity of our grief works to move itself out, evolving into more of a shadow over time. It is in our best interest, even when it doesn't feel or seem like it. Just like when we hear *that* song, or bump into *that* picture, years after the breakup.

When our sexuality is the site of grief (for instance, post-prostate cancer surgery, mastectomy, or when navigating fertility struggles and/or miscarriage), we are asked to allow those feelings to surface within its context, as part of the experience. Can you trust its wisdom? Trust yourself and/or your partner(s) to move through it alongside you? Can it be part of the expression of your sexuality now rather than something to shut down, a "problem" with the sex itself? Sex isn't always about pleasure, sometimes it's simply about survival, reclamation, and deep healing.

The Last Word on Death

If we are collectively engaged in the process of "dying before we die," shedding our ego, our identities, our stories of ourselves, then perhaps sex grants us a glimpse into what exists in this mystery realm, into the pleasure to be had in pure, unburdened, unscripted connection. Maybe sex becomes *the* place to understand who we are outside of the multitude of identities we carry, in a definition-less, abstract, kaleidoscopic universe that exists within us, hidden amongst our socialization. Our "humanness."

Much like sleep, sex offers to cradle us in its great nothing everything.

15 Sexual Trauma

Talking about trauma raises trauma in the body, heart, and mind. This book is your experience, for you; a place to do the learning you need at this moment in time, at this place in your life, love, and relationships. Please allow that intuition to guide you through and honor its message; giving yourself full permission to slow, stop, skip over sentences, paragraphs, the entire chapter. Maybe you'll be ready to revisit those parts at some point, but that's of no consequence today. The greatest thing you can do for yourself when healing from sexual trauma is honor or yield to your own boundaries, even if that is followed up with questioning and curiosity. Anxiety may be an important indicator that a boundary is needed, or at least that we have cause to slow down and zoom-in.

Speaking of slowing and stopping, it can be helpful to hold in mind a stoplight when moving through the material. Move slowly and keep "green," "yellow," and "red" in mind, slowing (yellow) when discomfort emerges, stopping if and when the discomfort continues building (i.e. we've entered "red" territory).

Possibilities and Protection

Claire's first sexual experiences:

1 10 years old: close lipped kiss – excitement, sparks, anxiety, racing heart, inner conflict (*Was that OK to do?*).
2 11 years old: make-out session – excitement, sparks, pleasure, sexual arousal, longing, desire.
3 12.5 years old: make-out with manual touching of vulva – nervousness, pleasurable sensations, self-conscious, gentle, sexual arousal, tension in pelvis.

DOI: 10.4324/9781003369080-18

4 13 years old: oral sex – reluctant consent, nervousness, sexy, erotic, disconnected, tense.
5 16 years old: penetrative sex – anxious, self-conscious, excitement, arousal, confusing, performative pleasure.

With your teacher (yourself) being given little information to work with around sex, every sexual experience growing up and into young adulthood was rich in terms of learning. Many of our first encounters hold a mixed bag of feelings as we grapple with our wants versus our "shoulds". Experiences of sexual trauma and abuse get folded into that process, but the information acquired is elevated to the status of paramount as sex becomes something that coincides with stress, threat, or danger, something the body learns it needs to protect our hearts and minds from. And it only takes one time.

The list above reflects the shadow left behind by the complex emotional experience of one cisgender female, Claire, as she navigates her first sexual experiences. Unlike learning to drive (our go-to metaphor), which once initiated we generally return to with some regularity, sexual experiences can be few and far between in the younger years, making the experiences that do happen hang heavy in our memory. Even when sexual experiences *are* happening with greater frequency, much as they might as we move into our teen years, challenging encounters often embed themselves in long-term memory as we visit and revisit, or as is sometimes the case, work to forget or distance ourselves from the step-by-step replay of what our mind recognizes as a developmentally significant event, a reference point, something to be logged as safe or unsafe to approach again. We can imagine what experiences Claire may feel excited about exploring again, and which she may feel nervous or even avoidant of in the future. Let's explore one potential path.

As Claire becomes involved in other sexual situations and romantic partnerships, she finds that oral sex is something she attempts to distract partners from. She notices her anxiety escalate and her pelvic floor clench as partners begin to kiss lower parts of her body. A few times she has tried to tolerate these feelings in her desire to please the other, moving deeply into thoughts about work or the TV show she loves in order to manage the emotions, allowing the interaction to transpire without communicating discomfort. Flash forward and she is a year and a half into a relationship with an honest, caring partner. They have an adventurous, exciting, and tender sexual life and connection, and yet the anxiety connected to oral sex remains. She is confused by these feelings and is fatigued by their intrusive nature. "Why am I so anxious about this? I love and trust this partner!"

The ways in which we protect ourselves, react to, simply cope in the face of intimacy, eroticism, sexual energy, and/or our own sexual arousal and functioning were important and wise at a point in time. We can simultaneously appreciate that protective device and also notice the ways in which it has overstayed its welcome and want it gone. Getting real, trauma is not something that ever fully leaves us, we are never "cured" from or able to fully erase the imprint it leaves behind. Consequently, the conversation is never done, as it reveals itself in different ways depending on what is going on in our lives, the kinds of intimate connections we cultivate, and the quality of the relationships we hold with ourselves and others. This is hardly regression when it does surface, it's an opportunity for further progression and, in some circumstances, can be a sign that it's safe enough now to do this version of the work. And the good news is that like anxiety in general (and often they are *truly* one-and-the-same) our relationship to it can evolve and change in a way that lessens its power, presence, and influence. The you of today can learn to deeply and pro-foundly embody new information and learning that alters the course of your life and puts you more solidly in the control seat.

What Constitutes Sexual "Trauma"?

> Trauma is a wordless story our body tells itself about what is safe and what is a threat. Our rational brain can't stop it from occurring, and it can't talk our body out of it... Something in the here and now is rekindling old pain or discomfort, and the body tries to address it with the reflexive energy that's still stuck inside the nervous system.
>
> (Menakem, 2021)

Trauma, from a therapy lens, is an emotional injury (and/or a spiritual or "soul injury" as Menakem writes), a response that has lasting psychologi-cal and physiological consequences and influence on the developmental trajectory of the person or persons involved. The lesson the body receives around what is "safe and what is threat" alters our nervous system and the ways our bodies respond to our environment. Trauma is often caused by a physical event, like abuse, assault, an accident, a medical procedure, but it doesn't have to be. Historically we've regarded trauma as a particular event or series of events of a certain magnitude, easily distinguished from the wide variety of struggles and painful experiences of life by virtue of its threat to our survival. We now understand that trauma is complex, perva-sive, and can be the result of:

- Behaviors;
- What we witness;
- Perception;
- Ideas;
- Larger systems, institutions, cultural norms;

- War and history;
- Confusion and neglect;
- Racism, bigotry, xenophobia, oppression in the present, compounded by historical imprint and shadow;
- A pandemic;
- A one-time event, experienced chronically, an accumulation of different kinds of experiences that reinforce the same feelings and ideas;
- Something blatant, overwhelming, and easily recognizable – something insidious, hard to detect, and covert.

Trauma can be carried through the generations, potentially traveling through our DNA; but also via attitudes and belief systems or handed to us in an instant. It can be physical, or void of touch entirely. It can be about self-betrayal or being betrayed by another. We can feel trauma in the loss of ourselves, from being erased (individually or collectively) or from hiding who we are. We can feel trauma from other people telling us we've been traumatized, whether that matched the lived experience or not. It can be found in a mistake.

The consequences can be felt individually or collectively as:

- Limiting or completely immobilizing.
- Deep pain, sorrow, and anger; the feelings involved can be mixed; it can hold both pleasure and pain, or it can come void of these feelings or any feelings whatsoever.
- Situational or generalized.

Resmaa Menakem, author of *My Grandmother's Hands: Racialized Trauma and the Pathways to Mending Our Hearts and Bodies*, explains:

> Unhealed trauma acts like a rock thrown into a pond, it causes ripples that move outward, affecting many other bodies over time. After months or years, unhealed trauma can appear to become part of someone's personality. Over even longer periods of time, as it is passed on and gets compounded through other bodies in a household, it can become a family norm. And if it gets transmitted and compounded through multiple families and generations, it can start to look like culture.
>
> (2017, p. 39)

Whatever the origin story or stories, sexual trauma (trauma of any nature) has lasting, long-term consequences for how we love, share, and express ourselves sexually as traumatic events fold themselves into our learning, our schema of the world, our understanding of safety (in connection, our bodies, relationship, society). We're often signaled to its presence with anxiety, panic, fear, and its web of related feeling states.

Does this all still sound terribly abstract? It is (and don't be fooled, very little isn't when it comes to our psychology). Learning and attention give it greater definition; feeling and understanding provide healing.

Trauma and the Body

The emotionally injurious nature of trauma is in connection with and informed by the physiological impact of the event, namely the completion or interruption of our body's trauma response.

Let's look at this in parts:

- Defining trauma and the trauma process in the body;
- Safety (coming back into the body);
- Boundaries;
- Inner child/adolescent/young adult (making meaningful contact);
- Awareness + healthy risk taking = growth: How to move forward.

Defining Trauma: Fight, Flight, Freeze

To understand how physiology, emotional processes, and the healing of trauma, or stored energy (stress, panic, and anxiety) in the body, unfolds for humans, it's useful to look at the similarities and differences in the experience of our mammalian counterparts. As self-aware, self-conscious beings, the suppression of our primal instincts following a traumatic event (which often looks or feels like the desire to cry, move, break down) in favor of social norms and adherence to the "shoulds" of human behavior can impede resolution of the trauma response, though in trauma's case, with long-lasting, complex consequences. By looking to understand the operation of the trauma response in its natural state, without the intervention of the human mind with all its training, rules, and socialization, we can learn to return to our symptoms and challenges in new ways, tapping into alternate possibilities for healing.

Trauma and the Animal Body

Moving away from our connection to earth's body has had far-reaching consequences for all realms of our health and well-being (sexual, spiritual, psychological, emotional, physical, mental). The more we adhere to rigid rules and ideas about how to work, behave, and operate within our bodies, the less we give ourselves room to honor, appreciate, and even simply understand how our bodies try to keep us safe, sane, and healthy. How many of us have judged someone dancing freely to a band or performer at a festival or community celebration? We may think something along the lines of "*How embarrassing, it's like they aren't even aware of themselves.*" We know dancing is good for our bodies, and anything that is good for our bodies is good for our mental and emotional health, our bodies *being* us. So, what are the ideas implicit in this judgment? That control is better than expression? How, then, does that influence our desire to dance next time the opportunity presents itself for us, even when alone or in the privacy of our own homes? How can we learn to trust our instincts when we're busy repressing and/or shaming them?

When thinking about trauma, nearly every aspect of the cycle *is* instinct. It unfolds without conscious input or management, an orchestrated, built-in response mechanism enabling the body to do what is required to keep us alive and mitigate the damage to our systems and psyche. Many of us are familiar with fight or flight as our primary survival responses when faced with threat. When working with sexual trauma, however, by and large we are/were interacting with a third, slightly lesser-known response called our "immobilize" or "freeze" response, an altered state of consciousness whereby the body goes limp or stiff, unable to move or take action whilst the mind is extremely alert and attentive. Faced with threat, the body and mind work together almost entirely offline, to understand what our options are in the moment. If fighting or fleeing are not possible or likely, in a split second the body moves into freeze, without our rational mind's ability to orient and organize, without conscious clarity whatsoever. By and large sexual trauma is trauma that occurs in contexts where fighting and/or fleeing is not available to us and we are working with the creative ways our system springs to action to separate us from the experience, our bodies, and emotional overwhelm. The body works to protect us from physical pain and injury, while the mind works to buffer the emotional and psychological consequences of the event(s).

Where Do Things Go Wrong?

Say a cat catches up with a mouse in its immobilize response and grabs it by the tail with its teeth. The cat then decides for whatever reason (very often boredom) not to play with this mouse any further, dropping it to the ground, only to saunter, unruffled, back to its cat castle. The mouse, still in the freeze response, senses the cat has made its leave; it is alone. If we were watching from afar, one of two things might happen:

- The mouse darts up, hyper-alert, with a big burst of energy and runs away to safety. That burst of energy being an expression of the fear and adrenaline that it came into immobilize or "freeze" with. The mouse moves through and releases that stored energy and tension, completing the survival response in the body as it runs, the nervous system re-regulating and moving back into homeostasis. The trauma response is complete.

- Alternatively, if the mouse no longer perceives active threat in its environment, we might notice that it begins to shake, moving into full-body convulsions, legs and arms outstretched, lapping the air as if imagining running away in its own mind. Its breathing might look labored at first, short and quick, but as it moves through the shaking, the body begins to slow down, and with it the breathing becomes increasingly deep and steady as the animal regains homeostasis, emotional equilibrium, and physical release (parasympathetic function). From there, it is able to hop up, steady itself on its feet, and continue on its way; system regulated, mind still, physiology at baseline. The trauma process is complete and, therefore, the animal is not *traumatized* but is different moving forward, traveling with its lessons from the experience (Levine, 1997).

Humans move through this differently. For one, we are creatures of habit, consistency, and routine. We like to get to know our partners so that we know what to expect and can begin to trust, just as we like to understand ourselves so that we can know what to expect from our own experience and can feel relatively in control over how we process our feelings and navigate emotional challenges. When we reach the release phase of the trauma cycle, when the threat has passed and the body and mind are making movements back toward equilibrium, we resist or attempt to suppress the body's need to move out that stored energy, which can look and feel like "out-of-control" behavior or expression. In humans, the release phase of the trauma response can show up as anger, crying, yelling, yawning, shaking, flailing, muscle contractions, and so on. Rather than allowing these feelings to spill over, moving themselves out of our system, running their course both emotionally and physically, we handle them much as we handle the sensation of needing to cry when we would rather not: we fight it, we push it down (e.g. tighten jaw, hold our breath, contract stomach and gut). Not understanding what is happening in the body, not recognizing a feeling and/or level of intensity, is scary for us humans. It is challenging to trust that something we don't understand is for our benefit, hard to even conceive of it as anything other than an unwelcome intruder (Levine, 1997).

What Informs Our Responses When in Fight, Flight, or Freeze?

Through this lens, it is useful to shine a light on our very real cognitive and physical limitations or "inhibitions" when in this state; the ways we are able to exercise control, and the ways we are held back from it, and why.

When in fight, flight, or freeze, the body shuts down systems that are not necessary in the moment in favor of those required to help us survive the situation. To break them down:

- The right brain is activated while the left is deactivated. Our right brain is intuitive, emotional, visual, spatial, tactile, while our left brain is sequential, linguistic, analytical:
  - Without the sequencing capabilities given to us in the left hemisphere, we cannot understand and create coherent plans for the future (both the immediate and beyond). Therefore, the ability to conceptualize how to protect ourselves rationally is inhibited.
  - Without our linguistic and analytical brain online, forming sentences, deciphering how to navigate the interaction with any skill (or even at all) verbally is not available to us. That is the felt experience of not being able to speak or yell for help is very real.

- The body goes limp or "stiff" as blood rushes to our vital organs. Our ability to "fight back" or run away, even if we could choose either of these options, is not physically possible as our muscles are reacting with tension and stiffness ("freeze") or full release (limpness).
- The mind dissociates, taking us to another place or another perspective that feels removed mentally and physically. We cannot make decisions, even if we had the ability to actively strategize on our own behalf, about our body if we're not "in" our bodies. Dissociation is a dream-like state, a place meant to feel removed, such as when we engage in a fantasy or blank out while driving on the highway. It is non-linear, abstract, and often disorganized.

When recalling traumatic experiences, hindsight can be cruel. The reality is that panic is immobilizing, fear is immobilizing – these emotions on their own create barriers to clear and strategic thinking. Add to that the mechanisms at play in the body and the neurological and physical selective shut-down that takes place, and we have quite literally been removed from our faculties. What we do in the face of these experiences is by and large, simply and truly, all we could have done. Resistance to this idea is something we need to look at in an ongoing way. Does it connect back to our desire to control, to make sense of behavior that doesn't follow the stories we carry about ourselves? *If I only had done A, then B would've been the outcome. I can't believe I didn't do A, I'm an A kind of person!* Or could it be connected to a long history of self-blame that is hard to shed, even in the face of new and important information that challenges its existence? *I can understand rationally that it was not possible for me to do A, but I just can't feel it.* Or are we looking at the situation as if the "you" of today, in a fully regulated state, was the version who went through the experience? Is it hard to separate the "you" of today from the "you" of that time?

Once we've arrived on the "other side" of the event (which can represent an entirely new experience of self), the "you" of that age was left to process and make sense of the overwhelming event, with all of its complexity, without a map, without understanding of trauma processes or physiological response. This is a major task for a fully grown adult, a monumental responsibility at any age. And yet we do it as best we can, able to preserve vital aspects of who we are and how we love (because we all do). We'll return to this shortly.

To summarize:

Neurological and physiological limitations and shut-down +

Developmental perspective and knowledge held by the person at that time +

Silence after and/or harmful reactions from caregivers +

Lack of training or conversation about how to take care of self on the back of a traumatic experience +

Isolation and disconnection =

I did what was available to me, my body and subconscious acted in my favor, I did not have meaningful access to safer alternatives.

Safety

Feelings of safety within and as oneself in the world exist and continuously evolve on a spectrum. Sexual trauma adds to the conversation by communicating that the container within which we live, breathe, dream, and love was not (or is not) able to protect us from harm, and at the extreme that our bodies can in and of themselves attract the harm we fear. This is an incredibly anxiety producing way of moving through the world, and many of us know nothing else (Haines, 1999).

What we want to invite in, in terms of our healing, is a sense of relative safety; it need not be perfect. We want to create the conditions under which safety is alive enough for us to understand its presence, enough to risk slowly releasing into it. We want to understand the control we have now in terms of the people we invite into our lives, how we navigate the various situations (sexually and otherwise) that we find ourselves in, and our relationship to trust and boundaries as we move forward in connection with others. As Staci Haines (1999), author of *Healing Sex: A Mind–Body Approach to Healing Sexual Trauma*, describes, identifying and cultivating safety happens internally and externally.

Internal and External Safety

It may seem obvious, but assessing our external environment for safety can be tricky, informed by our past (shocker), the degree of familiarity we have with various kinds of experiences.

Have you ever been to a party in high school or beyond where there were people partaking in various levels of risky behavior, from doing drugs, to driving recklessly – just generally ignoring the law? What else did you notice about the crowd? One person totally at ease, laughing and having a great time? One person in the corner, clutching their bag or drink, tense and visibly uncomfortable?

We all equate safety with different ingredients, and what one person reads as precarious, another might find familiar and therefore neutral, or even comforting. That said, depending on our past and the kinds of situations and events that were normalized in childhood, our assessment of safety might be unreliable, as our emotional experience may deliver "ease" when the situation is troubling on paper.

As I sit where I am right now, what in my environment lets me know I'm safe (if that's something I feel right now)? What do I notice that contributes to that feeling? What elements are important ingredients for me in general? Do I notice a few basic or "key" ingredients that seem to satisfy my internal criteria? Is my brain collecting a lengthy list?

If our internal sense of connection, our "tether to self" via the conversation we participate in with sensation throughout our day, via the witnessing and challenging of thought content, and via the movement into and through emotion, is tenuous or something we work to busy ourselves or distance from, internal safety is not possible. This is changeable! And we want to move slowly so as to assure we aren't reinforcing our trauma or, by virtue of pushing too far, reopening the trauma altogether.

How do we cultivate internal safety? We slowly and very gradually come back into the body, into sensation, and therefore into ourselves. Haines refers to this process as "emotional sourcing," and we can begin this in one of three ways.

(If during these experiences, you find yourself feeling disoriented, make sure you have objects around and in your immediate environment that are grounding, or that help you come back to the present moment. This can be a calendar, a clock, pictures from a recent experience and/or the people in it, an object you can reach for or hold onto, or even a song or podcast that you enjoy today that can act as a tether to your present life and interests.)

1 Sensations: Find a place in your environment where you will be undisturbed, a place free from busyness and distraction, and make yourself comfortable in a seated position (this can be on the floor or in a chair).

See if you can notice the sounds in the air, the feeling of your weight releasing into the furniture. Take a few deep breaths, release your jaw and shoulders, slow your breathing down, release. When you're ready, gently hold one of your hands in the other. Use the active hand to slowly caress the other, very slowly, noticing the textures of the skin, its warmth or coolness, the feeling of the tiny hairs that occupy the top of the hand, and the harder parts of the knuckles that make up the fingers. As you caress, come into the body and slowly scan for areas where you can identify sensations or places that feel more "still" or settled. What do you notice there? Warmth? Openness? What happens as you stay with the sensation(s), noticing how they shift and move as you continue to slowly caress your hand? If you find yourself getting uncomfortable or overwhelmed, simply return your focus to your hand and the feeling of your skin against your skin. If you can slowly return, if that feels available to you, great! Continue to explore sensation for three minutes or so. If not, and you feel inclined to listen to what might feel like a boundary, great! You can return another time and approach even more slowly or simply stay with the hand the entire time, practicing this form of connection to sensation first. Either way, you have begun!

2 Memory: Begin in the same way as #1, finding a comfortable position in a peaceful setting. Take a moment to settle, noticing the sounds in the air, releasing your musculature, taking a few long, deep breaths. When you're ready, see if you can bring forward a memory that represents happiness, presence, calm, comfort, or peace. Bring it to life in as much detail as you can: Who (if anyone) was with you? What did the space around you look like? Was it noisy, active, or quiet and slow? Were you outside? Was it hot, cold, or somewhere in-between? As you interact with the details, coming back into this experience in as full a way as is accessible today, how do you know it represents peace, or calm, or happiness? What in your body gives you this information? What sensations accompany the experience? Can you notice them more fully? Where do they live? How would you describe them? Breathe, release your jaw, release your shoulders, and see if you can return. How have these sensations shifted? How have they moved?

3 Object: If a memory feels challenging, see if you can locate an object that is meaningful to you, that you associate with love or thoughtfulness or care. Retrieve the object and place it next to you while you settle into your safe spot. Take a few deep breaths and allow the weight of your body to fully release into your seat. When ready, place the object in your lap and rest your hands on it in a way that feels physically comfortable. Keep eyes open in a soft gaze and think about where this object came from, what it means to you, and what it represents as you notice the feel of it against the palms of your hands. What let's you know it's

special? How does your body convey its meaning? What emotions surface as you look upon it and how do you understand them to be what
they are (love, gratitude, openness)? Where do these sensations live?
Can you interact with them? Are they expandable? Shrinkable?

If it feels like yellow or green light territory, see if you can approach this
experience more regularly, even in bite sizes. As you do so, the need for a
memory or object will fall off, and you will be able to come directly into
sensation in the body without their assistance. This means we're building
safety and embodiment! Once we have become familiar with sensations we
associate with calm, settled feelings, they become our secure base, or place
to approach challenging memories, or experience *from*, and then return *to*!
The more intimately familiar we are with these sensations, the more present they become in our lives. The more connected to sensation we feel, the
more learning and understanding are available to us, the better equipped
we are to take care of ourselves.

Boundaries

Boundaries are protective, period. Knowing when to exercise and let down
our boundaries is critical to the success of our relationships, the ongoing
development of our sexual life, and to our sense of comfort and ease living
in our own skin. They keep relationships intact, our sexual life evolving, our
sense of comfort and ease living within our skin available. Boundaries are
our way of honoring ourselves and our experience, of caring for who we are
and understanding what is required to stay in connection with others.
Boundaries are the walls, roof, and structure of the house that provides
shelter from the storm, while safety in bringing forward our vulnerability
(i.e. knowing when we can let our boundaries down) allows the light in.
Will we/can we react to challenging experiences where our boundaries were
violated by swinging to the other end of the spectrum? Of course. Will we/
can we inadvertently perpetuate the message that our boundaries don't
matter, and therefore will not be considered, even within ourselves? Yes
also. When it comes to the work of healing from sexual trauma, it can be
best to err on the side of the more bounded initially, allowing our body and
mind to understand that this is available to us now. Not only that, but we
will exercise and reinforce them if necessary, and check that they work (i.e.
will be respected by those around me). How do we determine where a
boundary is needed? How do we prevent the roof from being ripped off our
house? Connection to sensation and increased awareness of body. How can
we learn when a boundary can be loosened or edited? Checking in and
self-reflection each and every time our bodies communicate anxiety, fear,
discomfort, or are ill at ease.

What Can a Boundary, or Need for One, Feel Like?

- Overwhelm;
- Tension;
- Anxiety;
- Disgust and repulsion;
- Anger and agitation;
- Clenching and recoil;
- A sense of resignation, acquiescing, placating;
- Excessive giggles, jokiness, or inclination to get silly;
- Intellectualization;
- Intense focus on an unrelated object, aspect of the environment, or thought;
- Dissociation or feeling of disconnection (through thought spiraling, tuning out, or feelings of detachment from situation, feelings, and/or body);
- Profound tension in the body (any part).

This list is incomplete and is not meant to suggest that if we experience any of the above, we "have" to set a boundary. This is for you to determine based on your relationship to these elements in the moment. Overwhelm might feel OK if you understand it to be healing versus scary, part of the build of arousal versus an ingredient there to thwart it. Differentiating between the two can take time and practice, so go slow and be patient with yourself! Patience offers information, a new layer of revealing, and access to the kind of information that allows us to identify our limits and places of openness in a more present and therefore meaningful way. Patience cultivates safety, enabling possibility.

Coping, Avoidance, and Compulsion

Marcus: I'm the problem.
Therapist: Wow, let's not beat around the bush then!
Marcus: Well, it's true, though. I'm why we're here.
Therapist: Tell me about it, if that feels OK for you.
Marcus: Sex is just something that isn't super easy for me. I'm like, high maintenance I guess you could say, I have a lot of requirements and things that are off limits. I think it's too much sometimes for Charlie. Consequently, I don't think either one of us really wants it much anymore. I don't really have a super high sex drive to begin with, but Charlie has stopped trying to initiate nearly as much.
Therapist: Is that your version of things, Charlie?

Charlie: *I wouldn't say Marcus is "the problem," but yeah, I think sex has become like, this hard thing in our relationship. I feel like I'm doing things wrong or that I might do something wrong that will make him uncomfortable, which then makes me uncomfortable and nervous. I haven't had a lot of experiences sexually outside of Marcus, so I'm not sure if it's me or some of what he's been through, or both?*

Therapist: *Before we dig into what both of you bring into this relationship in terms of your sexual history, Marcus, can you talk about these requirements you've mentioned? Things that are "off limits"?*

Marcus: *Yeah, sure. I just, the conditions have to be right for me to feel in the mood or up for it or whatever. So, I need him to show me a lot of physical affection during the day, and then I need lots of making out, but I don't really like him to make eye contact with me. I also like to have the lights on but dimmed, I can't have the lights totally off. I don't really like a lot of focus on me. I'm like a service top.*

Therapist: *Charlie, when you say you're afraid you're doing things wrong, are you referencing operating according to the parameters and requirements Marcus just spelled out? Or is it something different?*

Charlie: *No, that's what I mean. There are a few other things too, like he only likes a certain kind of touch, it can't be too soft and he doesn't like a lot of dirty talk. There are just a lot of things and I want to make sure he feels comfortable with me and like he can trust but it also can feel like a lot of pressure.*

Therapist: *Sometimes when we've had challenging or even traumatic experiences with sex, our sexuality can become something that needs to organize itself around the pain, the memories, and the ways in which our bodies hold and remember those experiences. It creates a system where a lot of control is needed in order to provide enough of a sense of safety to remain engaged and able to access any pleasure or connection whatsoever. Does this resonate with you at all, Marcus? Am I off base?*

The creative ways our psyche has worked to cope with our experiences all organize themselves around control. *If I control my setting, the circumstances, your behavior, where I permit and prohibit touch, how we interact, what mood I'm in, then I can avoid my fear, aversion, overwhelm.* Some versions are more blatant, as Marcus and Charlie demonstrate, other versions are control in disguise, like avoidant or compulsive sexual behavior, low or no sexual desire (yes, low or no desire *can be* one means of control – often led by our subconscious), minimizing our experience (*"others had it worse"*) and inhibiting sexual response, among others. We can fantasize about our experiences, eroticizing our fear and powerlessness in order to understand them more deeply, create a new or alternate ending, reclaim a sense of control over the story. We can dissociate or "check out" when in the midst of sexual energy or our own vulnerability, our brain's creative way of removing us from real or perceived danger.

However our coping operates or has operated, it was important and wise. We will never fully understand how our brains, our bodies, protect or mitigate harm, but we can understand, simply in our learning about "fight, flight, and freeze," that they do, they are, even when we can't see it. Our job is to notice where the coping is no longer needed or where it has become problematic, and to help it move along.

Inner Child/Adolescent/Young Adult

Central to our healing in this arena is our ability to direct compassion towards and take tender care of the version of ourselves that lived through the trauma. This means letting go of or transforming any self-blame we may be carrying, however that may show up, and in whatever degree that may be present for us – releasing ourselves from the would've, could've, should've and the deep shame they inspire. They are (i) not helpful at best, (ii) detrimental to our self-worth and ability to embrace deep intimacy and sharing freely in an ongoing way at worst. They are misinformed, reactions from the perspective of this younger part that have been held in place by silence, disconnection, and lack of access to meaningful information.

(It can be useful to note that sometimes letting go of self-blame means acknowledging something harder: that we ultimately have very little control and, sometimes, none at all. If you feel yourself reluctant when conceptualizing a different relationship to self-blame, simply bring curiosity to that reluctance. *Is there a part of me that feels safer thinking I could've controlled challenging experiences? What consequences does that belief come with? What control do I have now that might allow me to let go of places where perception of control harms me?*)

Armed with the information described, aware of the very real physiological, psychological, emotional, and developmental limitations that version of yourself was contending with, can you begin to sense a distance or separation from them? Can you access their tenderness? Can you simply sit with the image of them in your mind's eye? What is it like to make contact with this shift, even if it's subtle? Can you stay with the feelings this brings to the surface? Can you release your jaw, shoulders, abdomen in the presence of them? It is absolutely OK if none of this is not available to you right now. The more you learn and allow yourself to be with and think about sex, your body, and relationships in new ways, the less your brain or psyche will try and protect you from addressing the most vulnerable version of your sexual self, from visiting the experience or experiences that person represents. Engaging with sexuality, even as a concept, in an ongoing way *is* breaking down the associations that keep our sexuality tightly bound. Whenever we sit down with the topic of sex, our sexuality surfaces and is paired with the feelings that come along with the learning, whether that be relief, curiosity, neutrality, and/or confusion. All of these feelings are more approachable than panic, all begin to layer different stories.

One boundary that we can start reinforcing with ourselves today is the one that protects us from further internalization or "the taking on" of misplaced blame or anger, if that is part of your experience. Even if we're not there yet, working in an ongoing way to understand that our bodies did not betray us, regardless of how they responded, is pivotal in freeing up real room for new experiences, self-trust, and the felt sense of love and connection we all deserve. This can look however you want, but it need not involve any real imagery of those involved. We can begin to "hand back" the anger, shame, and guilt we feel to a nameless, shapeless, blob in our mind's eye, and then continue to direct it there as it surfaces. It can sound like this:

I've carried this long enough; you can have it back. It's been yours all along.

Returning to Now

Our relationship to our younger part is something we want to nurture and attend to regularly, addressing that part's confusion, supporting the grief, and acknowledging the fear as we understand ourselves in new ways through our individual and shared healing (the kind of reciprocal healing that happens in partnership); and then our relationship to ourselves, this version of "me" in the present, is what we're addressing when engaging sexually. This can look like:

Day-to-day interaction:
My partner places their hand on my thigh as we are watching a movie on the couch, and my instant reaction is to recoil.

- "I" attends to "younger I": "*I know touch on this part of the body has meant danger for us in the past. I am in control now, we are safe. It's OK to feel nervous, and they can rest their hand there.*"

Sexual experience:
My partner moves to touch my thigh as we are kissing and lying next to each other in bed, and my instant reaction is to recoil.

- "I" attend to "me" in the present: "*It's OK to feel these feelings, they can stay. I am safe with this person, safe with myself. I'm going to release my jaw and breathe. My partner can have their hand there, I can pause or slow down whenever I need to.*"

Awareness + Healthy risk taking = Growth

The body will tell you what it needs if we slow down enough to listen. Sometimes what it asks is to demonstrate safety via the pairing of "letting go" with experiences that build on each other progressively. Other times, however, it asks for something entirely different, as a means of completing the trauma response that has lived in our bodies, waiting for an opportunity for completion. Remember the mouse and its movements, the big energy that it traveled through, the many ways animal bodies release and come back into homeostasis? When the body and mind understand that our context is safe enough to finally revisit and complete this process, these stored reactions can come online. Suddenly we may find ourselves inclined to yell, or run, or hit, or cry. Instead of pushing these inclinations down, keeping them trapped in our bodies, compounded more deeply into our muscles, translated as tension and hyper-vigilance and anxiety, might we risk allowing them to come forward? Call we follow their lead and let our bodies kick, or cry, or move more *deeply into* tension in order for it to move out? You are you, a human governed by rules and scripts and a brain that is aware of both; you are also that mouse, a being within an animal body, with a wisdom that attempts to work in our favor, should we let it (Levine, 1997).

(Sexual trauma deserves our deep and thoughtful attention and care. We deserve, our sexual or intimate connections deserve, to feel less controlled by our past. This information is a starting point, but the real work happens in therapy with a skilled and compassionate sex therapist. They will be able to hold your hand through the process, illuminate where the snags live, help provide the grounding and scaffolding necessary to move through stored emotion, and bring us more intimately back to ourselves. Our wounding happens relationally, our healing wants the same.)

In case you've never heard this from anyone, whatever happened should not have happened to you or anyone else. It was not OK and it created a pain that stays. *And,* you are and always have been whole and complete just as you are. Worthy of loving, just as you are.

You are a million universes more than the stories you've traveled through.

Racism, Trauma, Worthiness and Sexuality: Dr. Candace Hargons Interview

Dr. Candice Nicole Hargons (C) is an award-winning associate professor of counseling psychology at the University of Kentucky, where she studies sexual wellness and liberation. She is the host of F*ck the System: A Sexual Liberation Podcast and How to Love a Human, a liberation podcast that asks people with multiple marginalized identities what the world would be like if it loved them. She has published over 50 research articles and has been featured in the Huffington Post, *the* APA Monitor, Good Housekeeping, Women's Health, Blavity, Cosmopolitan, *and the* New York Times.

Paula Leech (P): In getting to know you online, I stumbled upon all this work you do around racial trauma. How would you define what that is?

C: It's the enduring response that people of the global majority have to racism: the cognitive, emotional, and somatic responses. So, you can have an immediate response, that's not racial trauma but, based on how intense or severe a racist stressor is, you can move into racial trauma in that those symptoms are long-standing, changing the way you think about yourself. Racism can change the way you think about worthiness, change the way you appraise your own value; you may start to buy into this human hierarchy if you're experiencing racial trauma. It changes you emotionally, so the stress that you're under means that maybe your capacity to hold or be with emotions has changed. And then there's somatic responses that lead to psychophysiological disease, so we see a lot of health disparities in people with racially marginalized identities and some of them start with the somatic response of "I'm holding my breath when I walk into this room," or "my sympathetic nervous system is activated when I experience a microaggression," or "my body is tight and tense so eventually my body won't allow me to relax anymore," those pieces altogether with the precipitant of racism, a racist stressor of any type, that's racial trauma.

P: How does racial trauma differentiate itself from our classic trauma symptoms that we talk about or think about? How do folx identify the imprint of it within themselves?

C: There are so many areas of overlap because it's trauma. But where it comes from, what is the trauma? Can other people relate to the trauma? Those are the differentials. You might have everyone experiencing COVID-19 as a trauma and people are like, "yes, that is traumatic. Whew!" And then you have people who are members of the Asian diaspora who are experiencing the racial trauma of how COVID-19 was racialized and antagonistic towards them, and then minimized by huge portions of the population, "no, it wasn't about that," invalidating their experience. Those are the two components: how people experience the trauma, how it started; and whether people are willing to agree that it's trauma.

P: How does racism prevent us from accessing pleasure and connection with others?

C: I developed this construct called "pleasure worthiness" to amend the construct of pleasure entitlements because I think entitlements come with "I will get what I think I deserve at all cost," whereas worthiness is, "I am deserving of, I'm worthy of" but it has to be more consensual and originating from your inherent sense of self. And what I found in my research is that for black people, 90% of the sample out of almost 500 people reported that they're extremely worthy of pleasure, so I think there's some resilience and resistance in seeing yourself as pleasure worthy in systems that try to annihilate you, in systems that sexually stereotype you and in systems that constrict your knowledge and capacities around sex. So, I'll say racism gives people of the global majority, racially marginalized people, something that they have to bump up against as they're coming to understanding their sense of pleasure worthiness or remembering (because I think kids tend to know and then we socialize it out of them). I think that racism assigns a set of "these are the only people that get to be valuable," and then anybody who's outside of that narrow window of value or credibility or beauty or desirability or worthiness (in any way that we think about worthiness), must fight against those impositions. But I see the fight, I see the fight happening.

P: What are your thoughts about the role that anxiety plays in this picture? What clues does it give us in terms of the trauma that we carry with us, the areas that we need to investigate with regards to our own sexuality, and our own experience of embodiment?

C: We talk in some of our papers, about sexual anxiety from the lens of black women and being afraid to disclose that you have sexual anxiety because you believe you're supposed to be strong, and that people have that expectation that you can handle anything. So, even if you do get the courage to share it with someone, they might just be like "noooo, not you! Haha! You're too strong for that," which is different from affirming a person's inherent worthiness, and I think sometimes the two get conflated. Being able to empathize, notice, and name, "this experience of anxiety is real for you, you have the resources, and I'm gonna help support you in how you recover," that's one part of it. And this connects to fear of telling partners, but also fear of talking to health care providers, with health care providers being known to minimize the pain of black women or ignore it altogether.

Sexual anxiety has a physical cost too. Not only do you feel exhausted but then if you think about genito-pelvic pain disorders like vaginismus, those are correlated with anxiety! So, if you fear that you will be in pain or that if something happens you may get into that loop of preoccupation or rumination again, then your body clenches, your genitals might clench, or you might struggle with arousal because you can't take the brake off.

P: Well, and that raises the question of what the body must register for our sexual functioning to come online, a sense of safety …

C: Most people that I know, when I think about being in community with black people and even for some people of Asian diaspora or Latino people, they don't even expect safety. It's not something that they believe really exists. I know I don't. I think safety is a social construction that I don't have available to me most of the time. That's a tough pill to swallow for people who feel like there are safe spaces, or safe spaces can be created, but it also feels liberating for me because that means, for me anyway, I don't have to engage in specific behaviors people think should afford you safety. I get to just be, and then recognize that, like any other being or human in the world constantly up against things that might harm me, some day they may and some day they may not be as harmful.

P: lAnd we think of it as black and white, you're either safe or not or you trust or you don't and these things always exist on a spectrum …

C: They're dynamic, yeah.

P: Very dynamic! And when sex is so much about releasing into, and releasing into our own vulnerability, there's a prerequisite there in terms of a relative amount of trust, or a relative sense of safety that we have to construct, how do you help folx cultivate those qualities? How do you talk about it?

C: I frame it more as willingness to be courageous. So, let me back up a little bit, when I say I think safety doesn't exist, I think protections exist and I think the more privilege we have the more protections are in place, but protections don't guarantee safety either because sometimes protections are transactional, right? So, even from your lens as a white woman, there may be more socio-cultural protections in place but what do you have to give up to be protected under the system of patriarchy? What do you owe patriarchy for its protection? Protections exist, safety, on the other hand, not so much. But are you willing to be vulnerable because it will benefit you or be mutually beneficial anyway? Do you have the capacity for courage in a moment knowing that sure, you could be harmed, even if it's not an intentional harm. So, the decision to be with someone, to engage sexually, to open yourself up to your sexual life after trauma or during trauma (while you're still experiencing traumatization), is a choice. "Do I have the capacity for this? Can I choose courage? Can I hold compassion for myself if I can't choose courage today? Will that be ok?"

P: It can be so tricky because our brain and our body can be on such different pages around things, right? We can find ourselves in an experience of, "I wanna choose bravery, why won't my body let me?" How do you address that?

C: I love mindfulness practices and I know that there's a lot of research to support what having reverence for what your breath can do for you: how you hold breath and expel breath can be one small thing that people feel they have control over. Because sometimes it can be like, "do I have control over my body? Is my body gonna betray me?" Deep breathing can be a part of that connection process, a meditation practice can be a part of that process, having a practice of attuning to your body before you're asking it to enter a sexual experience so that you notice what your body's experiencing. There are plenty of us who might experience arousal and not notice it! Do you take time to notice what arousal means in your body before you're in a shared sexual moment or during a solo sexual moment? Can you engage in masturbation or solo sexuality in ways that help you to recover that courage (if that's what you want) so you're sexually self-aware, attuned, where your mind, body, and spirit are in the process and it's not rushed, doesn't have to be rushed, and you can extend compassion to yourself if you're not there yet?

P: I love the idea of engaging with your body, yourself, before moving into a partnered sexual experience because it feels like that gives us such an opportunity to practice bravery on our own terms without the audience of someone we're invested in, concerned about how they perceive us or experience our body. So, it gives us the practice of the bravery piece and cultivating connection to sensation and the body.

C: I find my clients have a hard time with solo sexuality and affirming themselves. I ask them "when you're engaging, how do you care for and talk to and about your genitalia? How do you hold yourself? Do you rush through the moment? Do you make it a practice of self-reverence and take the time that you need?" and they're like "I don't know ... I feel awkward," and I'm like "Sure, ok. Because I didn't necessarily expect it to feel comfortable. So, are you gonna do the uncomfortable thing? Would you like to?"

P: Yes! Last question: Racism in the world, something that we live and breathe as a concept; how does it touch everybody?

C: I think that one of the ways it impacts everyone, the people who are targets of racism and the people who perpetuate racism, is that there's this comparison group when you invest in racism, if we're using a binary, black people are at the bottom of the comparison group and white people are at the top and everybody else is somewhere in the middle depending on their proximity to whiteness. To be at the top of that racial hierarchy means that you're also writing yourself out of all the things you said that those other groups are. So, if you think about white people in Puritanical America, Victorian era American history saying, "these are the savages, these are the people who are hypersexual, these are the people who are lascivious, that's them. We are pure, and pristine, and moral over here." And it's like, you're this little, tiny ass bubble over here, missing the menu of good sex, this whole menu that you've made pejorative and that you've used to create this artificial hierarchy. So, instead of being able to realize the pleasure and liberatory potential of these sexual decisions and experiences, now you feel shame because "I shouldn't have wanted to do that because I'm white, or I shouldn't've liked this because I'm moral." It's a constriction on everybody having to contend with all the boundaries you put on what it means to be white or what it means to be good or what it means to be pure.

P: Real implications for embodiment for everyone when this exists as an organizing principle for how we do culture, society; consequences in terms of sexual liberation for all.

C: Yeah, absolutely.

P: How do people heal from racial trauma? How do we liberate ourselves sexually from your perspective? What are some of the building blocks?

C: That's the main question I'm answering in my work, the whole function is the "how." And so, if you think about practicing liberation as opposed to getting there in your lifetime, then you reduce the stress of urgency, which is a white supremacist value. Everyday I'm gonna practice a bit, a tiny bit if that's all I have, is just fine. Today I'm going to tell my sexual self that it's OK to have the desires that I have. I'm gonna write down my desires and talk or journal through where they came from, think about what negative messages have been associated with them, and create or hypothesize about positive things I can associate with them instead, small things. But it also can be in how you experience sex with someone else, so how do you ask what turns them on and what turns them off? What is pleasure for them, without judgment or shame? How do you invite them to treat you without judgment or shame too? Those types of conversations with a partner, your sexual communication, can make a really big difference.

But at the top of this, with all the systems, you have to be willing to resist systemic oppression and that looks like how we choose neighborhoods and schools, that looks like how we construct the neighborhoods and schools, that looks like are you advocating for policy? For comprehensive sex ed in the public and private school systems? Are you talking to religious and spiritual leaders about their homophobia and their negative ideas about trans people? Are you going to your political officials and asking them to affirm the humanity of trans people, sexual minority people, and people of the global majority? Are you doing that work with some regularity? And while you do it, are you taking good care of yourself because it is exhausting, it is, but if we're going to realize liberation, sexual liberation isn't in isolation. It's like, you can't have regular therapy over here and then sex therapy over here and it not touch, you know? So are we talking about all people having access to housing and food and healthcare? 'Cause if we're not talking about that, we're not talking about sexual liberation.

P: What I'm hearing from you that I find so powerful is, all the way through, from the bedroom to the larger context, bravery in order for liberation is the thing. We have to be brave in order to be vulnerable, we have to be brave in order to confront the systems that we're embedded in, we have to be brave in order to be free.

C: And it shouldn't be, I wish it weren't. I wish you didn't have to be courageous because there weren't things to fear. But until we get there, yeah, courage is going to be necessary and compassionate courage. If this was a moment when you were too afraid, then you can still love on yourself and maybe the next moment you'll have a bit more internal resources based on that love, to do that thing you were afraid to do the last time.

P: Is there anything that you feel is important to touch on that we haven't discussed?

C: For me it's always a question of, what type of evidence are you going to need to recognize or remember your inherent worthiness? 'Cause everybody's going to need a different type of evidence, right? Based on how they were raised, their identities, etc. But to really find that out for yourself, if you're not already there and to move toward collecting that data, taking a scientist's mind around it, "Well, if I knew this, maybe it would help me practice that more or believe that more." And then approach that thing, have curiosity about it, and see where it takes you. If it doesn't take you there, keep going, and if it does … great! Show somebody else how to do it.

P: Instead of collecting evidence for all the other awful things we collect evidence for.

C: We collect evidence, all the time! So, what argument are you trying to support?

Note: Dr. Candice Hargons referenced two of her publications in the conversation: Hargons et al. (2022) and Hargons and Thorpe (2022).

16 Sex as Pathology (Fantasy, Porn, Kink)

- *You're self-medicating through sex – I better get on antidepressants.*
- *You're being unfaithful to me by watching porn – I've betrayed my partner and must stop consuming erotic media.*
- *You're masturbating too much – I must be "too sexual," I need to cut my masturbation habits in half.*
- *You're using sex as escape – Sex is only for intimate connection; I need to find other means of relief and release.*
- *You're objectifying me when we have sex – I need to hide my attraction towards my partner.*
- *Your kink is a trauma response – If I heal my trauma, my kink will go away (do I even want that?).*
- *You shouldn't care about sex so much – I need to push away my sexuality.*
- *Casual sex is reckless – I need to shut down my desires.*
- *You're a sex addict – I need to abstain.*

Landing on a "should" or a conclusion around something can simultaneously kick up distress and provide relief. Counter-intuitively, the anxiety of sitting with uncertainty, ambivalence, and conflicting ideas and feelings, including our own insecurity, can feel more challenging than deciding something is wrong. If it's "wrong," I can try to do something different, take action, or ask (or even demand) that *you* do something different; even if that ask is enormous, even if it's not rational or even possible. As an arena of human life occupied for all of us by varying levels of shame and confusion, sexuality is particularly susceptible to this process. The more rules we give sex, the more "shoulds" we add, the more we trick ourselves into thinking we understand it and therefore can do it "right," and if I and/ or my partner can do it "right" my shame, confusion, anxiety, and insecurity will be resolved. In the name of safety, we have effectively made less room for authenticity, honesty, curiosity, and pure, unbridled intimacy.

DOI: 10.4324/9781003369080-19

Diagnosis

We have an entire book devoted to helping us give definition to our mental and emotional struggles, called the *Diagnostic and Statistical Manual*, or the DSM. This text is meant to help clinicians group together a cluster of symptoms, give them a name or "diagnosis," and provide a path forward in terms of treatment, a way of conceptualizing what "help" will look like. On the plus side, having a name for something, alongside the treatment "package" that can come with it, can be immensely helpful, for both the client and the therapist. It can give us a way of understanding ourselves, our behavior, and putting it all into context which can be normalizing and relieve the sense of isolation that comes with the unknown. It can open doors in terms of real medical and therapeutic options for people whose diagnoses present significant and constant barriers, making it challenging to function or achieve one's goals.

They also have the potential to be limiting. For both therapist and client, a primary risk in diagnosis is the way it shapes how we see the struggle moving forward. If we land on a conclusion, how invested are we in continuing to learn about the challenge with wide open curiosity, and the openness and attunement we think about when conceptualizing the role of the therapist? With the exploration influenced by the diagnosis, to lesser or greater extents we begin to use a filter in terms of how we continue to learn about the struggle. If I've been told I am a "sex addict" in couples therapy, it is likely that my partner and I are going to abruptly switch lanes from open "wide net" inquiry to attempting to understand all behavior through the lens of "addict," including how my behavior evolves moving forward. Just as in science class we work to prove a hypothesis, "*You thought about masturbating after making love yesterday? That was your addiction.*" "*You felt inclined to watch porn after making love yesterday? That was your addiction.*" "*You felt deep shame about your desires, ones you've carried with you since you were a young kid? That was your addiction.*" "Sex addict" is a prime example given that, despite our best efforts, we do not have a lengthy list of diagnoses to refer to when it comes to sexual behavior. "Addict" becomes a sort of catch-all for a plethora of misunderstood and/or challenging sexual proclivities, desires, and activity. Lack of sex therapy training, understanding, language, and our own sexual wounding combined place most therapists in the same position, with one label to reference when working with sexual behavior that feels "outside the norm" (which can be an endless, exhaustive list when it comes to sex).

Talking about and exploring sexuality requires having an intimate and comfortable relationship with the topic and our own challenges in this arena. Therapist and author Doug Braun-Harvey (2016) references what he calls "premature evaluation," or the tendency by many therapists to jump to conclusions (often *a* conclusion, "sex or porn addict") about what might be going on out of their own discomfort with the topic at hand, therefore bypassing the need to ask more probing questions and venture into increasingly private places with the client. If health professionals, people trained to be thorough and brave when it comes to the collection of personal information are doing it, rest assured most of us are too.

This in mind, greater understanding is a must. Let's provide some much-needed depth and exploration around a few commonly misunderstood behaviors, struggles, and aspects of our humanity that get grouped under the sex addiction umbrella, or simply pathologized, and determine if the "shoulds" and conclusions we've carried, connected to them, thus far are worthy of continued travel. Let's normalize some normal behavior so we can see more clearly when we've gone off track or when our relationship to our sexuality truly has become cause for concern.

Fantasy, Porn, and "Sex Addiction"

Taylor (32-year-old, trans/lesbian, Irish-American woman) and Amelia (29-year-old, cis/lesbian, second-generation Caribbean woman) have been together for four years. The first two years were a long distance relationship as Taylor finished up her degree in California, while Amelia lives in Philadelphia, where they're both from and where they ultimately met. Two years into living together, Amelia discovers pornography on Taylor's computer that was out on their bed and is horrified. She describes feeling betrayed by Taylor, that watching porn feels like cheating, especially in light of their virtually non-existent sex life since moving in together a year and a half ago, a sexual life and connection that Amelia so desperately wants but Taylor has seemed to be disinterested in. To add insult to injury, Amelia is completely confused by the content of the porn: a mix of cis/straight "dick worship" scenes alongside lesbian porn that features cis women with big breasts and much bigger bodies than Amelia has.

Taylor: *I honestly don't know why I watch it; I just always have despite trying to stop when I get into relationships. I know it's not right. I love Amelia and would never want to hurt her! I'm so ashamed, this is all so embarrassing. I'll do whatever's required to fix this.*

Therapist: *Are we on the same page about what "whatever's required" means? What are your goals in coming to therapy? Amelia, I wonder what your thoughts are on that?*

Amelia: *Well, I don't know ... I just want to feel like Taylor wants me, that I'm enough for her.*

Therapist: *And how would you know that Taylor wants you? What would she need to show you or do?*

Amelia: *Stop watching porn for one.*

Therapist: *OK, and what about masturbation? Are you comfortable with Taylor masturbating?*

Amelia: *I mean, not really. She could just masturbate and fantasize about the porn she was watching, and it would be like the same thing.*

Therapist: *So, I'm hearing porn, masturbation, AND fantasy are problematic. It's feeling to me like the issue isn't really about porn at all, are you getting that sense as well? Where might we begin here?*

The above scenario (porn versus masturbation versus fantasy) was inspired by Marty Klein's (2016) work in his groundbreaking book, *His Porn, Her Pain: Confronting America's Porn Panic with Honest Talk about Sex.*

Fantasy

When anxiety moves in to show us what might happen, the catastrophic scenarios that could, or just might, or most assuredly will come to life, we are engaging in fantasy (in this case, a form of prediction). When anxiety moves out of the way, illuminating other possibilities, potentially successful or benign alternative outcomes and scenarios, we are also dealing with fantasy. Our reality passes through our psychology, interacting with our carried stories about what life is, what to expect from it, helping us understand how to deal with what unfolds and where to go. How often are we and where to go. How often are we running through and predicting how we might feel and perform differently if we just had one more cup of coffee? How many of us have envisioned a life in an apartment, condo, or home we were looking into renting or buying? Fantasy shows up in ways both big and small, to lesser and greater extents depending on the scenario, enabling risk taking (e.g. *asking that person out because they were super nice and funny online and I can picture us at dinner having easy conversation and enjoying a laugh so I'm gonna go for it*) and keeping connection and chemistry alive (for better when it comes to the fond stories and memories we visit about our long-term partners, and for worse when it comes to that ex that we just can't shake).

Within our long-term relationships, we can place our partners in fantasy space on occasion or even in an ongoing way to differentiate, re-encounter the spark, and revisit the stories that helped develop feelings of love and/or lust to begin with. We are often required to intentionally dig up old narratives to bring this all to life (e.g. *we're parents in the grind of the day-to-day but behind that they're also an artist, a great cook, so intelligent*). Fantasy is part of what it means to have a brain, an inseparable part of how we think things through, part of the literal definition of conceptualization.

When it comes to our sexuality, fantasy draws inspiration from limitless sources, and most of the time without our conscious input. We are capable of eroticizing everything: shame, trauma, jealousy, memory, power, guilt, abuse, joy, longing, objects, situations, people, places, roles, rules, oppression, race, and gender. We then place this eroticized content, experience, or memory in a context where we can interact with it on our own terms and from differing vantage points – and we have fantasy. Even when we're awake and fully conscious, our fantasies are abstract, imagination space, dream-like territory, weaving together themes from our present and/or past, helping us work through feelings, create or maintain balance, understand ourselves and the world around us, and ultimately helping us meet and/or feed our wants, needs, and desires in safe and creative ways. Just like children play with themes of death and violence to understand them more fully, fantasy in adulthood accomplishes the same, taking us to seemingly strange or troubling places to process them more deeply, weaving them into our understanding of the world, helping us articulate or clarify our relationship to them in a more embodied way. This process can feel confusing as fantasies can hold seemingly contradictory experiences alongside one another. We can simultaneously know that something is wrong and not an experience we would ever desire for ourselves in our lived reality and enjoy or derive pleasure from interacting with the concept of it in our fantasy world. That is *I can enjoy playing with ambiguity around consent, or even lack thereof entirely in the scenes I visit in my erotic mind, and very much require consent in my lived experiences and relationships.*

Fantasy allows us to step into past experiences, or variations of past experiences, and re-enact key elements that were painful, overwhelming, or even traumatic in order to gain a greater *sense* of control over the stories and the imprint they've left, understand the experiences from a different lens, process individual elements, and move through the associated feelings on our own terms. This is possible for both overwhelming or confusing experiences from our past, and also in relationship to overwhelm or confusion that exists in our present context. Placing challenging experiences in fantasy context buffers some of the pain and fear involved in living that experience, allowing us a reprieve from the enormity of those challenging feelings and the presence they take on in our lives.

Fantasies = Our Truest Desires?

With all of this in mind, it can be anxiety provoking, problematic, and sometimes entirely off-base to assume that our sexual fantasies reflect our deepest, most profound desires for our reality, or a deeper truth about who we are. Even when that content seems very translatable to our relationships, A + B does not always equal C. Let's play out a hypothetical (and very unadvisable) scenario with Amelia and Taylor that illuminates the complexity here.

Therapist: *Sometimes our sexual relationships can become as routine and formulaic as doing the laundry: we do the same things, visit the same or similar behaviors and routes to pleasure on autopilot, never really bothering to ask ourselves if this is still doing it for us. One way to introduce some novelty and creativity is to share your fantasies with one another. Even if you can't locate a specific current fantasy of your own creation, can you recall one you've enjoyed in the past or even think of a scene in a movie that you found or find exciting or hot? What would it be like to share this information with your partner? How might you think about bringing it to life with them?*

Amelia: *I would be very interested in hearing Taylor's fantasies, interested and a little scared. As hard as it is for me that she imagines herself in scenarios that don't always include me, I would like to understand what turns her on and how I can be a part of it.*

Taylor: *Me too. We've never talked openly about our fantasies and I'm sure I could do a better job at being more of what Amelia needs in this relationship. I would love to hear what she is thinking about that turns her on.*

Therapist: *In that case, Amelia do you have a fantasy you'd like to share? No pressure of course, you can always think about this for next time.*

Amelia: *Well ... ugh, this is oddly hard to talk about! I don't think about this so much anymore, but ... I used to fantasize about wandering into the changing rooms after a game and, um ... finding the cheerleaders all disrobing. A few approach me and, well ... we begin hooking up with the rest of the cheer squad watching. Bah, it's so strange saying it out loud!*

(Amelia looks over at Taylor sheepishly, while the Therapist nods at Taylor, prompting a response.)

Taylor: *Wow, I don't know how to react to that, honestly. On one hand, it's exciting to hear her talk about something she gets off on. On the other hand, I'm sitting here feeling super confused and insecure. Like, if you're into girls with cheerleader bodies, who are young and sporty, that's not me at all.*

If fantasy is dream-like in its make-up, then why do we take them so literally? Why is this especially so when it comes to our partners? Is it true that our fantasies can be literal representations of our desires for reality? Sure! Most of the time, however, we are dealing in *themes*, the vast majority of which are hard to grasp, or challenging to uncover at all. Maybe Amelia is into whatever Taylor is imagining when conceiving of the "cheerleader body," or maybe Amelia is into the idea that she is desired, and not just by anyone, by a group of people generally thought of as desirable themselves. Perhaps high school was a challenging time in her life and hooking up with the cheerleaders (who typically held a sizeable amount of social status in most high schools) feels like vindication. Maybe Amelia is into being watched, and the cheerleaders are easy material because they're on a team, and typically all together. Maybe she likes to revisit a more youthful time in her life via this fantasy. How old is the version of her in this scene?

We can dissect and analyze down to the detail and still not be able to pin down exactly what this fantasy represents for Amelia and what the specific ingredients are that make it so supremely erotic. Sharing our most private fantasies, therefore, requires that we go through the process of sifting through the content and distinguishing what aspects of the scene we wish to bring into not only our lived reality, but the reality we share with our partners, and what aspects we wish to remain with, comfortably in our safe, confidential, mind space.

Amelia: *I actually don't think it was about "cheerleader bodies" per se, although it was mostly white girls with rich boyfriends who seemed to get on the cheer team. I think maybe I wanted those girls, the "cool," popular, straight girls to want me, like really, really want me. Talking about this now, I think it was a power thing! I think I constantly fought seeing myself as a poser and perpetual outsider as one of the few queer, black girls at the school.*

The Benefits of Fantasizing – About Other People!

I wake up to my partner each day, we live together, share responsibilities for the house, we play together, share a social life, we raise children together, we navigate the struggles we bring home from work together, and share in family occasions and holidays together, we grow together, navigate grief and hardship together, are accountable to one another, watch each other age and change and evolve, we explore intimacy and sexuality together. Sometimes I need to imagine not being together, being free and wild and sexual with other partners in other places to feel the desire to want to fuck together.

We recognize we love our favorite food by interacting with other foods: a variety of flavors, textures, settings, and arrangements that highlight what is so incredible about the unique combination of ingredients and sensations that make that favorite a favorite. We would lose sight of what is so spectacular about a really great taco (for example), if we didn't have other experiences with other foods to compare it to. In fact, over time we might begin to thoroughly dislike that taco and each individual element if exploration of and experience with other foods were not an option. We live through and play out the same effect in our relationships with agreements and parameters to guide the way and protect what we define as sacred intimacy, monogamous or non-monogamous. We move through the world interacting with and getting to know the landscape around us, including noticing other people's bodies and physicality, cultivating connections, and having experiences that allow us to come back to our partners with fresh(er) eyes, recognizing their uniqueness in subtle or not-so-subtle ways. This is one way we enable ourselves to continue to identify what we appreciate about what makes our partners "them" while simultaneously getting to know them intimately, deeply, and personally in a way that can seem to erase the definition between us. Our fantasies provide yet another avenue for us to back up in order to come forward. They remind us of our separateness, of our partner's separateness, and place us in contact with sexual differentiation, or the imagining of ourselves being sexual with others in order to learn and understand who we are sexually for ourselves. This has huge benefits for our partnered lives – if we can learn to enthusiastically welcome our own and our partners' honesty, evolution, and ongoing development into the bedroom. The more we can hold the door open for change, open communication, and negotiation, the less stagnant or avoidant our sexual lives become.

Now go have hot sex with a ghost in your head and come tell me what you learned.

Getting Needs Met

When we watch a movie, we're engaging in fantasy. Video games? Deep in fantasy. Books and our favorite tv shows? Fantasy! What do you love about the shows you frequent? The characters you become attached to? What does visiting these shows do for you? What does it put you in contact with that is meaningful to you now, in your current life and context?

We take for granted how much we respond to our own personal wants, needs, desires sexually and beyond through content that exists in media or text. We fail to recognize how interacting with stories rounds out our lives, providing depth, putting us in touch with different experiences, different lives, different feelings. We interact with our own sexuality, our own eroticism each and every time we watch sexual or romantic chemistry exchanged between characters on a screen or brought to life within pages and text. Our sexuality, desire, and even feelings of arousal live and breathe and take up space in nuanced and not-so-nuanced ways, weaving themselves into the stories we step into, whether explicit in nature (porn) or not. Fantasy, then, represents so much more than the scenes that play themselves out in our own minds, of our own creation, as simply a version, one slice of our fantasy life.

Clara (cis/het female) is a 41-year-old mother of two young children. She lives a busy life trying to juggle her work, various projects she's taken on, social and familial obligations, and toddlers, but despite the exhaustion that can take a toll she is content with her life. Clara has also been married for 15 years. They share a strong connection and a loving relationship despite a lot of the erotic spark having faded substantially over time.

Clara stumbles upon a new series that catches her eye on Netflix one not-so-late night after putting the children to bed. She makes her way through episode after episode and cannot stop. The show, a gay high school romance series, has awakened feelings in her that have lied dormant since dating. Chalk full of steamy chemistry and eroticism between the main characters, and loads of conflict and barriers to their love, she is transfixed. After binging the season, she revisits it again and again, fast forwarding to her favorite parts. When she's not watching it, she's listening to the soundtrack. She laughs with friends about her obsession, but what is actually going on here?

Clara asks herself the following questions.

- *Am I attracted to these teenage boys?*
- *Am I strange for enjoying gay sexuality as a straight woman?*
- *Does this mean anything for my marriage?*

Clara discovers the following through her exploration of these questions in therapy:

- *Am I attracted to teenage boys?* Yes, but in what context? Clara is able to identify that she doesn't feel attraction towards teen/young adult cis boys/men in her everyday life. She doesn't notice younger men when around them, it's just not a thing. When Clara imagined or tried to place herself in the scenes with one or both characters, it felt jarring. A "yuck" moment. What are the feelings of attraction made of, then? So immersed in the story, Clara is brought back to her own high school years, a time that was challenging for her and a time characterized by deep longing for romantic and sexual connection. When watching the show, she is seeing the teen boys through her 16-year-old eyes, tapping into the desire she felt for young men like the characters, both in terms of physicality and personality. As if revisiting and meeting the deep wants of that version of herself, the excitement and energy that is kicked up while watching the main characters interact sexually has everything to do with the mix of both grief and longing for a time that was simultaneously incredibly lonely and painful, but also exciting, full of mystery and potential. In these scenes, the teen version of her comes alive again, bringing forward butterflies and electric energy, feelings that are less present in her current reality.

- *Am I strange for enjoying gay sexuality as a straight woman?* Our fantasy life is fantastically, wildly queer! There is a blurring of the lines we perceive for ourselves in our reality when in fantasy space. If there wasn't, straight/cis people would likely not feel inclined to watch straight/cis porn. Instead, we might spend our time watching videos of the gender/sex we're attracted to in our day-to-day masturbating or hooking up with others of the same gender/sex. Clara's enjoyment of gay sexuality would actually make more sense as someone who is attracted to primarily cis/male bodies and people! When watching straight/cis porn, the arousal wraps itself around and is connected to images of penises and vulvas, the "masculine" and "feminine" and neutral aspects of the scene. We are interacting with and finding arousal and excitement in it all, without implication for our lived reality and the very real feelings that we uncover and that give us important information about who we are attracted to, what our gender is, and who we want to love in reality. This is not to say that if we have someone who hypothetically identifies as a cis female who partners with cis males but finds herself fantasizing about other cis or trans females that there is never any implication for her reality with that in mind. Sometimes our fantasies point to truths that we have a hard time seeing or reconciling with the realities we exist within; sometimes they are simply play space, dreamlike abstractions. We get to determine which is which.
- *Does this mean anything for my marriage?* Clara feels content in her marriage, happy with the life and connection she shares with her husband. She is bumping into a hard truth we all have to contend with in relationships: we will not and cannot have everything we want. Our partners will not and cannot meet all of our needs. It is possible to both be happy and crave other feelings, other experiences, and to want to revisit aspects of life that aren't as present or that are entirely absent. Clara doesn't want to change or renegotiate her monogamy. These feelings and experiences are alive and vibrant in her solo sexual life and allow her to step into new relationship chemistry, new love in a way that fulfills that want in as full a way as is possible given her desire to

keep things status quo, to keep her marital agreements solidly intact and operational. It fills that cup in a safe, but real enough way. Say her husband were to suddenly feel threatened by these feelings, insecure about her engagement with them, and so determines he wants her to stop watching the show. One potential consequence might be that the longing that she was working through and fulfilling would eventually dissipate with lack of inspiration and she would return to existing within the feelings associated with and inhabiting her marriage. Another option would be that the feelings, without an outlet or something to connect to, moving them along, enabling a want or desire to be met, would become stronger and more compelling. On the "risk trusting and let go" versus "distrust and control" continuum, I think we can agree that one end of the spectrum is generally a better bet.

Our fantasies (including the fantasies we consume through television shows, movies, fiction podcasts, and porn) round out our lives and put us in touch with elements we need at any given moment, day, or chapter in our journeys. Taking away, forbidding, or demanding less often only inspires more desire for more. Getting curious about it's role and function if the frequency of engagement becomes problematic, places us on a more meaningful path towards understanding and if necessary, change.

Fantasy and Consent

When having sex with my partner, I find myself jumping from a moment with them, to fantasies of my co-worker. This happens like ping-pong the entire time! I'm not sure if it's my ADHD or what, but I feel weird about it. I don't like having basically added a third to our time unbeknownst to my partner, but I also feel like I'm violating my co-worker by sexualizing them in this way. It makes it hard to be "casual" and "chatty" with them the next day. How do I make this stop?

Can we cheat or "micro-cheat" with our fantasies? No! We get to fantasize about anyone at any time without shame. Why? Because the people that exist in our fantasies are not real people! When we engage with a fantasy about our boss, for example, we are taking the internal visual we have of that person and projecting qualities, stories, and ideas onto them in our imagination play space. They are not real, they are not them, they are actually – us! We are the characters in our fantasies because we are actively making them up. They are our stories, feelings, and pictures puzzle-pieced together. In this sense, consent is not required. This goes for our memories as well. Our memories are ours, to visit and revisit, elaborate on and embellish in fantasy form as often as we like. This can feel weird, of course, but it is the reality of living life with and alongside other people. Those experiences get placed in memory storage for us to interact with in whatever capacity is interesting or useful for us moving forward. The person in the memory is, once again, no longer them in reality; they have become brain content, a character held together by the pieces of memory we can grab that become interwoven in story, projection, emotion. Betty Dodson (1996) first introduced this idea in her infamous book, *Sex for One: The Joy of Selfloving*, explaining how we play all the parts in our fantasies. There is no separation from ourselves in the content of our own creation. I am both pursuer and the pursued, the dominant and submissive partner, myself and other, or others.

Fantasy as Intrusion

What if we are on the receiving end of a fantasy that we find disturbing? That we cannot seem to shake? The important factor here always is whether we find ourselves compelled to act on our fantasies, to bring them into our reality. If that is the situation, seeking out a therapist is a necessary and important step. If bringing it to life is something we can rule out, the most valuable thing we can do to help a fantasy along its way is to stop resisting it, to return back to the way we receive and interact with dreams. The fantasy is likely visiting you for a reason: potentially helping us work through challenges in life, past or present; touching on themes, feelings, and/or abstract representations of things that are hard to grasp and interpret with any clarity. We are also capable of being simultaneously shocked/repulsed and aroused at things that are off limits, horrifying, and/or forbidden. Releasing ourselves of any personal attachment to, or responsibility for, the fantasy, conclusions about selfhood connected to it (e.g. *I dreamed about cheating on my partner so I'm a bad person*), and sense of identification with it can unhook the anxiety that it gets tangled up in that then keeps it solidly in place, stuck in our life and orbit. *Why am I having this fantasy? What does it mean? Am I a bad person? Maybe there's a reason for it – I'd better return to it to find out. Oh god, I just did it again, I must really want this, I must really be bad.*

But I Don't Fantasize About Explicit Sex!

If we erase the entire fantasy-sharing conversation between Amelia and Taylor from the beginning of this chapter, and imagine instead that although Amelia doesn't watch porn, she frequently enjoys imagining romantic encounters with her celebrity crushes that involve long walks, deep conversation, and profound emotional connection. How might the conflict look different? When attempting to draw out the fantasy landscape of both partners to normalize erotic fantasy as a process (because porn *is* one form of fantasy and fantasy *can be* pornographic), these kinds of examples are often given as less threatening and more permissive than literal oral or penetrative sex with no demonstration of care, romantic connection, or love between partners. Why might this be so? If we take the fantasy of penetration with a strap-on as an example, what makes imagining that particular act with a stranger more threatening to a relationship than the fantasy of love connection between the partner and someone else? Much of this has to do with our socialization and what we learn about what sex is and has to offer us based on gender norms.

- Socialized female = emotional expression, trust and openness, nurturing, vulnerability = encouraged in everyday life and relationships (family, friendships).
- Socialized male = emotional expression, trust and openness, nurturing, vulnerability = sex.

When sex is the primary source of our most basic relational needs and wants (connection, love, acceptance, intimacy, vulnerability, nurturing, and care, etc.), then sex is going to be on the mind – a lot! Sex is going to be a driving force, celebrated and sought after with enthusiasm and grieved deeply and desperately when absent. The images, the porn, then, represent so much more than just the behaviors it demonstrates, in the same way that long walks on the beach hand-in-hand do.

Fantasy Wrap-Up

Fantasy is woven into our reality, nearly every facet of our day, and has been practiced since we were children. It is simply too complex a system to attempt to shut down, even selectively. Instead, can we attempt to accept our fantasies in their absurdity, edginess, transgressiveness even? Can we give ourselves full permission to invite them in, rather than try and fight them out, kicking up anxiety, taking us away from our partners, and from our sensual and sexual experience? There is no need to do anything with them at all unless they begin to ask to be taken beyond the fantasy realm, unless we are truly tormented by their content. They are an offline, processing, reorganizing, reorienting, balance-creating, control-granting, play place and tool. They are half our active input, half subconscious material. Let them visit, let them be, let them go.

Porn

Porn gets a lot of credit for a heap load of problems that extend far and beyond sex. It has single handedly been told to: ruin marriages; light up and feed addiction centers in the brain; change how penises respond to intimacy and sensation; create a "slippery slope" in terms of problematic or compulsive sexual behavior; incite violence; objectify women; and on and on. Some blame is warranted for some of the list items above; but how do we adequately address anything when it's blamed for most everything? It's an easy target for partners in relationships when looking to blame something external (which we will always look to do to absolve the pain of responsibility), for turbulence we encounter around our intimacy and beyond! As Dr. Marty Klein reminds us, porn is fantasy put-to-screen. This is reflected in the broad spectrum of sexual content that porn encapsulates. If through fantasy we approach the unapproachable, interact with the forbidden, work through trauma, play with power, manage and process feelings, be someone else, practice or rehearse, gain a sense of control, and so on, then porn demonstrates exactly what has gone on in this realm for other people and what other people imagine it's made of. This is precisely why porn can be problematic: some things are better left in the safe container of our own imaginations. Our fantasies are not politically correct and porn illuminates that. Can we do that differently? Absolutely! There is a wide variety of ethical and feminist porn available on the market. But as decades have gone by with a vast variety of pornographic content readily available, it has become a meaningful part of people's solo sexual lives, embedding itself in our erotic routine and imaginations, often from our early, most formative years onward. Our developing sexuality feels drawn to it, not only because it's forbidden, breaks rules, and is something our adults want us to stay away from (the ultimate draw), but also, and very importantly, because porn can be a useful tool as a vehicle for self-exploration, a way to find ourselves in other people, a route towards greater learning about our evolving eroticism, and a means for connecting with, understanding, and creating spaciousness and ease in our bodies.

So, *is* porn a problem? *The* problem? Is the porn I watch shameful? Is it cheating? Will it cause people to want to cheat? Is it bad for relationships? Can we stop this train, putting a halt to the consumption of erotic media even if we wanted (*genuinely* wanted) to? Do we need porn when we have fantasy? Do we need porn when we have love?

What Porn Is and What Porn Isn't

Amelia: You're watching porn instead of having sex with me.
Taylor: It's not like that ... ugh, this is such a frustrating conversation every time! It's not like a replacement for you. It's different!

Amelia: *I get that getting off to massive penises and huge tits and asses is different than having sex with me, that's obvious!*

Therapist: *Can I interject for a moment? Taylor, this idea that porn is not a replacement for Amelia, can you talk about that further?*

Taylor: *She just fights me when I talk about it.*

Therapist: *Let's just try again. Amelia, can we try this again? [Amelia nods, reluctantly.] Let's see if we can all slow down a bit, soften up our defenses, and listen to understand each other like we're on the same team. Because we are, right? [makes eye contact with Taylor and Amelia to confirm]. Taylor, when you're ready.*

Taylor: *It doesn't feel like a choice between the two most of the time. When I watch porn, I'm usually taking a break from work, or I'm super tired but want some relief. It's easy for me, and it can be quick. Or however long I want it to be.*

Therapist: *As opposed to sex with Amelia.*

Amelia: *But that's not fair! I'm not asking for a multi-hour sex fest here. Who ever said I wouldn't be down for a quickie?*

Taylor: *That's what I can't seem to get across. I love being intimate with Amelia, but it involves much more from me. Not that she puts anything on me, I just feel like the expectations I have for myself are that I need to be attentive, be loving, give pleasure, cuddle, or be affectionate after, and so on. As the eldest from a big, Irish family with four siblings, I don't know how to not overly attend to others. Even a "quickie" involves so much more than I regularly have the capacity for in the midst of works stress and our insanely packed social life. I really love her, AND I just wanna zone out and have a freaking orgasm. That's all.*

Watching and masturbating to porn and making love to or having sex with partners are experiences that frequently get conflated, placed under the same umbrella of human experience. As such, it is often imagined that one can, and often does, replace the other, meaning that we get our sexual needs met through porn. Which brings us to what "needs" sex satisfies to begin with.

- *What porn is*: erotic images designed to kick up arousal in the body leading toward orgasm (or not).
- *What partnered sex is*: inherently vulnerable experience involving expression, sharing, communication, care, and (frequently) investment in the other and their experience of us.

When viewing porn, we have full control over the content of the porn, the duration of the porn, how we engage with and navigate sensation in our bodies, when to pause, stop, or even shut it down entirely and move on with our day. When stepping into partnered sex, control is shifty, elusive, and makes itself most readily available in the respect and care category, rather than the emotional, sensory, arousal category, as intimacy is inherently risky and involves co-sculpting experience with another person with vulnerability at the center (i.e. shedding control in favor of authenticity and surrender). We cannot control how our partners feel about what they are experiencing with us; we cannot control how our own bodies, hearts, and minds respond to the interaction; we cannot control what our own vulnerability brings to the surface. In other words, we have far less control.

Enough Is Enough

When you watch porn, or fantasize about other people, it makes me feel like I'm not enough for you.

We are enough as individuals, as people. We cannot be "enough" to fully satisfy our partners in all ways in an ongoing way, long term. This is altogether impossible as we've learned from how nuanced and evolving our sexual wants are. Our partners cannot be everything to us, fulfill every desire and need, nor us to them. We choose to stay because we are happy "enough," satisfied "enough," fulfilled "enough." Fantasy in all forms (porn, movies, TV, daydreams, stories) takes care of the rest.

Porn helps us visit the stirrings of our erotic imaginations risk free, in the same way fantasy does. We can approach the unapproachable, visit another life/be another person, practice for "moves" in the bedroom with our partner, with the added benefit of other people having done more of the work for us, helping us enter into the fantasy in a more immersive way with real imagery and real human beings.

Additional Challenges: Our Relationship Narrative

Remember our myth busting list from several chapters back? Our Disney vs. Reality reckoning? Let's review:

- We meet and find "the one."
- Partner should meet all our needs: sexual, emotional, spiritual, etc.
- Healthy, "good" relationships should be easy (i.e. devoid of or very little conflict).

- Similarities are the most important indicator of compatibility and a sign of closeness:
  - Should enjoy similar things, share the same values, have similar goals for the future;
  - Finish each other's sentences – "two peas in a pod" – very little differentiation.
- No secrets (i.e. no private life).
- No more attraction or feelings of lust for other people. Physical attraction is "very important" initially, then something we should feel shame for caring about as relationship progresses.
- No solo sexual life (or very minimal – but what does that look like?).

Based on these ideas, what must watching porn (or even masturbating and/ or fantasizing for some) mean for my relationship?

- They're no longer attracted to me/my kind of body;
- They long to cheat, have cheated, or are likely going to;
- The porn *is* cheating;
- They're a sex addict;
- They have a secret life;
- I'm inadequate, inexperienced, not good enough;
- They don't love me or care about my feelings;
- They are selfish: they "get to have their cake and eat it too."

Myth Busting

Let's go through some common concerns that surface around porn and challenge their validity. Of course, it is important to consider your personal responses to the myths described: locating your perspective today moves us towards behaviors that align with our current understanding uniquely.

1 *"They're directing their sexual energy toward porn instead of me."* Suggests there's a limit to our erotic potential, a limit to the amount of desire and eroticism we can tap into. We are capable of cultivating end-less amounts of sexual energy, even in the absence of erections, orgasms, or lubrication (i.e. physiological responsiveness).
2 *I can't compete with the "porn body."* "Porn or no porn, every man and woman (person) has to figure out how to feel ok with themselves when they don't look as good as others, have as much money as others, or have children as well-behaved as others. This is the fundamental exis-tential task of all people who want to enjoy life, and porn didn't invent it" (Klein, 2016, p. 111).

3 *Porn treats women as objects, my partner must be objectifying me too!*
Porn treats *people* as objects, because objectification is a core element of physical attraction for many, inseparable from our experience. We may enjoy the object (e.g. physical appearance, qualities, characteristics), which often leads to exploration of whether we enjoy the other aspects of the person (personality, interests, hobbies, values), which may or may not lead to love. We interact with the whole person in partnered sex (our stories about who our partner is, feelings about those stories, shared history and connection) *and* engage with and have a relationship to our partner as object in long-term relationships. Extracting that complexity from the shared atmosphere is impossible.

Turning to Porn to Feel

Lily (29-year-old, cis female) grabs a coffee at the local crowded coffee shop she frequents and calls her friend immediately after to talk gossip about the pretentious customers she encountered in the parking lot. She gets to her lunch break at work and calls her dad to get advice on a challenging situation with her boss (and to vent a little). After addressing the challenging situation, she confides in her colleague about the bravery it took to stand up to her superior. She gets off, heads home, and gives her partner the Cliff Notes (summary) while snuggling on the couch.

Mark (30-year-old, cis/male) grabs a coffee at the local crowded coffee shop he frequents and then sits in traffic, anxiously trying to get to work on time. He arrives to his lunch break and strategizes with himself around a challenging situation with his boss, formulating a plan, amping himself up for the confrontation. After addressing the challenging situation, he replays the scenario over a few times in his mind, analyzing his words, the words of his boss, trying to reassure himself he did that just fine. He gets off, heads home, and gives his partner the Cliff Notes (condensed breakdown of the day) while snuggling on the couch.

If we return to our understanding of socialization for the examples above (namely that people socialized male are largely trained to hide their vulnerability, only display or express anger, frustration, or jealousy, and figure out solutions rather than ask questions or ask for help), and combine that with what we understand about the parasympathetic nervous system and sexual stimulation/orgasm as self-regulating mechanisms (catharsis, achieve emotional balance and homeostasis), who would we guess might masturbate and/or watch porn more? It's easy. And this is not always specific to gender socialization! There are different ways of interacting and being in relationship to emotion based on culture and heritage, family and history, and a multitude of other factors.

If we imagine Mark initiating therapy because he masturbates to porn three times a day, would we be surprised? When Lily feels free to move through, express, and process emotional experience multiple times a day in connection with others, the sensations associated with Mark's experience stay in his body, translated into tension that accumulates as he continues along. Perhaps masturbation and fantasy (i.e. porn) help him stay alert, focused, able to function in his job, giving him physical and emotional reprieve and release. Perhaps they help him stay regulated rather than panicking or sitting with mounting anxiety. What would happen for Lily if she suddenly couldn't share with her friend, dad, coworker, partner? If she didn't have "pallet cleanser" moments of connection and expression throughout her day? What would happen for Mark if we asked him to quit masturbating and watching porn?

When moving through our emotions (i.e. releasing tension) is not available one way (vulnerability and emotional sharing in conversation), our physiology and imagination (often with the help of explicit media to bring us further into the fantasy element with efficiency) provide an alternative that won't get you high, isn't bad for your health, and that we can generally attend to quickly and efficiently. This is built into our design – maybe *by* design?

If we find ourselves watching porn constantly, filling all the little spaces in our day, taking up meaningful space in our relationships in a way that creates real and palpable distance, it is important to check in: *Am I primarily or even exclusively dropping into and feeling my feelings through my sexuality? Why am I needing fantasy, escape, regulation to this degree? What am I attempting to escape from, regulate, or release? If I want to have less eggs in the "porn" basket, can I learn how to cultivate connection, expression, and release in other ways? What might I need to change to make my reality more "me," or more rewarding?* Learning to explore other avenues in favor of meeting the needs porn and masturbation satisfy, which often requires undoing primary aspects of our "training" and socialization, may not scratch the itch in the same way, but it can make porn less compelling as the sole source of an important part of our self-care. Our sexuality takes care of us in a wide variety of ways, there is complexity in all of it, worthy of being explored and understood. What sexual behavior "means" for one person, what it addresses, does not apply to all.

No More Porn

What happens when we focus on porn as the problem? What is missed when one partner "sends" the other to work on quitting their habit on their own? Do we understand what might be challenging about their intimacy, their romantic and emotional connection? Is porn helping one partner stay in the midst of neglect, conflict, illness, and so on? Is performance anxiety a struggle? Pressure (internal or external or both) to "do things right"? Is engaging in fantasy regularly, or even very frequently, helping them cope with depression or struggles in their reality? Wouldn't that be important to know and work with? How would we identify it if we're more concerned with images on the screen and their representations? When confronted with the reality of our partner's solo sexual life, attraction to other bodies, scenarios, experiences, what are we really talking about? What do we risk in avoiding this exploration? Insecurities, shame, and confusion on the part of the partner, but which are also present in the relationship as a whole. We miss the opportunity to look at our own attachment history and wounding, the challenges we face when real intimacy reveals itself, the associations and predictions that make partnered sex hard. We miss the opportunity to understand the relational dynamic in a meaningful way, identifying places where partners miss each other, feel hurt, or are backing away. In short, centering porn in the conversation is a distraction from much greater, more meaningful exploration! Once the porn is gone, the challenges it brought to the surface or illuminated remain.

Porn and the porn industry itself are tricky and problematic (they can be exploitative, degrading, dehumanizing, etc.). Watching erotic media as a way of moving ourselves deeper into letting go, into homeostasis, is a different topic entirely. Let's not conflate the two.

> "Go to war with your sexuality, you will lose and end up in more trouble than before you started."

Kink as Shame, Kink as Cure: Interview with Abbie Nederhoed

Abbie (A) is a licensed clinical social worker and a therapist who specializes in kink, non-monogamy, and alternative relationship styles. As an educator, Abbie seeks to share from lived experience, bringing additional insight from their mental health and sex therapy training.

Paula Leech (P): What is kink?

A: Any "non-conventional" sexual practice. Someone once applied it to a literal definition of a kink outside of sexuality, like a bend or a knot. So, this is like a bend in your sexuality. Trouble is, what is "conventional"? Someone could say "I like being choked," or, "I like being spanked," and then many people nowadays might respond with "That's not kinky, everyone likes that."

P: The criteria keep changing as things become more "normative."

A: Right!

P: From there it seems very likely that different groups have different definitions and within those groups there's variance. With such a shifty conceptualization, it seems like the perfect breeding ground for shame. Do you think shame is something that everyone encounters when bumping into aspects of their sexuality that fall outside of their understanding of that rigid "norm" that we are referencing?

A: Unfortunately, I think it is something everyone encounters; my own belief is that it doesn't have to be that way. I have a friend that was raised in the kink world, in the leather community, their parents are leather contestant holders. Did they experience shame around kink as they came into it or was kink just normalized? Did they experience shame if they realized they *weren't* into kink?

P: Could the kink actually be "I'm vanilla?"

A: Or could we change the narrative for shame to not exist if we talked about things openly growing up, embracing and normalizing a multitude of sexual expression, or are we still going to get it from a social community world standpoint as inevitably behaviors get categorized and judged relative to others. And is that just always going to exist because it's really hard for it not to?

P: How might you describe what most don't understand about what kink is and is not as it relates to our sexuality? Are there any myths to dispel on a general level?

A: On a general level I think what you most often see is "This is abuse." This brings us to consent. On a generalized level, like for people new to kink, I'm personally not a huge fan of enthusiastic consent because I think consent's allowed to be complex, but maybe informed consent is a good place to start. To actually *give* informed consent, you have to know yourself well! The intensity and depth that goes into conversations around kink, I don't have in a lot of other places in my life. But I think people just see the surface of things and label it as abuse when they don't know everything that has gone into creating that thing. I think kink is also a really good place for predators to hide, which then contributes to all of the stereotypes it's been given.

P: I'm wondering if you wouldn't mind giving a glimpse behind the curtain in terms of what gets discussed around consent? What does a typical negotiation process look like?

A: So, if I was going to negotiate with someone brand new, and hypothetically we're negotiating some rope [a form of bondage, also known as Shibari], I have to know what's within my risk profile. For example, if I'm tying someone new, I probably won't suspend them in the air the first time, I'm going to ask to keep things on the ground where I know it's safer. I have to know about them: where it's OK to touch on their body, where not to touch (I'm still going to ask permission before touching your body). I have to know where it's OK to put rope, we have to talk about fluids (so if you're doing any mouth rope or crotch rope, those are things that you could risk fluid transfer, so we talk about that). We talk about nerves, so as a bottom you have to understand where nerves live in your body and what impingements may feel like; you have to know if you've had any previous nerve damage. We'll sometimes talk through what's going to happen, the whole scene. Like, "We'll do this, and then this, and this is how we'll end." We're going to talk about what we each of us need afterwards, and if we don't align on any of these things, is there room for compromise or to be able to say "Hey, I don't think we're a good fit for playing together," and that either of us can say that at any time. I have to know what I'm looking for and what they're looking for out of this scene. Are there any possible emotional triggers? Are there any possible physical triggers? And it's OK to say "I don't know" to those questions because a lot of us are still learning and exploring, but we can also negotiate into that, "What're we going to do when this happens?" Or at least, "What're we going to try," "What're we going to do when something goes wrong?"

P: It's so involved, and my brain goes two places simultaneously, it's like: in terms of creating a safe context for surrender, going through this conversation we're getting to know so much about one another and our limits and each other's bodies beforehand. It really creates the scaffolding necessary to freely explore, as a real celebration of boundaries and respect for all involved. Also, where I go is: I can imagine people feeling like the conversation/negotiation takes a lot of the excitement out of it, like when we talk to couples about planning sex nights and they respond with grief over the lack of spontaneity.

A: I love spontaneity too, I love not knowing what's going to happen and I don't want to know every detail of the scene. It really depends on how much you know and trust the other person. What I say to people that I may be negotiating with for the first time is, "Hey, I'm really connection based, so here's what I'm willing to negotiate within my risk profile, and here are some things I would be OK not fully negotiating for a first time." And then, do *they* want those things negotiated? With people I'm very established with, going into an experience I'll say "Hey, this is my mood, this is the connection I'm looking for, here are the things we've pre-negotiated, let's go." But that took all the talking and getting-to-know in previous experiences to get there.

P: What if we did that across the board, even in vanilla sex, where there is just a lot more conversation in the beginning and then we could loosen a bit as we moved along as opposed to just very little or no conversation at all, at any point? Would we have the kinds of associations many of us have with sex? Would a lot of the challenges people bump into be there if we learned to communicate around it with such skill and detail, and as directly and honestly as you're describing?

A: We get caught in this narrative of "this is supposed to be mysterious and I'm supposed to not tell you what I want," and I'm like "if you actually got your wants and needs met, wouldn't that feel really fulfilling?"

P: Once we make peace with our kinks, and for many people that looks like finding community and coming out of isolation, how can we partner with them toward our healing? Can you give an example or examples of what that looks like?

A: We can partner with our kinks to continue to engage in acceptance of self. We can partner with our kinks to practice being in our bodies and experience emotions. Kinks can become a safe place to experience emotions that have been shamed/not allowed/we don't have experiences of seeing that emotion portrayed safely. An example of this can be someone doing an impact or spanking scene – we can go through an entire range of emotions in a structured setting (container) that we created with another person. It is normal to feel anger when experiencing pain, even if it is pain we consented to, so a scene can be a safe place to experience anger without needing anyone to fix it or change it, we can scream and yell/release and create safety in those actions in ways that don't cause harm to other people.

Mindfulness practices don't always click for everyone. Some people have a harder time naming their emotions in the moment, and what may be easier for them is identifying the physical sensations they are experiencing. I have learned that rope bondage can be a great tool for learning mindfulness. You have to be risk aware and in your own body and notice things like, "Am I experiencing circulation loss or could this be nerve damage (you have to know the signs of each and what things to look for in your body, 'Is this tingling, is this numb, is this only happening in two of my fingers versus my whole hand')?" These body scans we do in rope can be a great mindfulness practice, they help you identify good pain vs bad pain, what is harm vs discomfort. For example, someone has rope on their body and it is being maneuvered in a way that compresses their body into an uncomfortable position that may even hurt a little bit. They do a body scan and notice none of the pain is pain that would put them at risk of harm in that moment, they can then decide, "I want to stay in this position a little longer and be curious about it, explore the discomfort. Can I breathe into it? Can I find other parts of my body to breathe into? Can I make a micro-movement with my body that may shift the discomfort?" It creates a space for the person to explore and play in their own body. Once you've done that a lot, you can start to translate that skill to emotions or experiences: "This emotional experience I am having is really uncomfortable, it hurts. I am having anxiety, I am noticing increased breathing, it feels like my heart is racing, my chest is heavy, this is really uncomfortable, but I am noticing that I am not at risk of harm in this moment by this emotion, so, can I explore this a little bit more and be curious?" Or the opposite might be happening: "I am noticing that if something doesn't change quickly then I am at risk of this emotional experience harming me – this is not a safe emotion for me to experience in this moment and I need to get out of it."

P: Seems like not only profound connection to other people that you're speaking to, but intimate connection with self, the consequences of which directly and powerfully impact the other areas of our lives: our emotional intelligence and attunement, our connection to physical body and wellbeing, our ability to interact with thoughts and emotions in new and curious ways. Seems like what you're describing, when approached as carefully and thoughtfully as you've described, would only lead to a deep sense of self-trust. What could be more healing than that?

17 Sex and Porn "Addiction"

If you look up "sex addiction" online, odds are you'll find you are one. Assessments and infographics list characteristics common to "sex addicts" that are vague, moralistic, and pathologizing of sexual expression, experience, and behavior that has nothing to do whatsoever with compulsivity or the experience of being "out of control." Examples include:

- Watching pornography (so, a substantial portion of the planet).
- Frequently thinking sexual thoughts or having sexual urges/feelings (so my "addiction" was at its peak when I was 14?!).
- Excessive masturbation (How much constitutes "excessive"? Where is the line?).
- Compulsively engaging in fantasy (we do compulsively engage in fantasy all day every day – some of which is sexual).
- Hiding aspects of your sexual life and behaviors (Are we talking about cheating here? Or simply fantasies and behaviors we engage in on our own that we don't share with our partners because we can't and usually don't share everything?).
- Sadistic and/or masochistic behaviors (Is consensual impact play or degradation, for example, addiction? Regardless of frequency?).
- Having caused someone emotional pain with or as a result of your sexual behaviors (this is dangerous: there is a huge difference between violating someone's overt and clear sexual boundaries and experiencing hurt or pain as a result of disapproving of someone's solo sexual behaviors and habits. This criterion is, again, far too vague).

Based on a list like this, nearly any sexual behavior or struggle can find a spot under the addiction umbrella, alongside a treatment methodology (sex addiction treatment) without further investigation into what the client understands their struggle to be, mean, or how it actually manifests.

DOI: 10.4324/9781003369080-20

What is it you want me to understand about you, OR importantly, what is it you want me to understand about your partner, when you say you/they have a porn or sex addiction?

(Braun-Harvey, 2016)

Adem (cis/het, 23-year-old male from Turkey) recently relocated with his family to Las Vegas, Nevada for his father's work and to begin a master's degree at UNV. Despite speaking English fluently, Adem finds himself feeling overwhelmed with culture shock and out-of-sorts and out-of-place socially. He struggles to strike up conversation with peers at school and feels self-conscious about his English, resulting in a great deal of isolation and loneliness.

Devoutly Muslim, Adem initiates therapy out of shame and guilt for his recent behavior around porn, the viewing of which, to any frequency, is at odds with his faith. He finds himself watching sometimes up to five times a day, a drastic escalation from his typical porn use at home in Turkey (a few times a week). He is completing his studies, although sometimes with difficulty, and finds himself easily distracted and eager to get back to viewing porn. He pursues therapy for his "porn addiction" and accompanying anxiety and depression.

According to the kind of criteria listed above, Adem certainly qualifies as a porn addict. If the therapist is in agreement, what might treatment look like? We know that the focus would be on porn, his relationship to porn, and on managing or shifting his frequency of viewing erotic media (sometimes via abstinence). Yet, if we look more closely there are a few key details even in this extremely short description that are important to bring curiosity to:

- The resistance he feels around pornography as it relates to his faith and how that shows up in his body. Is there an erotic element to engaging in something "off limits?" How much of a role does it play if so? How much more enticing is an experience when we're working to resist it? What has this looked like for him?
- How has the anxiety about who he is as a result of betraying his faith, and what it means to him that he views porn, embedded him in a cycle of porn use that self-sustains. That is *I can't watch porn I'm not allowed; I watched porn, I must be a bad person; I might as well watch it again, I'm a bad person.*
- Adem's isolation and disorientation and how it coincides with the uptick in his porn use/desire to escape into fantasy.

Is Adem's behavior "out-of-control" or does it make sense given his circumstance? Can we begin to comprehend how challenging and destabilizing it might be to relocate to another country, away from everything familiar, and start anew? How might our reaction to his story shift if he was simply watching a lot of TV each day, eager to get back to his shows after a day at a new school, in a new culture, with entirely new people that he may perceive he does or does not fit in with? Porn use (i.e masturbation) provides the added benefit of release, the catharsis experience that helps us self-soothe and recalibrate. Why wouldn't that be appealing? In deciding Adem "has a problem" are we setting him up for more struggle (added shame and guilt, which can translate to more profound depression and anxiety compounding that which is already fueling the behavior)? Might this desire pass as he acclimates, finds community, makes friends?

What Are We "Addicted" to?

Defining addiction is tricky even as we apply the term to substances. Does one need to be drinking all day, from the time one wakes until one falls asleep, for example? What about someone who only drinks at the weekends but is a binge drinker, to the point of blacking out every time? Despite the relative ambiguity, one thing is clear as we reflect on these particular questions: alcohol is the problem. When it comes to sex, things get blurry.

The argument for and against including "sex addiction" as a diagnosis in the *Diagnostic and Statistical Manual of Mental Disorders* (DSM) has been an ongoing and polarizing one. The American Association of Sexuality Educators, Counselors, and Therapists (AASECT) released a statement that posited the following:

> AASECT recognizes that people may experience significant physical, psychological, spiritual and sexual health consequences related to their sexual urges, thoughts or behaviors. AASECT recommends that its members utilize models that do not unduly pathologize consensual sexual behaviors. AASECT (1) does not find sufficient empirical evidence to support the classification of sex addiction or porn addiction as a mental health disorder, and (2) does not find the sexual addiction training and treatment methods and educational pedagogies to be adequately informed by accurate human sexuality knowledge. Therefore, it is the position of AASECT that linking problems related to sexual urges, thoughts or behaviors to a porn/sexual addiction process cannot be advanced by AASECT as a standard of practice for sexuality education delivery, counseling or therapy.
>
> (www.aasect.org/position-sex-addiction)

The statement itself divided the field, where certified sex therapists and certified sex addiction therapists found themselves overtly and publicly at odds, and the debate/conversation continues to this day. This seems like a fairly simple argument to resolve: What does the research say? Well, research supports arguments in favor and against sex and porn addictions, and they exist in abundance. We can quite literally find compelling evidence (and podcasts and blogs and entire social media profiles devoted to both causes) for either argument, a common dilemma for relationships trying to navigate these waters. Yet, over the years the inclusion of "sex addiction" or "sexual compulsivity" or "out of control sexual behavior" in the DSM has been repeatedly denied due to, as AASECT stated, a "lack of empirical evidence." This has been joined by shopping, working, and internet use on the list of contenders for the addiction title, who have ultimately and repeatedly been rejected for inclusion as diagnosable disorders as well. The symptomology of "sex addiction" is regarded as symptoms of other disorders: that is anxiety or obsessive compulsive disorder (severe anxiety). According to David Ley (2014), author of *The Myth of Sex Addiction*, in the "Rationale" section of DSM V's workgroup's discussion, the clinical need for inclusion of a diagnosis was based on "demand" from consumers and providers to recognize and diagnose the significant amount of people seeking and receiving treatment for "out-of-control" sexual behaviors.

So, is sex an addiction? How are we collectively conceptualizing what sex is and means in order to understand what its addictive qualities might be? We might assume an expansive understanding of "sex" will be comprised of four major ingredients:

1　Physiological response: our sexual response and arousal cycle.
2　Emotional experience and expression.
3　Thoughts and fantasy.
4　Behaviors: literal tongue on body, hand on skin, penis in mouth, etc.

Can we be addicted to our own, built-in physiology that we've been inhabiting and exploring since childhood? To feelings or emotional concepts we experience within ourselves? To the literal behaviors involved? It would be false to claim that as humans we aren't moving through our day searching for happiness, experiences that bring us satisfaction and peace. When we can look to ourselves, to our own bodies and sensation to provide an experience that touches on these themes, why wouldn't we? Meditation provides benefits for many, a sense of connectedness, peace, and stillness. Can we become addicted to meditating? What makes meditation different from self-touch?

What We "Use" Sex for

What are your motivations for engaging sexually with yourself or others on any particular day? More than likely, your response would vary depending on the events of day, state of the relationship, mood, level of energy, and so on. And guess what? We get to have a list of reasons each time, an honest one, shame free! Even if we are looking for straight-up big-bang sensation and pleasure, we do not escape connection, sharing, vulnerability, and so on. Even if we tried, attempting to show up for sexual experience with "shoulds" attached to our intentions wouldn't work. Our psychology, emotionality, wants, and desires would find their way in. The nature of what sex asks of us, what sex is, is present with us regardless. So, let's return to a few of the statements from the beginning of the previous chapter, and take a closer look at motivations generally thought of as negative when it comes to sex so we can make peace with their inherent existence in our intimate sexual lives and experience.

- *Using sex to "self-medicate"*: Sex feels good, which is the appeal! We gravitate toward things that feel good, experiences that allow us to move into pleasurable feelings and sensations. It is on our mind, a primary motivation all day every day. How can I feel more comfortable? I can't live without yoga class at least three times a week. I can't wait to put my feet up and listen to a podcast on the couch when I get home. Are we self-medicating when we snuggle up with a super soft blanket? When we curl up with that podcast? Release into yoga? I guess it would depend on your definition of what exactly it means to self-medicate. Sex is not a substance, sex is a complex experience that we hold within us, that we can access at any time. You cannot "medicate" with who you are. We find comfort, pleasure, exploration, and sensation within ourselves all the time, and we call that coping, creating balance, or stabilizing ourselves.
- *Using sex as escape*: Sex is an experience that can hold seemingly contradictory feelings, experiences, and ideas in the same place. We can approach sex to both escape and feel connected at the same time (e.g. in escaping the version of ourselves we inhabit in our day to day, we are more able to connect with our partners). When we reference surrender, isn't this precisely what we're talking about? Sex helps us detach from our daytime brains, social norms, scripts we inhabit, and step into an emotional, abstract, primal space. It is meaningful to many of us because of the sense of balance it creates in how it can uniquely fulfill so many of our wants and basic needs as human beings for intimacy, connection, and love in one place. It is escape and we need it to be.
- *Using sex to feed addiction (i.e. sex as an addiction)*: – Truly out-of-control sexual behavior, the kind where we're getting in trouble with work, unable to function and accomplish meeting our basic needs, and completely neglecting our relationships (we have to be careful with this one, because how different people define "neglect" can vary drastically), is fairly rare. Most of the time, what people are labeling as addiction is in reality simply problematic behavior that we feel a level of discomfort with on an individual level. At its most benign it can be used to describe someone who is simply a sexual person, more in touch with this part of

who they are. What we understand as true compulsivity has its origins in anxiety, or obsessive compulsive disorder, the true underlying cause in need of treatment.

Self-Harm vs Self-Care

There are exceptions to everything. For some, porn use can be truly problematic. There are those for whom sexuality feels and is wholly and entirely out of control. Most of us, however, are accustomed, have been trained, to find fault in our own sexual behavior and desires and those of others and therefore can bump into opportunities to do so frequently. There is a lengthy collection of "shoulds" waiting for us around every turn. What separates the kind of behaviors we gravitate toward in order to feel good, regulate our nervous systems, and stabilize unsteady emotions like meditation, exercise, watching a TV show, even having a glass of wine from self-touch and masturbation? What is the difference, truly, between being an avid runner who goes for runs twice a day to let off steam and feel connected to the body, and watching porn with the same regularity, give or take? On a philosophical level, this has everything to do with the values we hold around sex and what it means to be sexual, to prioritize our solo sexuality in any meaningful way. Armed with the very real and important differences between watching porn, engaging in fantasy, and partnered sex, knowing what we know about what these things do and do not provide us in terms of our basic wants and needs, let's break this down:

- *Running*: connecting with the body, engaging in emotional and physical release, interacting with pleasurable sensation ("runner's high," etc.), breaking up the different parts of the day (palate cleanser), taming stress, escape, doing something meaningful just for us.
- *Watching porn*: connecting with the body, engaging in emotional and physical release, interacting with pleasurable sensation, breaking up the different parts of the day (palate cleanser), taming stress, escape (moving into fantasy realm/story), doing something meaningful just for us (playing, evolving our understanding of our sexuality).

We view running as a form of self-care. Is engaging in our solo sexuality not accomplishing the same goal? If we free ourselves of our hang-ups and hard-wiring around what it means to be sexual, and particularly sexual on our own and with ourselves, isn't this fulfilling so much more than what is listed above? Providing balance and differentiation? Self-exploration, learning, and understanding?

Part III

Divorcing Anxiety from Your Sex Life

Actionable Steps

Now we get to work figuring out how to stop working at sex. We will:

- Train ourselves to secure the parasympathetic nervous system's position as primary in its relationship to the sympathetic nervous system, and how to respond more effectively when we do find ourselves in "fight or flight" or stress/fear/anxious territory (i.e., sympathetic nervous system activation).
- Practice letting go of tension in the body and in the mind, over-and-over again; and carving out and reinforcing new associations with sensual, sexual, and/or erotic energy and simulation.
- Begin to understand what is possible when we diminish, minimize, or even completely eliminate anxiety from the body, mind, and our relational dynamics sexually.
- Make room for the natural function of our sexual response cycle to come forward, keeping the chatter of our minds from hijacking our sexual functioning and the unfolding of arousal, orgasm, and potentially ejaculation (for people with penises), however those elements manifest today.
- Learn what it takes to feel rewarded from sex, every time, and how to cultivate real, honest intimacy with ourselves and others with ease.

Expect anxiety to greet you as you step into this part of your journey – it will and we want it to. We want to continue expanding our understanding of what it's made of and what barriers it presents. Resistance will only keep it in place. Still, identifying and processing some of the reasons for our anxiety, as we did in Part II, won't eliminate activation of it in real time. Rather than try and turn away, we are going to attempt to allow the feeling to be, turning toward and deeply learning what else it has for us, while communicating to the body that it no longer needs to protect us in

DOI: 10.4324/9781003369080-21

this way: we no longer require its warning, communicating safety (only if you truly are), and readiness for change (only if that feels true for you).

If you're partnered, it's useful to understand that unless they are reading this book alongside you and you're talking the chapters through, the relational anxiety that develops around sexual struggles is not being thoroughly looked at or addressed and, therefore, will still exist to some extent. Change on the part of one person does have an impact, however, and the new ways that we are able to come into our experience and make different choices in the face of anxiety that gets kicked up will prove useful. A new level of familiarity, self-knowledge, and presence in the body can't help but help!

You will feel stuck, or as if progress is elusive at some point in your journey (this is inevitable). If partnered, the relational dynamic is often a primary source of anxiety in the bedroom. Without proper guidance and a watchful, trained eye, we risk reinjuring ourselves, deepening or leaving unattended major wounding from our pasts, creating greater distance and misunderstanding in relationships. Given these factors, and the very real limitations to the kind of work available in a self-guided way, it is important to move through the experiences in the following pages while consulting/working with a trained, credentialed sex therapist. The American Association for Sexuality Educators, Counselors, and Therapists is a great resource and has a "find a therapist" tool that can help you locate certified sex therapists or sexual health professionals in your area. We deserve to get the most out of our healing, we deserve a full sexual and intimate life of our choosing.

18 Taking Responsibility

In Part II we dug deeply into some of the forces that make us "us," our "training" in sex and intimacy, the very real and important players, memories, relationships, systems, and overt and covert messages that exert varying degrees of influence behind the curtain of our sexuality. Were there chapters that were more impactful than others? Why? Were there areas of confusion, conflict (which is OK!), or even pain? What was it like to sit with those feelings? What "ah-ha!" moments surfaced for you? Answering even one of these questions means that we've gained greater understanding of ourselves sexually and intimately. Understanding fills in the spaces the unknown previously occupied. The less unknown territory there is, the less anxiety there is, or the ability for anxiety to create stories we trust.

Meaningful learning happens when we tie content back into our own lives, relating it to our story, reflecting on its unique manifestation in our own experience. Simply digging into research doesn't pack the same punch. To elaborate on, and then *reinforce*, this learning, we will put knowledge into action.

- Step 1: *know* and *think* about things differently.
- Step 2: *embody* them.

The tasks below give us some footing, or a starting point, in terms of consolidating information, providing scaffolding for how to implement a new mindset or frame for sex and intimacy in our day-to-day experiences, and introducing strategies we can bring with us into our sex. Many of these tasks seem basic and logical on the surface, but they require constant practice and reinforcement as our history, practiced processes, and associations surge to the surface in the heat of a moment. We will follow them up with exercises designed to bring us more deeply into our bodies, sensation, and towards the resolution of specific sexual struggles: our Basic and Advanced Practice chapters.

DOI: 10.4324/9781003369080-22

The tasks that follow are our way of beginning to take greater owner-ship. *This sexuality, this sex, this sexual and intimate life, is mine. I am no longer placing it upon others to figure out, myself to perform, or allowing it to be controlled by ghosts of the past. And it starts now.*

Fundamental Task #1

Perspective shift.

When working with couples, one of the first items on the agenda is to shift the lens from focusing on what the other person is doing and trying to control them, to focusing on what we are doing on our side of the street, working to understand and manage ourselves. The same logic applies to sex. The best way to be present with our partners is to be present with ourselves, that is *without worry, ego, anxiety, and pressure, I am freed up to be profoundly connected to my own experience, and to ask for what I want, set boundaries around what I don't, and to be more presently attuned to and with you, no barriers.* By saturating ourselves in our own experi-ence, we can befriend our own pleasure, bringing our sexual functioning solidly and happily online. Sound selfish? To zoom in further, *when we're in the company of significant levels of anxiety in a sexual experience, we can find ourselves:*

1 Abandoning what we want and need for the goal of pleasing our partners;
   Or
2 Becoming so consumed in how to get and stay aroused that we inadver-tently neglect meaningful presence with our partners in the experience.

In one scenario, anxiety gets projected outward (*Your pleasure is my responsibility, and I am desperate to get it right*), and in the other, inward (*Maybe if I do this I'll stay hard, that's not working, I'll switch to this*). Neither brings forward sharing, revealing, or connection; and both require holding on rather than letting go. We're left with crumbs in terms of inti-macy, a one-sided experience at either end that leaves one, or likely both, partners hungry. Learning how to cultivate deep connection and intimate understanding of our own sensory experience, arousal levels, emotional landscape, and thought process enables release into these aspects that we then get to share with our partners, giving them permission to do the same. The connection we hold with our partners then gets accessed in a greater way as another element of absorption, with no intimacy barriers, no anxi-ety, to keep us back from the power of those feelings. From there, we can ask for what we want, instruct when needed (because we will need to), and free our partners up to do the same. No more head work, no more guess-ing, no more trying to figure things out that are not our responsibility, or getting frustrated and resentful when our partners are unable to intuit what best pleases us!

Let's begin with an exercise adapted from Gina Ogden's *The Return of Desire: A Guide to Rediscovering Your Sexual Passion* (2011) that will allow us to begin connecting with and taking responsibility for our own sexuality and sexual experience. This exercise can be done partnered, whereby each person will go through it individually and then share with the other. Alternatively, it can be done on your own, if single. Both configurations come with great learning and insight.

Grab a piece of paper and create two columns; the header on the left side of the paper will read "I turn myself on when," and the header on the right will read "I turn myself off when." This may sound backwards and you might be saying something to yourself like *"but I don't turn myself on when my partner yanks my hair, they do that."* Yes, your partner has literally taken your hair in their hand and pulled it, but it is what you make up about that (*they're so powerful and full of passion for me*), what you associate that action with (*that kid I had a crush on in sixth grade who'd tug at my ponytail to flirt with me*), and the themes it touches on for you (*being wanted, flirted with, controlled*) that make it erotic. That meaning-making aspect was all you and your brain at work. That is you've effectively turned yourself on! Now, when thinking about the ways we turn ourselves on, cast a wide net. Things on the list can include behaviors, scenes, and visual input that are explicitly "sexual," just like *I turn myself on when you yank my hair*, or it can be situations, behaviors, experiences that make us feel connected to ourselves, comfortable in our own skin, and therefore more open or even enthusiastic about sharing sexually with partners or inviting in pleasure for and with ourselves! This can sound like, "*I turn myself on when I go for a long run after work*," or "*I turn myself on when I get up before the rest of the family and get to be in silence by myself*." So, let's begin here, returning to the "I turn myself on when" column, and jotting down whatever comes to mind. No overthinking, but stream-of-consciousness style.

The challenge is to really sink into this investigation/exploration. After you've identified the low-hanging fruit, sit and see what else surfaces.

When you feel you have finished, check in with how you feel. What was it like to go through this exercise? To take responsibility in this way? Remember, this is just a starting point. If grief comes along with this process, allow it forward while holding alongside it the knowledge that you are actively in the process of uncovering more in terms of learning, and with that understanding what is possible in a much more expansive way.

Now switch columns, and shift gears into "I turn myself off when." This can mean anything that takes you out of sexual experience or energy with yourself and/or partners, anything that makes you feel lousy about, uncomfortable with, or simply disconnected from yourself, and therefore less open or eager to share body/heart/mind sexually with others. Examples might include, "*I turn myself off when I focus on your breath and what you might've eaten for lunch rather than the softness of your lips (something I used to be obsessed with),*" or "*I turn myself off when I am thinking about how you might be judging my penis,*" or, "*I turn myself off when I've made no meaningful 'me' time in my day.*"

It is very common to have a very challenging time answering the questions at all, let alone creating a list. That's OK! This is an activity that simply gets us started in terms of shifting our lens, which is the most important task, and is something to add to as you move along. Keep the list nearby for this purpose!

Fundamental Task #2

Taking care.

Peter: I feel like my opinion doesn't matter at home. I feel like a door mat most days. It's hard to feel confident and free in the bedroom when I just don't think my partner respects me anymore.

Mira: I gave birth to our baby just over a year ago. My partner has been super patient and there's a part of me that wants to have a sex life again also, but then I look in the mirror ... I don't recognize my body, I haven't showered in days, my hair is a mess, and I'm covered in crusty breastmilk and spit-up. I walk away feeling so far away from even remotely sexy, I just kind of separate myself from those feelings and hope that things will one day change.

The bedroom is an extension of our day, an extension of the relationship we've had with ourselves that day. Even when we're very skilled at shifting gears and stepping into a different mindset with sex, it is impossible to completely wall ourselves off from ourselves. Today is the day to begin taking notice of how you treat yourself and making edits. This will only feel meaningful if the edits you make aren't superficial or untrue. For example, if you really do believe you aren't an interesting person, telling yourself you are won't work. We will need to challenge the block there in order to find the right way of editing that premise to make it more trustworthy (even if it's a matter of degrees). *When did I arrive at this conclusion about myself? What evidence tells me that it's true? More importantly, what evidence is there to suggest it may be untrue [look closely because our brains are trained to prove hypotheses so it will scan for evidence in support automatically, without collecting evidence on the opposing end]? What does it mean to be interesting? Is anyone really "uninteresting," or are some people more closed off or less inclined to share themselves? If I don't know who I am enough to share, how can I get to know? What experiences can*

I bring into my life that may help me learn more about myself in order to share more with others?

Fundamental Task #3

Identify and work through the hidden "no's" we communicate to our sexuality that prohibit our physiological "yes."
That thing you do (you know, *that* thing) to get yourself off? It is invited. That fantasy or memory that really lights you up? That too! Your sounds, smells, lubrication ... it's all welcome. That super edgy kink or extreme scene you visit in your mind to "get you over the edge?" Great, come on in! Not always, or even rarely ever in a literal way, but all parts of who we are, they are welcome in the ether, in the orbit of the experience, in the fullness of intimacy that wants to visit those involved. When we try to shut ourselves out, walling ourselves off from ourselves, our body understands this experience as boundary setting or "no's." Our sexual functioning follows. Sex asks, "*Will you allow yourself to be 'you' in this experience?*"

- My fantasies: *I don't feel comfortable fantasizing about other people when with my partner.* (No.)
- My sounds and movements when aroused: *They're embarrassing and "unsexy."* (No.)
- Interaction with my vulva: *Masturbating feels dirty, I don't do it.* (No.)
- Asking for what I want: *I feel squeamish talking about sex, it's fine if they just do what they want.* (No.)

"Sexuality, can I have an orgasm (if that is the desired outcome) with this partner please?"

Can you identify the ways you're blocking out or editing your sexuality from the experience? Why are certain elements or aspects not allowed? Can you begin incorporating small risks, allowing more of yourself in? How might it feel to include more contact with yourself, *for* yourself? If we have a difficult time being "with" ourselves (including our own body, sexuality, feelings, expression of emotion), we will have a hard time being with another. We don't need a full list of "yes's," but we certainly want enough to make the "no's" less heavy or substantial.

- My fantasies ... *are allowed to be with me and bring me further into my arousal and into connection with myself and my partner.* (Yes.)
- My sounds and movements when aroused ... *I discovered my partner really loves. I feel comfortable letting myself moan.* (Yes.) *I still feel self-conscious about letting them really "see" parts of my body.* (No.)

- Interaction with my vulva ... *is part of what it means to share myself and my pleasure with my partner. It also helps them understand what parts feel good to be touched.* (Yes.)
- Asking for what I want ... *is tricky but I try. I can get anxious when I can't find the words, but I'm trying to practice.* (Yes.)

"Sexuality, can I have an orgasm with this partner please?" Ah, there you are. Yes, let go!

Fundamental Task # 4

All sex is intimate sex: no more bad or good categorization.
If we approach sex as a good/bad, pass/fail endeavor, we invite anxiety and shame in. If we assign blame to the success or failure of a sexual experience, we invite anxiety and shame in. If we make sex a high stakes, high pressure game, we invite anxiety and shame and avoidance and low desire in. Approaching sex in this way sees sex as a task, a challenge, and a performance. It disregards what is at the heart of really good sex for most: intimacy. If we consider intimacy, characterized by sharing and revealing which is inherent in sex, can we ever really fail? This is the mindset we want to cultivate now. An attitude of "*I am going to show up and discover what I need and want from sex today, right now, with myself and/or with my partner. No matter what happens, I will have shared myself and potentially been shared with as well.*" Whatever is revealed to you reflects who that person is that day in their vulnerability, their openness. This is sacred and worthy of our consideration, care, respect, and protection.

Can you imagine letting go into your sexuality, feeling the emotions and release that can come with that experience, allowing your "other" to witness this journey, only to be told that the sexual experience "didn't go well" because they didn't _____ (fill in the blank), or worse because you didn't —— (fill in the blank) (orgasm, maintain an erection, ejaculate after the desired period of time, etc.)?

Let this be the end of judging an abstract, emotional experience based on concrete or behavioral elements. Success *is* sharing.

Who cares that we didn't cum, it felt so good to make out. The way we kissed tonight felt more intense than it has in a long time. I loved feeling that from you.

Fundamental Task # 5

No more show stopping moments (i.e. learn how to pivot).
We are drawing a line in the sand: no more reinforcement or creation of negative or challenging associations when it comes to your sex life. Whether

you're partnered or not, everything we do moving forward is in the spirit of protecting your sexual life as a sanctuary. That means, if you lose your erection, ejaculate sooner than you'd like, are having discomfort with penetration, and so on, you are pivoting rather than shutting the experience down, and there are a wide variety of ways to do this.

- Behaviorally (e.g. *that felt so good, I couldn't hold myself back. Can I focus on you now? What would bring you there?*).
- Emotionally (*I can feel my body getting anxious. Can we slow down and hold each other for a moment? I just want to breathe in your arms*).
- Even in terms of style or pace (*I love when you take control like that so much, it gets me so hot. Let's slow down so I can pace myself*).

There are exceptions to this. When we feel overwhelmed, scared, checked out/ dissociated, or simply like we are participating in something that we really don't want to do, it is critical that we honor those feelings and experiences and pause or stop. If partnered, can you stay connected as you navigate the feelings that are surfacing? Even if this looks like holding your partner's hand as you turn the rest of your body away to regulate or move through emotion, that is a great starting point. Our wounding happens in relationship, and then we move into ourselves as individuals to try and make sense of it and manage its consequences. As such, the most powerful healing happens relationally as well, communicating the message to the mind/body now that this relationship with this person is safe. *I can bring my healing here as well*. When this is not the case, and things have simply not gone as expected (say we did ejaculate earlier than desired), we learn to pivot, and with confidence.

Refer to the Pivot Playlist at the end of this chapter for ideas on how to expand your individual and shared repertoire.

Fundamental Task # 6

Inviting in the "no" leads to more "yes" (boundaries are our friend).
Inviting in the "no" leads to more "yes." Truly, if we feel we can't say "no" to an experience or specific aspects of it, we will either avoid the experience entirely or end up engaging, pushing past our own boundaries, and therefore potentially creating challenging associations that shove desire underground. If sex is routinely a five-step process, including initiation, the unfolding of the sexual script, after care, and then some clean up, how on-board for the five-step routine are we going to be after a particularly challenging and exhausting day? For some of us, that routine *is* the relief from it all – the big exhale; for others, it's just too much. If we feel like our partner can hear our limits and not internalize them as rejection, we are freed up to both put those limits on the table and describe what

exists around them, what "yes's" and perhaps even "maybe's" exist outside of or within our "no's." It might look something like this:

Partner A: It's Tuesday night, our time to connect. What would feel good to you tonight?

Partner B: I would love to make out for a while and have you hold me. It's been a super stressful day, so that sounds perfect. Does that sound OK to you?

Partner A: I'm game for making out. Penetration feels super hot to me also. Is that on the table at all for you?

Partner B: No, I'm really just up for a good make out session and snuggle.

Partner A: Cool, follow me.

Would Partner B be inclined to offer up any suggestions at all if they feel like they will:

1 Experience pressure (real or perceived) to go further during the experience?
2 Hurt or upset their partner by being honest about where they are at?

Most of the time the answer is "no." We will simply avoid sex entirely if sex can only mean one kind of experience, or series of experiences. If we can trust that we can show up with our honesty and have it received, we are just much more likely to engage. It's that simple! And more sexual engagement often leads to more sexual engagement.

A key component here though is authenticity. We can't say we're OK with hearing what our partner(s) is/are up for and then get frustrated when it's not what we want and demonstrate that frustration via more distant connection or half-presence in the experience. We can express our feelings honestly with something like *"can't say I'm not slightly bummed, I have been craving going down on you all day, but I'm happy just to be close to you, so let's go."*

If you've collected a number of experiences where "that thing you love" has not been available or has been bypassed, a conversation is in order. It can look something like this:

Partner A: I've noticed that you've been less into me touching your breasts lately. I miss this experience with you. Is there something that is making this less approachable in our experience together? Is there something I can do to make this more comfortable for you?

Fundamental Task # 7

Give yourself and your partners an "out." Accept disappointment in the short term for desire preservation in the long term.
To expand on Task #6, if partnered sex feels like a lot of effort to make sure our partners orgasm or have pleasure at our own expense (e.g. *I'm tired of giving my partner oral but I have to stay here and continue despite my discomfort for as long as it takes to get them off*), then we *will* avoid sex or feel less inclined to approach subsequent experiences. This is how sex goes from being something approachable to something we have to "be in the right state of mind" or mood or have enough energy for. If we can give ourselves and our partners a way of getting out of a situation, and the shared understanding is that we engage in experience as long as it feels OK to us, and then we pivot or ease into conclusion, then sex becomes approachable in a much more regular way. What does this mean? Allowing disappointment or frustration to be a part of the experience, knowing that a bit of disappointment in the face of your partner's desire to pivot is preferable to the erosive quality obligation has on our desire long term.

How sexy might it be to have a partner turn to you and say the following before a sexual encounter:

> *This shouldn't have to be said, but I want you to know explicitly that you do not need to feel obligated to do or stay with anything in this experience together. If you get tired, bored, or want to switch things up at any point, please let me know. I can tend to any disappointment I may or may not feel in favor of your comfort. I can get myself off if needed. I know how to take care of myself.*

How sexy might it be for someone to hear that from *you*?

Fundamental Task #8

Learn to have sex with yourself (i.e. masturbate!).
You are your primary partner in sex, even with other people! Understanding how to have sex with yourself comfortably and with an exploratory mindset is a key ingredient in what makes for comfortable, uninhibited sex with others. Luckily, learning how to cultivate this relationship is profoundly healing outside of the bedroom as well. It means creating comfort with being vulnerable with yourself, with accepting and exploring your own body. It means learning to trust yourself and your instincts, it means reclaiming physical and emotional territory that has felt judged, used, wounded, or shamed, or worse.

Staying away from self-touch means keeping a distance from what our sexuality looks like, feels like, and how it operates today. It means depriving ourselves of the meaningful learning that we can then take to our partners (because it is our responsibility to do so). Lack of understanding about our bodies, our desires as they evolve, our curiosities, inevitably leads to discomfort or awkwardness, an intellectual puzzle to solve rather than something to experience. Again, feeling the breeze as you cruise down the highway necessitates familiarity with the car, its buttons, its quirks, your relationship to the machinery.

Experience with self-touch can include orgasm or not. It doesn't matter which, since our definition of sex isn't limited to orgasm or any particular kind of sensation (i.e. it doesn't always need to include "pleasure" sensation). The shift we want to make here has to do with attention and attunement, noticing what your body and mind are doing as you touch, and rewinding the tape after. *What was the quality of sensation in my body today? Where did I feel it most? Did it come with noticeable emotion?*

Concurrently, it may be fun to play with some intentionality in terms of the different kinds of experiences we can cultivate with ourselves. Variety of experience only translates to greater learning.

- How might I engage in sensual touch with myself? (Sensory exploration, embodiment, and learning.)
- How might I make love to myself? (Connection to self and self-care/love.)
- How might I fuck myself? (Accessing play and pleasure for play and pleasure's sake.)

Fundamental Task #9

Uncomplicating consent in relationships.
One of our primary goals is to eliminate guess work and the stress and anxiety that come with our desire to predict in order to do right by our partners (*"They probably won't like this part being touched since it didn't get them off last time, so I'll avoid touching here,"* or *"They felt some pain at different points in the past when I've touched these parts, I better work around these areas and maybe even places nearby"*), or even just "do sex" right in general. Talk to your partner about what implied consent looks like in your relationship if you're at that point in its development. *Are there behaviors or experiences that exist outside of the implied domain? If so, are they off-limits entirely, or do I simply need to ask before engaging them?*

When our understanding of what lives under the "implied consent" umbrella changes, it is that person's job to communicate the change to their partner, and the partner's job to yield (e.g. *"I know that butt grabbing has been something I've been OK with in the past, it's gotten uncomfortable for me now a few times, so I'll need you to ask before you grab, OK?"*).

Sometimes, depending on our relationship with sex, even after being in a relationship for a long time, implied consent can only exist in certain spheres, like in day-to-day affection, or on the weekend when free from work stress. Sometimes we need the scaffolding pre-negotiation provides in order to feel at ease enough to play. Despite how "unsexy" that might seem, it makes room for possibility, versus skipping this critical step and holding on, living in our headspace, rather than dropping into our bodies, and trust, and sensation, and connection. Can we can make this a fun game? Sure! Can you text each other throughout the day? Spelling out your "yes's"? Texting one "yes" item at a time, every few hours? Can you play a game of "guess my green lights" before diving in? The chemistry and/or playful energy that gets kicked up by this back and forth can buffer the part where we put definition to our "no's" or "red lights."

Fundamental Task # 10

Let an inherently emotional experience be – emotional.
One of the most challenging elements in working to free ourselves from anxiety in a sexual experience is the task of letting go of trying to fix or shove out the feeling, as we often try (and fail) to do in our day-to-day lives. First, it doesn't work, and second, the tension and resistance this challenge kicks up often results in more anxiety and greater disconnection. Allow the anxiety to be there, allow all the emotions that surface to take up space. Let. Them. Be. If feelings are invited and not perceived as threatening, they move through with greater ease, and we feel more free in the midst of them. Part of what our sexual functioning does is help us do just that, move through what gets in the way of homeostasis, of our sense of well-being (thank you, parasympathetic nervous system!). Does anxiety effect our behavior? Yes. If I can be anxious, stay connected, and have that met with tenderness or care or even eroticism (if that feels OK), is my anxiety likely to stick around? No. When this is our relationship to our feeling states, they are experienced as helpful visitors, providing information while creating spaciousness in our minds, hearts, and bodies, when allowed.

Fundamental Task #11

If at first things are – awkward, try, try again!
Expansion is clumsy, and learning takes practice and perseverance. Sex is no exception. Did you try on a new kink with a partner and find it was a bit of a mess? Well yeah, it is likely to be! Rather than run away screaming

because sex is never allowed to be awkward or messy or anything but amazing (sense the sarcasm?), we must return if we're truly interested in learning something new, experiencing what it has to offer. We are stiff when stepping into a new skill, situation, or role. We can feel uneasy when we don't know what to expect, which often puts us in our heads, on high alert as we orient ourselves, take in the information and learn. Ease comes with practice, ease comes with repetition, ease comes with time. With ease comes possibilities, but ones we must earn.

Fundamental Task # 12

Eroticize yourself.

In Chapter 16, we visited the idea that we are constantly in relationship with fantasy, including with our own fantasies about ourselves. Do you envision yourself as a sexual person in your mind's eye? Do you see yourself as desirable? As an attentive and curious lover or sexual partner? If the answer is "no," then it's likely you are currently or have played an entirely different movie in your head about what sexual experiences with you might look like, feel like, be like for others. Returning to visualization as a tool, let's practice regularly playing out an entirely different scene, starring ourselves, in our own mind's eye. Draw upon media for examples if helpful, put yourself in the place of an actor you're watching in a show or movie. Imagine what it might be like to actually live out that scenario.

When we practice placing ourselves in erotic or sexual scenarios in our fantasy or imagination space, we not only help our body understand and practice (in its own offline way) what we are looking to express, exude, or feel, but we also begin to create a sexual self-concept that includes ease, desirability, playfulness, and intensity (or adjectives of your own choosing). When we understand what it might actually look like to get curious about our partner's pleasure, when we have a style or approach to engaging that we have a template for in our imagination, we experience greater ease in embodying these concepts, in making them ours and folding them into our experiences. What this isn't is an exercise in applying a script or formula, practiced in our mind to be played or "acted" out with another. This is an experience of placing ourselves in multiple erotic scenarios in our own mind, and imagining how we might embody ease around them. What that might look like, feel like, be like. Can you play out (in detail) the following?

- A slow, sensual experience;
- A playful, light experience;
- An intense, passionate experience;
- A curious, exploratory experience.

If this is a real challenge, that's OK. Use information from Task # 15 (Getting to know my eroticism) to draw inspiration. Can you find examples in media that feel true enough to life for you? Do you have experiences with partners to reference? Documentary-style pornography can be helpful here as well, preferably even media that depicts real partners "making love" or having a sexual experience. To add further utility to the exercise, see if you can imagine experiences that highlight different sexual behaviors or forms of sexual play. Can you broaden the menu in your own mind's eye, making it easier to pivot in real time?

Fundamental Task #13

Teasing out "needs" vs. "wants."
We look to sex to satisfy a plethora of needs and wants, each with their own weight and each with their own *perceived* availability outside of the sexual relationship. The differences between partners in terms of the list of wants and needs sex satisfies reveals itself as desire discrepancy, an inevitability in relationship. If for one partner, sex is perceived as the only place that satisfies the *need* for intimacy, vulnerability, release, nurturing, and the *want* for adrenaline, eroticism, validation, a sense of power and control, then they will likely feel a compelling "pull" or deep desire for sex, versus their partner who gets the needs listed above met in friendship, with family, and simply turns to sex for the unique experience of having those needs addressed with their partner, alongside some wants. For one partner, sex is supremely important as the source of basic needs we look to address as humans, for the other, it is a special and distinct form of connection, expression, and play that represents intimacy in this unique relationship.

Why is it important to tease out your wants and needs when it comes to sex? Because if we understand what eggs we put in its basket, we can help our partners understand our relationship to it with greater insight. We are also able to determine if we want to make choices that allow more meaningful access to the experiences that feed our basic needs outside of our sex. That is *"if I only let myself be vulnerable and nurtured in sex, can I challenge myself to step into these experiences with more regularity outside of the bedroom? What might that look like? Do I need to practice?"*

Fundamental Task #14

Tending to your training
This task means navigating complex feelings as they relate to our upbringing and the lessons we were exposed to and internalized from primary people in our lives, who often (but not always) tried their best. If it's

helpful, focus on the lesson rather than the people. That's what matters most of the time; for example:

> If Lana's parents value the family image of "perfection," placing tremendous pressure on her to get A's, attend church regularly, dress properly, and seek out other "high-achieving" friends in order to receive their love, then Lana is likely to approach sex as another thing to accomplish, something her ego needs to "do right" in order to gain connection. With that much on the line, sex will be stressful – who is she outside of what others tell her to be? Does she know how to let go and enjoy just for enjoyment's sake?

The lesson is "project perfection," something her parents learned or were given in their own way as well. *How do I release this ideal? How can I provide myself with support as I move out of goal orientation and into my body? Can sex teach me about the "me" underneath it all?*

- Can you name any themes you're working with, like "being the best?"
- A lesson learned that your body is trying to alert you to?
- What is the message and how can the "you" of today counter it (this requires ongoing thought and effort)?
- What do you want your fear, your anxiety to know as you reapproach your sex life (with yourself and/or others)?
- Can we relay our message without trying to push up against it or force it out? Honoring its wisdom?

I understand what you're trying to alert me to, anxiety, I feel you, and I am safe. I no longer need your warning. Thank you for trying to protect me all these years, you can stay but so can I.

Fundamental Task #15

Getting to know my eroticism: if fantasy life feels elusive.
Our sexuality is moving alongside us each day, influencing how we interact with others, what we long for in terms of connection, motivating what we gravitate towards for sensory stimulation, fantasy content, and the level of closeness we feel comfortable with in our relationships: platonic, familial, and romantic. It can be challenging to identify its presence because it is so deeply woven into the fabric of who we are, because of the rigid ways we've chosen to define it, and often because of the ways in which we turn away from it out of fear, pain, shame, and guilt. This is good news in terms of ongoing sexual self-discovery and exploration. For those of us who never got to explore what pleasure feels like for our own sake, what it

means to safely let our own curiosity lead, and to truly release in the presence of another, fantasy can feel particularly elusive. *How would I understand what I might be interested in if I don't even understand my sexuality to be mine whatsoever?* We get to turn that around, starting now! Our sexuality is always waiting for us, to explore, understand, and embody (if we so choose).

Remember when we discussed how watching TV shows and movies *is* actively engaging in fantasy? We are participating in the story, relating and reacting to the characters, escaping and finding aspects of ourselves as we go. Despite our sexuality maintaining a constant presence in our lives, it becomes more palpable, more distinguishable when we are interacting with erotic, sexual, and/or romantic content (coming to life in particular and distinct ways dependent upon sexual orientation, e.g. gay, straight, asexual, and in combination with our unique complexity). In other words, when watching our favorite TV show and one of the characters is kissing, sharing an intimate moment, or rolling around in the bed "having sex" with themselves or someone else, our sexuality responds, emerging and kicking up feelings and reactions that are distinct and important and revealing. Is there a movie or episode of a show you can revisit that depicts sex, or romantic intimacy, in whatever capacity you feel comfortable with? As you watch, tune in: to your body and physical sensation, to your thoughts and any chatter that surfaces, and to your emotions and any complexity that reveals itself there. Anything and everything is welcome: discomfort, tension, curiosity, excitement, or even stillness, disconnection – all are useful, and simply the starting point in your development. Revisit this exercise with the same scene multiple times, tunning in with the same gentle attention each time, taking note of any subtle or not-so-subtle stirrings in your experience. Don't try too hard! The most meaningful information reveals itself when we allow ourselves to be "in" the experience rather than "in" searching or "in" effort.

Fundamental Task # 16

Understand initiation as a big, not-so-big deal

If the key ingredient to intimacy is risk, then initiation can feel like the ultimate game of Russian Roulette, especially with our sense of worth, of selfhood on the line. Can we appreciate how much bravery is involved in putting ourselves out there, asking for what we want, and making a real bid for connection, closeness, and play? We often turn to jokeyness, cuteness, and/or crass behavior to buffer the scary feelings that come along with stepping forward: "Am I enough for you? Worth loving? Are you attracted to me? If I show you my body, will you react with excitement or something else? Will that then confirm all of the harmful ideas I've learned from the world about my body/my value/myself? If I joke about it, then at least if you turn me down, I can blame it on the joke rather than who I am. Are you going to reject *me*?

It is important that we simultaneously appreciate the bravery that is required in an ongoing way to initiate intimacy, while also uncoupling our partners "no" with our sense of self worth. Rejection is a terrible experience and feeling, and one we all dread, but are *we* being rejected or is the experience being turned down (often due to fatigue, other things to attend to, or relational conflict)? Anxiety will gravitate towards one answer, but is it the most likely one? What question could we ask to find out? Will you be brave enough to ask?

Fundamental Task #17

"Should" clean up

What parameters do you give your sexuality to operate within? How do your "rules" get determined? Just like dating, when we approach sex with a very lengthy list of requirements, of "shoulds" and "should not's," we box ourselves in, and the other (often very quickly) out. We become so busy with our "shoulds" that we forget to attend to our wants, instincts, or feelings, consequently inhibiting expression, exploration, and our authenticity. Intimacy becomes lacking, sex risks becoming performative, and our sexual functioning is interrupted or unavailable entirely. A few guard rails can create safety, but if there are too many we become immobilized. Becoming aware of and bringing into conscious awareness our "shoulds" can facilitate editing, paring down, or shedding of the inhibiting rules and parameters that manifest as barriers to sharing, surrender, and arousal.

Respond to the prompts below with anything and everything that surfaces (don't overthink it) and then review these responses, taking a critical eye to their utility. Which of your "shoulds" serves you, bringing you into greater connection, freedom, sensation, and which keep you back? Can you pair your "shoulds" down to five or less? What is your new criterion for a "should" to exist in your sex life, within your sexuality, whatsoever?

- Sex should be (use adjectives) ———.
- Sex should feel ———.
- Sex should look like ———.
- My sexual life should look like ———.
- I should be able to ———.
- With my partner I should ———.
- I should look like ———.
- My arousal should ———.

- Orgasms should ———.
- My vulva should ———.
- My vagina should ———.
- My penis should (my genitals should) ———.
- My body should ———.
- My breasts should ———.
- My partner(s) should feel ———.
- My partner(s) should be ———.
- My partner(s) should communicate ———.
- I should communicate ———.
- For sex to happen, I should ———.
- For sex to happen, my partner(s) should ———.
- To initiate, I should ———.
- To initiate, my partner should ———.
- During sex, fantasy should ———.
- During sex, pornography should ———.
- Sex should happen like ———.
- Sex should end like ———.
- If I like something that is happening, I should ———.
- If I don't like something that is happening, I should ———.
- Aftercare should look like ———.
- My sexual wants should ———.
- My partner's sexual wants should ———.
- My desire should ———.
- My fantasies should ———.
- My solo sexual life should ———.
- My sexual values should ———.
- My sexual boundaries should ———.
- My gender should ———.
- My sexual orientation should ———.
- My sexuality should ———.

Fundamental Task #18

Center "reward" rather than pleasure.
With all this in mind, it's time to approach sex by understanding that it always has something to offer, it just might not be what you think it will be or should be or expect it to be. As a reflection of who we are, how we feel, what state we are in, and what we are needing/wanting at any particular moment, if we truly show up and shed the veneer, our sex will bring us back to an intimacy that's alive, and moving, and free from the past's shadow (the transcendent part). And yay for that! Imagine how much more sex we would be having if we felt we could be truly met, in our

authenticity, in our vulnerability, masks off, and even held there. If we knew that sex was *the* place we could breathe, let go, express, explore. We may not walk away having had the orgasm, having gotten wild, or adventurous or kinky *that* day. Perhaps we won't get what we go in wanting in every circumstance, but we will nearly always leave with what's needed if we show up, open up, and explore. If there is always reward to be had without pressure or the weight of expectation, what do we have to lose (can you imagine?!)?

Sex is an entire landscape of emotion, and you never know what your vulnerability might bring forward. Even when sex is about grief, pain, release, or catharsis, even when we're in the rockier areas of the landscape, it offers reward. Can we allow ourselves to meet and honor its depth? If that was our experience, our reality, would there be any desire to "perform" whatsoever? Would sex therapy have a place?

Pleasure is one feeling in a color wheel of emotional experience. The other shades offer beauty too. Pleasure is often the outcome of allowing the other colors to move through our bodies if we understand them to be passing through in our favor. Release *is* one powerful form of pleasure.

- I'm not feeling desire, but what am I feeling?
- I'm not about to cum, but I'm accessing _____ (connection, comfort, closeness, sensation, desire, fantasy, etc.).
- I'm not sure what sex has for me tonight, but I know it's something.

Pivot Playlist

Putting an end to show-stopping moments can mean pivoting to other behaviors or experiences. Add to this list as you expand your sexual menu to help your brain meaningfully understand options, storing them in long-term memory in a way that becomes easily accessed over time, a natural part of your interactions rather than an effortful one.

- ___ Self-touch (masturbation);
- ___ Stroking hands;
- ___ Hugging;
- ___ Kissing, cheek or face;
- ___ Kissing, closed-mouth;
- ___ Kissing, open-mouth;
- ___ Being kissed or touched on the neck;
- ___ Using breath to trace along a partner's neck;
- ___ Kissing or touching a partner's neck;
- ___ Giving hickeys;
- ___ Getting hickeys;

- ___ Tickling, doing the tickling;
- ___ Tickling, being tickled;
- ___ Wrestling or "play-fighting";
- ___ General massage, giving;
- ___ General massage, receiving;
- ___ Having chest, breasts, and/or nipples touched or rubbed;
- ___ Touching or rubbing a partner's breasts, chest, and/or nipples;
- ___ Frottage (dry humping/clothed body-to-body rubbing);
- ___ Tribadism (scissoring, rubbing naked genitals together with a partner);
- ___ A partner putting their mouth or tongue on breasts or chest;
- ___ Putting my mouth or tongue on a partner's breasts or chest;
- ___ Self-touch or masturbating in front of/with a partner;
- ___ A partner masturbating in front of/with me;
- ___ Manual sex (hands or fingers on penis or strap-on), receiving;
- ___ Manual sex (hands or fingers to penis or strap-on), giving;
- ___ Manual sex (hands or fingers on testes), receiving;
- ___ Manual sex (hands or fingers on testes), giving;
- ___ Manual sex (hands or fingers on vulva), receiving;
- ___ Manual sex (hands or fingers on vulva), giving;
- ___ Manual sex (hands or fingers inside vagina), receiving;
- ___ Manual sex (hands or fingers inside vagina), giving;
- ___ Manual sex (hands or fingers on or around anus), receiving;
- ___ Manual sex (hands or fingers on or around anus), giving;
- ___ Manual sex (hands or fingers inside rectum), receiving;
- ___ Manual sex (hands or fingers inside rectum), giving;
- ___ Ejaculating (coming) on or in a partner's body;
- ___ A partner ejaculating (coming) on or in my body;
- ___ Using sex toys (like vibrators, dildos, or masturbation sleeves), alone;
- ___ Using sex toys (like vibrators, dildos, or masturbation sleeves), with a partner;
- ___ Oral sex (to vulva), receptive partner;
- ___ Oral sex (to vulva), doing to someone else;
- ___ Oral sex (to penis or strap-on), receptive partner;
- ___ Oral sex (to penis or strap-on), doing to someone else;
- ___ Oral sex (to testes), receptive partner;
- ___ Oral sex (to testes), doing to someone else;
- ___ Oral sex (to anus), receptive partner;
- ___ Oral sex (to anus), doing to someone else;
- ___ Vaginal intercourse, receptive partner;
- ___ Vaginal intercourse, insertive partner;
- ___ Anal intercourse, receptive partner;

- ___ Anal intercourse, insertive partner;
- ___ Using food items as a part of sex;
- ___ Cross-dressing during sex;
- ___ Having a partner cross-dress during sex;
- ___ Biting a partner;
- ___ Being bitten by a partner;
- ___ Scratching a partner;
- ___ Being scratched by a partner;
- ___ Wearing something that covers my eyes;
- ___ A partner wearing something that covers their eyes;
- ___ Having my movement restricted;
- ___ Restricting the movement of a partner;
- ___ Being slapped or spanked by a partner in the context of sexual pleasure;
- ___ Slapping or spanking a partner in the context of sexual pleasure;
- ___ Pinching or having any kind of clamp used on my body during sex;
- ___ Pinching a partner or using any kind of clamp on them during sex.

Non-physical (or not necessarily physical) sexual activities

- ___ Communicating my sexual fantasies to/with a partner (use caution with this);
- ___ Receiving information about a partner's sexual fantasies;
- ___ Role play;
- ___ Phone sex;
- ___ Cybersex, in IM;
- ___ Cybersex, in chat room;
- ___ Cybersex, on cellphone;
- ___ Getting sexual images of a partner in my email or on my phone;
- ___ Sending sexual images to a partner in their email or on their phone;
- ___ Reading pornography or erotica, alone;
- ___ Reading pornography or erotica, with a partner;
- ___ Viewing pornography, alone;
- ___ Viewing pornography, with a partner;
- ___ A partner reading or viewing pornography;
- ___ Giving pornography/erotica to a partner;
- ___ Getting pornography/erotica from a partner.

(www.scarleteen.com/article/advice/
yes_no_maybe_so_a_sexual_inventory_stocklist)

19 Identifying and Managing Distancing Strategies

It feels counterintuitive to think of anxiety as serving a distancing function, attempting to alert us to and move us away from challenging feelings, memories, and potential outcomes, when the emotion itself is so profoundly uncomfortable on its own. Is the reality of asking that person out really as bad as sitting with this feeling? Much more often than not, the answer is no. This speaks to the compelling sources it draws from, the most uncomfortable and extreme examples of a similar event gone terribly wrong, as if to say *Hi, I'm here!! Enjoying your cruise? There's ice in the water. Remember the Titanic?!* We've become so accustomed to the feeling and trust it so completely that we run for the life vest and start counting the lifeboats before even thinking to question or look at it (*Hmmmm, I'm noticing I'm feeling anxiety. There's been a lot of change lately leading up to this cruise, I know I must be a bit thrown off. What might I need to help myself feel more grounded on this trip?*).

Anxiety asks us to step back to zoom in. We can take its presence as an indicator of a need to pause, check in, and look closer, rather than skipping these important steps, trusting its distrust and reacting. *What is this context or situation showing me about me? What do I need to do with and for myself to navigate this feeling?* Even when the source of the anxiety seems to be linked to another person's behavior (*My partner gets so frustrated and disappointed when I can't make them cum*), the only place to start is within (*What am I afraid might happen if they're frustrated and disappointed? How might I need to provide more information or advocate for myself here?*).

In your daily life, how do you react to anxiety when it surfaces? How do you react to it in social situations (if it shows up here for you)? How do you react to it at work? How do you react to it sexually? Some common examples include:

DOI: 10.4324/9781003369080-23

- Social situations: Alcohol, lots of talking, shutting down, performing or entertaining, leading with the ego (e.g. *I ran a triathlon last week, I was top in my age group. Oh, you're into music? I played the cello for 15 years*), becoming a chameleon (*I perceive these people to be super sarcastic, so I'll meet them with sarcasm as well*), over-disclosing.
- Work situations: Overperforming to control, underperforming to avoid, passive-aggressivity, aggressive-aggressivity, leading with the ego, taking an "expert" position, taking too much responsibility (quick to apologize), denying accountability, aloofness (detachment).
- Sexually: Skipping to the "action" (e.g. penetration for many); performing emotion, pleasure, orgasm, facial expressions; thinking rather than feeling; being jokey, giggly, or crass; sticking to a very specific sexual routine; trying to control or put all focus on your partner; attempting to manage specific conditions required to feel comfortable having sex.

Exploration opportunity:

- What is my anxiety blocking me from?
- How is my anxiety a boundary?
- What is my anxiety asking me to look at as it relates to my relationship to myself?
- What is my anxiety distracting me from?
- What is my anxiety distracting me with?
- How is my anxiety a reflection of unwelcome influences? Ideas, experiences, ghosts of people and relationships?
- What part or version of you does your anxiety represent?
- What is your anxiety's agenda?

After reviewing the answers to your questions, in addition to the learning we've encountered thus far, how might you answer these questions:

- How do I (or we) understand my (or our) struggle to be an intimacy issue?
- Even if there is a medical component at work, even if there is an identifiable issue concerning our biology, how can you locate an answer to this question?

Bridging the Distance

Right now, in this moment, I'd like to invite you to read through the following instructions and try them for yourself. They may seem simple, but depending on the hour, day, month, or year you've experienced, something as basic as slowing down with yourself can feel foreign, complex, or even silly. Anything that surfaces – boredom, even lack of information – is information, which is precisely what we're looking for: simple observation and learning, so it's all welcome.

Pause for 5–10 seconds, give or take, on underlined words: the amount of time is less important than the pausing and tuning in, so if you find yourself counting, simply pause and notice for a moment.

Sit back in your chair or bed, pause, and notice the activity of your thoughts while you pause for several seconds on this <u>word</u>. Can you see those thoughts? Breathe in, and then let them go (even imagining them floating away) on the <u>exhale</u> as you shift your focus to the coolness of the air moving through your nostrils as your body breathes back <u>in</u>. Notice, then let thoughts <u>go</u>. Even as some thinking lingers, or bubbles immediately back up to the surface (and it will), you will now actively shift your focus to your musculature or <u>body-at-large</u>, and release as you read these words. Start at your <u>calves</u> and gradually move up – <u>thighs</u>, <u>buttocks</u>, <u>abdomen</u>, <u>shoulders</u>, and <u>arms</u>. Pay particular attention to your abdomen and buttocks and then finish by releasing and resting at your <u>jaw</u>. Release further into your chair, bed, or whatever is supporting your body, release your musculature, <u>release your jaw</u>. Slow your breathing <u>down</u>. Release even <u>further</u>. Simply stay for a few moments once you're done looking at all the words in this sentence; notice what's with you and how you <u>feel</u>.

Feel that release in your body? Did you notice softening (even if it was subtle) as you asked specific parts of your body to let go of tension? This is our foundation. Thoughts aren't particularly obedient; emotions are the same. However, we aren't trying to control or shut them out; we are learning to let go: **let go of, let go into, release our attachment to (or let be)**. We can practice noticing our thoughts and letting them go, returning to sensation in the body. We can practice noticing our emotions (i.e. our emotional concepts) and letting them be. This is why "doing" anything at all with your emotions isn't part of the instructions, we're simply going to notice them when they arise and passively receive them, observing the accompanying sensory experience in the body, letting go into sensation.

We "release" instead of "relax." Although these two words can mean the exact same thing, relaxing can veer from releasing – in that it also conveys a state of being, a mentality, an emotion – though "releasing" is in fact simply a verb, an action word. This is precisely why we want to partner with release and ditch relax: releasing is something we can actively practice and have control over. We cannot make ourselves relax, and attempting to do so often backfires. Tension in the body? Release. Tension in the mind? Release the jaw, release the pelvic floor, release the shoulders, and the mind often follows. Again, **release the body and the mind follows** rather than the other way around.

Each and every time we release our musculature, even when we are experiencing challenging emotions like anxiety and worry, we are communicating safety to the body. Each and every time we release, even in the presence of sadness or shame, we are letting go into our feelings, effectively allowing them to move through us as they're meant to rather than strengthening them with engagement, resistance, or elaboration (unless moving further into tension, which helps us release the feelings out, as discussed in Chapter 15).

Setting the Stage

In order to let go we must feel the presence (even if it's vague) of a sort of internal "safety net" to catch us. If we feel like we will get swallowed up, or hurt, or completely overcome, we will move away from taking the risks required to release. We know when we fall into sleep that we will be safe in our sleep, that it takes care of us, and that it represents respite (most of the time). If sleep becomes associated with frequent night terrors, we will no longer experience it as a safe, restorative experience, which would then predictably change our ability to let go into it. What does this ultimately mean for healing sex? That we must locate or build on a sense of self-trust. The ability to know that our emotions – even though they can be overwhelming, and can feel like they will break us, though they won't actually do so – allows us to attend to ourselves in meaningful ways in the midst of them. Concerned about what might happen if you let your guard down and welcome feeling in rather than trying to manage or keep emotions at bay? Staci Haines, author of *Healing Sex*, breaks down the phases of emotional expression:

1 Sensations and emotions emerge.
2 As you attend to or turn towards the emotions, they intensify and increase.
3 Emotions grow to a point of fullness, like water about to spill over the top of a bowl.
4 Emotions release or are expressed bodily (depending on the emotion, they may be gentle or intense – as sweat or a blush, sob, shake, tremble, kick, laugh, yell, or becoming overheated or chilled).
  Staci adds an important additional step in the process:
5. Intentionally complete the cycle, drawing upon your internal emotional resources (or integration).

(Haines, 1999, pp. 176–177)

Item 5 is meaningful in terms of helping us connect with what the emotion carried (its stories, memories, associations, and predictions), and therefore what was processed or digested. Without it, we risk experiencing our emotions as intruders without any purpose, and therefore chaotic and destabilizing, thwarting the process of release. They then have the potential to linger, stirring up depression and agitation, as they were unable to be received without resistance and lacking that internal safety net. Like an interrupted sneeze. These emotions then reposition themselves inside the mind/body where they continue to collect more ammunition and wait for another opening for processing and meaningful release.

We can partner with our solo sexuality and practice this process in baby steps on our own. Releasing more and more each time we engage with ourselves builds that internal sense of trust that becomes our raft, keeping us afloat as we drift into an ocean of experience, exploration, and the unknown.

Boundary/Pacing Assessment

When approaching the individual and shared experiences outlined in "Basic or Advanced Practice," the visual and cue words of "green," "yellow," and "red" will express our internal willingness and potentially the pacing required to proceed and how we help our partners understand what parts of the body as well as specific behaviors and experiences are on the table, are "proceed slowly and with caution" territory, or are off limits entirely. The cue word will sometimes be sufficient on its own; however, when in "yellow" territory, we will often be required to articulate what kind of support is needed and/or if any boundaries need to be exercised as guard rails to navigate the experience.

Grounding Cue Words

Similarly to our cue words, when navigating the experiences to follow, and even when approaching sexual experiences outside of what is outlined in this book, we want to hold in mind one of two grounding cues:

1 Let go, release, surrender (slow down);
2 Release, breathe, reassess, reassure.

These groupings of cue words are what allow us to come back into the present, back into the sexual values and perspectives we'd like to embody, and back into care for ourselves when emotional intruders from the past, thoughts meant to distract and distance, and physiological tension surface.

Breaking down #1: Let go, release, surrender (slowly):

- Let go: Let go of thoughts and tension in the body – let it all go.
- Release: Release your musculature and weight into whatever is supporting your body, release your shoulders and jaw.
- Surrender (slow down): We are moving deeper into letting go here, whether that feels like surrender for you, or simply slowing down (our breathing and our touch).

Breaking down #2: Release, breathe, reassess, reassure:

- Release: Release your musculature and weight into whatever is supporting your body, release your shoulders and jaw.
- Breathe: Connect with your breath and consciously slow it down.
- Reassess: *Am I OK? Is this experience one that I want to continue to choose to have, even if it might be a bit challenging? Is it safe for me to continue?* Allow your rational mind to come online here to determine if the feelings, sensations, and/or thoughts that might be arising have their origins in what is happening in the present, or if they are reactions to and warnings from the past, or both.
- Reassure: If you determine you are OK to continue, say so internally before slowly proceeding. *I'm OK. This is OK. I can let go.*

These are foundational – as you move along, ditch, edit, and/or replace these groupings with cue words that are meaningful to you, ones that you choose. These particular words are important to connect with in the early stages of your journey as they are also action words rather than abstract concepts or emotional states. We want to hold action words as our grounding cues so as to embrace all of the complexity that we are, that sex is, and everything that we bring to our sexual experiences. In other words, we want to steer away from cue words that might indicate a desired outcome, like "be grateful" or "welcome orgasm." Call upon these cue words as often as needed to address the anxiety embedded in our sexual experiences. The more you practice, the more intuitive and "second nature" they become, the more space we create for ease and comfort as anxiety learns it's not needed.

Pressure and Progress

Pressure is a killer in the bedroom, as we've established. Pressure is one of the first things we look to diminish or eliminate in the spirit of "sex that's not worth wanting, is not worth having," and we can add to that: it "often won't happen at all (in terms of free, uninhibited sexual functioning)" if our bodies detect it in the mix. And yet, how do we get past sexual avoidance, how do we challenge ourselves in any capacity to break through the tension, fear, anxiety if we don't push ourselves a bit to do so? Is self-directed pressure a requirement for change?

Pressure is often externally induced: *I am doing this because I have to, or my partner will be unhappy with me.* Feeling "pressured" can lead us to push past our own personal boundaries, silencing our inner voice, and communicating to our body and mind that *I don't matter here.* For many of us, this reinforces messages that are tied to experiences of coercion, of trauma, something we seek to unravel in therapy. For all of us, this may lead to behavior or change that looks good on paper and in the moment, but that falls apart in terms of longevity. In this way, we can view pressure as a red flag, letting us know that perhaps we've lost ourselves and are no longer motivated for reasons that will lead to our desired outcome, toward ease with sex.

What we want to bring forward instead is bravery, which comes from within and has everything to do with pushing past our fear because of our own powerful internal motivations. When our defenses step forward and our anxiety attempts to immobilize us, bravery is what allows us to see what we're contending with, make an assessment, and then determine the degree of risk in the actions we take. It means tapping into another aspect of our experience that is bigger, more powerful, or more compelling than our fear. It is intentional movement in the presence of that fear. We find bravery from new understanding, healing, and motivation in the face of our brain's predictions. If we lose bravery, if we can't grab onto motivation, we risk stepping into pressure and other-driven motivations (which are flimsy at best).

Can you identify three primary reasons for engaging in this healing? Reasons that are only yours, just for you? How will you benefit from continuing your learning? Why is it meaningful to cultivate a different relationship to your sexuality, to yourself?

1

2

3

The sexual values I want to embody include:

1

2

3

20 Mindfulness and Sensate Focus

Mindfulness, for those of us who haven't cultivated a relationship to it already, can easily get lumped into the "good for me, I'll get to it later" category. Something that we understand to have benefits intellectually but that can live alongside skepticism about how impactful these benefits actually are in real time, in daily life. "Is it woo-woo or is it science?": confusion risks sprinkling fuel on the skepticism fire as we struggle to wrap our heads around a way of being that is said to cultivate more peace, calm, or joy, i.e., vaguely defined internal states, seemingly abstract and ungrabbable. This exists in stark contrast to that prescription that states *very* clearly what promises it can make and, very importantly, when. We want solutions and relief now, and why wouldn't we? There is frequently either the perception or the very real threat of a lot being on the line. This anxiety will lead us in the wrong direction. This anxiety is something we must get clear on, get underneath, and learn to meaningfully diminish in our sex.

"*How many sessions till we're done?*" (i.e. When will I reach the finish line?).

Sex therapy *can* be a quick fix, but more often it is a process of retraining that requires education, deep exploration, and practice. Having arrived at the practice portion of this version of a sex therapy journey, it is important to ask yourself if you're ready to:

- Adopt a new framework for navigating sexual experiences and intimacy.
- Take emotional risks (with yourself and/or others).
- Communicate much more directly, clearly, and honestly with partners (if applicable).
- Be honest with yourself about your progress and what is required in your process.
- Carve out room for practice in order help the body understand change in its own language, experientially and behaviorally.

DOI: 10.4324/9781003369080-24

Potentially most importantly, are you ready to take the time that this needs to take? To sacrifice a period of time outside of the status quo (which isn't particularly comfortable or optimal to begin with) for the potential of the rest of your sexual life? If we're engaged, attuned, curious, and honest with ourselves along the way, the work of change is much more efficient. Mindfulness will assure we don't miss clues and important steps in our progress, and we need not be skillful or practiced at it (although we will practice) to begin to recognize the changes it ushers in.

The results of regular practice are cumulative, like a muscle you exercise. Everyday effects become noticeable as our brains learn to interact with our thoughts and emotions without immediately identifying with them reflexively, noticing and making choices from that distance in-between "me and my internal world." Partnership with this practice is essential if our goals have anything to do with comfortable, pleasurable sex and ease in engaging with our sexual functioning. Without it we will miss important clues from the body, important disturbances from the mind, and emotional concepts that threaten to grab the wheel.

In terms of our sexuality, mindfulness is so much more than that breath: it is the life force that breathing awakens. Meaning that without it playing a meaningful role, we have a hollow experience, leaving everything to be desired in terms of chemistry, electricity, passion, arousal, and (as always) trust in our bodies as our minds are in another experience, anticipating the next move, and making a series of assumptions as we go. We will miss the learning that adds to our sexual instincts, kicking up chemistry, and revealing where we go astray. Mindfulness lets our brain know that we are here, in this moment rather than the ones before it, paving room for the kind of beginner's mind that unhooks and dismantles anticipatory anxiety, granting us access to our natural functions, securing the parasympathetic nervous system's place at the helm. So, is it woo-woo or is it science? Perhaps it's both.

Slowing Down to Speed Up

The way out of striving, thinking, controlling, and holding on, and into new associations that open us up, is by taking a slow, progressive rhythm that we can build on over time. It is practicing a new way of being over and over to communicate to the mind and body (and heart) that this difference is meaningful, and what to expect as the new baseline. It is comfort and sex, ease and sensuality, release and eroticism, over and over, carving out and forming new connections in the brain that relay an entirely new experience to the body. We want to take this slowly, mindfully attending to the learning, able to notice and work through the barriers that operate or reveal themselves both covertly and overtly. Again, the slower we go, the more progress we make. No amount of rushing or pushing past or through gets past our internal eye, and consequently new associations are not able to develop, sex continues to be challenging, and the healing work (on our own or in therapy) is an uphill battle. The more mindfulness is prioritized when it comes to our sexuality, the greater ease we'll find in the work required to inspire meaningful change. Befriend it, center it in your experience, and change *will* follow. It is key.

> *But does this mean that sex has to be slow and sensual every time? Is this a new "style" that I have to adopt? What if it doesn't sound sexy to me?*

No, no, and no. What we are establishing here is a baseline of parasympathetic nervous system presence, through which we can build energy, excitement, passion, adventure, fantasy, and action (if that's what's on the table). With the parasympathetic nervous system in the drivers seat, the sympathetic nervous system can play the supportive role it was born to play when it comes to sex. It's the difference between feeling safe and letting go into the thrill of the rollercoaster, hands waiving in the air as you scream with joy, and feeling like you've got a faulty seatbelt on, gripping the safety bars in fear as you tolerate the ride.

Defining Mindfulness

So, what *is* mindfulness and how do we apply it to our sexual lives? In a sentence, it is presence in the now, without judgment. It is open-hearted residence or "being" in the moment as it unfolds, without resistance, planning, or forecasting (which is different from anticipation). *When it comes to sexual intimacy, we are considering mindfulness in the context of sharing our sexual selves with others, allowing them to witness who we are in our eroticism, and inviting them to do the same.* Through this lens, mindfulness includes allowing fantasies that pass through, go-to behaviors or brands of stimulation, meaningful elements of the experience that enable immersion in our arousal to simply be and unfold as they will; it is presence with *your sexual self* with all its contradictions, inclinations (as they relate to ourselves), and longings. Moving out of this solo-sexual realm relationally involves:

- Communication (asking for what we want and getting curious about our partners' desires).
- Providing active instruction regarding how our partners can interact with and respect our unique and evolving bodies in this moment in time (and getting curious about how to interact with and respect theirs).

- Yielding to, holding an appreciation for, and exercising boundaries and consent (which can be implied, depending on the relationship).

Sounds simple enough? Or maybe simply complicated?

Below you will find a breakdown of the basic principles of mindfulness as spelled out by meditation expert and professor, Jon Kabat-Zinn. As you read through, try to consider your present relationship to these principles in two categories:

A My daily life (including work and social life, day-to-day tasks, relationships with others).
B Sexually (within your relationship to your own sexuality, and within your partnered sexual life, if present).

- **Non-judging:** Through mindfulness meditation practice, we become aware of auto-judgments, watching, observing, and therefore seeing through our usually unexperienced prejudices and fears, the labels we place on nearly everything we see, interact with, and experience, categorized as either good, bad, or neutral. Non-judging means openness to and the observation of emotions, thoughts (including judging thoughts), and sensations in the body as they pass through our conscious awareness, without pursuing or acting on them.
- **Patience:** "Patience is a form of wisdom. It demonstrates that we understand and accept the fact that sometimes things must unfold in their own time" (Kabat-Zinn, 1990, p. 23). Patience means allowing ourselves the space and freedom to have the experience we're having because it is in our reality, though unfolding nonetheless. "Why rush through some moments to get to other, 'better' ones? After all, each one is in your life at this moment" (Kabat-Zinn, 1990). Through patience we learn to connect with, be open to, and curious about each moment, accepting each one in its fullness.
- **Beginner's mind:** This is the willingness to see everything with fresh eyes, as if for the first time, outside of the stories and beliefs we've collected and carry around about the world. It allows freedom from expectations based on past experiences, paves the way to see things uncluttered, as they actually are.
- **Trust:** Learning to listen to, take responsibility for, and deeply understand our own being above the voices and influence of others. It moves us toward true embodiment as we learn to identify our wants with greater clarity and fully inhabit our choices and actions.
- **Non-striving:** "*I am going to control my feelings, chill out, and be more confident,*" introduces an idea of where you "should" be, suggesting

you're not OK as you are. Non-striving means separation from the goal-oriented mindset that permeates nearly every decision we make.

"In the meditation domain, the best way to achieve your goals is to back off from striving for results and instead start focusing carefully on seeing and accepting things as they are, moment by moment. With patience and regular practice, movement towards your goals will take place by itself. The movement becomes an unfolding that you are inviting to happen within you"

(Kabat-Zinn, 1990, p. 27).

- **Acceptance:** Coming to terms with the state of things as they are rather than wasting energy/time resisting or turning away from reality. Different from passive resignation, our willingness to see things as they are enables appropriate action.
- **Letting go:** Putting aside our inclination to elevate and attach (or cling) to some aspects of experience and resist or reject others. We let our moments be what they are and unfold as they may, including the thoughts, emotions, and sensations that inhabit them, and by doing so, we accept them and let them go.

Can we begin to imagine what our sex, our intimacy, might look like if we applied the principles above to our sexual lives? How game changing it might be to release ourselves of judgment, accepting and befriending each moment, one after the next? When sex asks us to let go, get vulnerable, express, communicate, exercise and respect boundaries, share, play, reveal, step away from our socialization and the stories the world has made up about what sex is and isn't, should or shouldn't be, and just – be in it, with it, moved by it. Mindfulness is the vehicle.

Stepping into practice doesn't require cultivating a "clear mind" or neutral thinking, which is a common misconception; nor does it involve attempting to block out or resist certain aspects of our experience in favor of others. It is awareness of the entire landscape, through a lens that permits letting go and letting be, allowing all emotional, sensory, and cerebral input in. Increased familiarity with ourselves is *the* way we identify any barriers that exist beyond conscious awareness while also strengthening the connection to our physiology. The end result? More control over how to pave the way for arousal, erections, ejaculation, and orgasm to unfold alongside greater ease and freedom. The shedding of the performative, fearful, frozen, and/or anxious version of our sexual selves and lives. Practice that is progressive, slow, and intentional is how we carve out and reinforce new associations, ones the body and mind can trust, and therefore durable associations that last longer than two weeks or a month, the window of time most couples describe change living within before we default back to our struggle and the system we've created around it.

Sensate Focus

How do we accomplish rolling mindfulness principles and embodiment into our sensual and sexual experience, breaking down old, negative, or challenging associations with sex and intimacy, and building new ones that help us stay and play in our parasympathetic nervous system? Sensate focus (SF) is a sex therapy technique developed by William Masters and Virginia Johnson to treat common sexual challenges. Through behavioral at-home experiences, SF helps us come into our bodies, sensation, and emotion while creating space from our thoughts, cultivating the ability to recognize the role our thoughts play in the experience: learning to let be thoughts that are welcome, and conversely let go of thoughts that are simply visitors passing through, carrying with them old narratives and stress. Through individual and relational progressions, we practice new responses to previously anxiety provoking or panic inducing situations or triggers, progressively pairing release with sensual and "sexual" stimulation and arousal. SF takes us from focus *on* sensation to immersion *in* sensation, the gateway into sexual responsiveness. More on the logistics in "Set-Up" in Chapter 21.

21 Basic Practice

A Few Important Notes before You Begin

Buy-In

When in doubt (because you will be – if not now, at some point in the journey), this is the section you can return to. It is your "buy-in" pitch; but it is only as effective as *you* make it. Add to the paragraphs that follow, write out the reasons you know this journey is important to you uniquely that you began considering in the last chapter, and why taking a risk and trying a different route is important for you at this place in your life. Revisit this section and continue to add – the more compelling motivations we can muster, the better.

We cannot communicate active no's to primary elements of our sexuality (different from no's around behavior and boundaries) (*no fantasizing about that, no asking for that, no being honest about that, no expressing that, etc.*), we cannot communicate a list of "shoulds" to our sexuality (*I should look like this, I should be performing like this, I should act like this*), and we cannot treat sex like a puzzle and experience to control and manage (engaging higher order thinking – communicating off-timing to the body), and ask our physiology for a yes (e.g. sexual functioning and orgasm). Our anxiety alerts us to these contradictions, the hidden forces at work behind the curtain. Now we know how to identify and address them psychologically, it's time to turn to the body.

> Having taken a deep look at my past "training" around sex and intimacy whilst developing my current sexual values, I have arrived at the place where I practice embodying new associations, helping my mind and body get on the same page behaviorally, where I take all of the learning I've done and apply it – meaningfully and durably.

Our conscious mind is useful in helping us identify the low-hanging fruit in terms of what our sexual anxiety is made of. Mindful embodiment practice (i.e. sensate focus) is *the* way to both learn more about and understand

DOI: 10.4324/9781003369080-25

what our conscious brain cannot identify, the deep players in the game, and then to move through them, paving the way for new or different messages to embed themselves. By learning how to feel and allow in rather than think and work to resist, we make room for the natural function of our arousal and sexual response to come online in the way it is designed to today. Learning how to meaningfully let go of control, allows us to paradoxically feel more in control as we come to understand how our bodies operate, how our arousal feels, and what emotions exist outside of the influence of anxiety. With this information in hand, we can be the wind in the sail moving the boat forward, rather than the crew working to secure the sail in the desired direction.

> *Medication that aims to "treat" sexual dysfunction will not address the underlying cause (though there's no harm in turning to it as a tool if called for). It cannot provide a liberated and dynamic sexual and intimate life on its own. It will not set me free sexually. Only I can do this, with myself, for myself, through deep inquiry alongside experiences with myself and a partner (if applicable). I can and will create new associations with sexuality and intimacy that reflect the kinds of attitudes, feelings, and values I want to embody now. This will come to be through slow, progressive experiences that pair release with sensual, intimate, vulnerable touch and closeness, over and over again. In this slowness, I will begin to see actual progress. It emerges, lives, and thrives when we allow things to unfold in their own time, speeding up at just the right time. Just like great sex.*

Additional reasons addressing my sexual anxiety and fear through mindful embodiment is important and (importantly) makes sense for **me**:

_____

_____

_____

_____

Buy-In Breakdown

To simplify just slightly, as a (or arguably *the*) melding place of all that makes us human, when we address, *really* address, anxiety within our sex, we change our relationship to ourselves in profound and lasting ways. How might learning how to let go of control in sex change our relationship to control in our jobs? Our day-to-day lives? How might more ease in emotional expression shift how we communicate in our important familial and friendship relationships? Will shedding the performance in the bedroom lead to more authenticity across the board? Perhaps. While we ponder those larger questions, you can be assured that if you take your time with the experiences included in this chapter, at minimum you will:

- Diminish anxiety: i.e. make room for desire and arousal.
- Pair release response with touch/sensory and then sexual experiences.
- Uncover stored feelings/memories/experiences held in the body in a grounded and controlled way.
- Build tolerance for, and then befriend, vulnerability.
- Practice embodied differentiation (e.g. being in "my" experience, speaking to what I want when I want it, identifying and then speaking to my boundaries, feeling into my sense of separateness so I can be connected).
- Learn about individual and shared sexuality in the present.
- Expand my repertoire.

Avoidance

Avoidance will be a visitor in this journey. Whether you're partnered or exploring individually, expect it to rear its head throughout. How you treat yourself when you bump into it matters. We are not in the business of shaming or even guilting ourselves for falling off schedule or failing to show up. In fact, this sort of self-treatment only risks making matters worse: it amplifies pressure and stress. Instead, we will be getting curious in the face of it. *What is it doing here? What information does it have for me? What is it trying to show me? What feelings can I identify that have brought it about? Fear, anxiety, concern? What might I be afraid, anxious, or concerned about and then how might I take a small step back in order to ease into the experience more slowly?*

Avoidance always carries useful information with it. We want to zoom in to understand how to decipher its message to better curate or adapt our process to fit us uniquely.

I may have simply had a particularly busy week and was truly tired, or I'm avoiding because I will be coming into contact with that part of my body, and the steps I'm planning on taking feel too big.

Repetition

In the experiences described, it is crucial that you're being honest with yourself with regard to readiness to move on to the next progression. We want to stay where we're at with one experience until you're able to:

- Notice what is happening in the body (sensation as it moves, tension, numbness).
- Observe thoughts and allow them to come and go.

- Notice emotions as they surface and let them be/manifest as they will.
- Identify and notice the dissipation of our mechanisms for coping with our own vulnerability (laughing, talking a lot, a quivering or jerky stomach, instructing, critiquing, rushing, etc.).

The more we can recognize our presence with ourselves, the more we can notice and practice attunement to the moment, our experience, and our sensations and feelings, the more deeply the body begins to register safety and comfort. We want this foundation of safety and comfort to be strong and meaningful; our physiology and the quality of anxiety present will show us when it is shaky and we're moving too fast.

You may also need to refer back to specific sections of Part I or Part II in order to reground yourself in ideas you want to embody. The ideas we come into this work with we have been carrying around for years, maybe even the better part of our whole lives. Exposure to new ideas that resonate can't be a one-time thing: it's insufficient in the face of deeply engrained values, beliefs, and messaging. Repetition can feel annoying and like a chore, but your brain and body will thank you for it.

Boredom

Slowing down with yourself and your partner (if relevant) in the way that sensate focus asks can be different for us, even potentially unusual. We simply aren't accustomed to it in the fast-paced, performance-driven world we live in. Consequently, the brain can find it hard to adapt, as many of us experience when sitting down to meditate. It can take practice to shift from getting lost in our thoughts, to noticing them; from resisting or trying to encourage emotions, to letting them be; from trusting our anxiety and avoiding, to approaching and staying. It can feel fruitless to have an experience where "pleasure sensation" is not the thing we are targeting, where we are inviting in all aspects of our emotional and sensual experience. Where we don't get a grade on our paper. Enter boredom. Boredom has a message, and it is almost always *"this thing you're doing has no utility or its value is not clear or important enough, so it's better to tune out, think about something else, or even judge what is going on as ridiculous or worse."* If boredom reveals itself (which it almost certainly will), get to know it as you would other aspects of the experience: *"What are the thoughts it's telling me are more important or worthy of my attention? Do I agree? What are the associated sensations in the body?"* As always, allow it to be, don't resist it, simply return to sensation in the face of it and release. Return to the "Buy-In" section above as needed, refer back to previous chapters, or review the sensate focus/mindfulness break-down to connect more deeply with your motivations for embarking on this journey with this degree of depth (i.e. with long-term, meaningful change in mind).

If boredom persists, it is a good idea to get curious about its role as a distancer, because it is one. *Why might my brain be creating distance from my body, my sexuality, my vulnerability, in this way? What is it attempting to protect me from? Do I require that protection in this moment?* If the answer is no, simply practice returning to *"I'm OK, this is OK, I'm staying here"* and release. The more we approach and reapproach the experience, the more our mind/body understands the experience as one of safety as opposed to danger, and the distancing methods the brain employs fall off.

Every aspect of your experience is useful, even the message of "uselessness" itself!

A Word for Partners

What is happening within your relationship is an opportunity for growth, understanding, connection, and expansion. It is critical that we step into that frame as we navigate this struggle, because anything else is very frequently overly simplistic and off-base, born from our own anxious mind (ill-informed even though our conclusions can feel very compelling and seemingly obvious). It is a chance to get really curious rather than defensive, because an attitude of openness and solidarity paves the way for progress and can inspire change in and of itself.

One strategy that we can safely dump right off the bat is any shaming, hostility, or constant and intense pressure to resolve the struggle. Anxiety, stress, and pressure all fall under the same umbrella and, with the sexual challenge very likely being anxiety-based, we are adding fuel to the avoidance and perhaps even resistance fire. If sexual trauma is part of your partner's history, we risk inadvertently reinforcing messages taken away from that experience, for example *"sex is not for or about me,"* or *"sex is something I have to do to get love."*

It is also important to understand that low desire is very frequently, if not always, part of the package. If you look closely at this, it makes perfect sense. We will not seek out experiences that are embarrassing, scary, overwhelming, emasculating, or that make us feel like we've disappointed someone. It's that simple. To *desire* an experience, we must do just that: anticipate the reward it has for us, the pleasure (including connection, release, escape, comfort) that we can sense is on the horizon with any given interaction. In no world will we long for, crave, seek out, and desire experiences (even sex) that bring shame, embarrassment, worry, and/or fear. It takes a while for desire to come back online, and you play a critical role in that process. Can your partner, can you for that matter, step toward your sexual life and know that you will be supported and held no matter what happens? Do you feel like your shared sexual life is dynamic and rich, able to accommodate the changes that life and aging and changing bodies and minds will bring? Can you feel confident and secure in the knowledge that, no matter what happens, we have shared ourselves with each other, and *that* is intimacy. If sex is something we can do right or wrong, if we get frustrated when our partners "can't perform," we are creating an unsafe environment for sharing, revealing, and connection. If we can provide reassurance that boundaries work (e.g. *what would feel good to you tonight? I can show up for that and not go any further*), if we can invite in the "no" without upset or shut down if it shows up (e.g. *feel free to say no at any point and to anything I might suggest*), we will have more engagement. This does not mean backing off entirely and waiting for them to approach: avoidance is a powerful force and will always attempt to assert itself. It simply means approaching with a different attitude, a different means of getting curious, creating a plan, and providing support.

How can I support my partner when things get challenging during sex itself? What does that look like?

The best way to understand what feels best for your partner is to ask them! *What feels good from me when anxiety kicks up or when things don't go as planned? Do you want me to "do" anything? What words are helpful, if any?*

Here are some tips regarding what generally does not work despite good intentions:

- **Do not** move into a parental position relative to the struggle. Meaning, resist the urge to say things like, "*It's OK ... you are so great at so many things and this is hard! Come here, come in for a hug.*" It sounds silly on paper, but it is very common, especially with folks who tend to be nurturers in general.
- **Steer clear of** passive–aggressive support (which often doesn't intend to be passive–aggressive whatsoever, but often ends up being received this way). For example, "*Don't worry, we'll try again next time! I'm sure you'll do better then!*"

Instead, try the following:

- **Treat it like it's no big deal**, but we must mean it! What is your definition of a rewarding sexual experience? What are the qualities inherent in it for you? Can you describe this for yourself in great detail? The more details that are available, the easier it will be for you to pivot and get excited about what else is available (because there is always other fun or comfort or forms of connection available). This can look like, "*No big deal! I'd love to move on to this,*" or "*here's what sounds good now, what do you think?*"

Self-Care Acknowledgment

All of us arrive in adulthood with sexual scars and bruising. We all have experienced shame and confusion in this arena of human life, built and informed by and from all the others. Our healing journey is our chance to introduce a different mentality, different attitudes and concepts around what sex is and means to us now, and to help them take up meaningful residence in our hearts and minds. At the core of this is honoring ourselves, our boundaries, our limits, our inclinations to pause, slow down, pivot, and change course. Below you will find examples of some reminders or mantras to carry with you throughout your process. As always, add to or edit this list in an ongoing way from your own perspective and with your own words to make them more "you." The more "you" they feel, the more powerful they become.

- *I am invited into my own sexual healing; it is available to and for me always.*
- *Any and all wants, desires, interests, and curiosities that surface are abstractions until I give them definition and decide where and if they belong in my lived reality. With this in mind, they are all welcome to surface.*
- *My experience matters. I have control now even if it wasn't available to me in the past. I will take care of myself and understand that this is critical to the sense of sexual freedom I feel. The more connected and cared for I feel within myself, for myself, the more sensual and sexual freedom I'll experience.*
- *I will hold myself tenderly throughout my process and with whatever it brings forward. The ease with which I express, receive, and experience love for myself and others is infinitely complex and ever-changing. Sexual intimacy is and asks permission to be allowed to be these things. I am OK just as I am in that complexity. I am not responsible if others I share myself with cannot understand that.*
- *Thank you to me for stepping into the bravery required to have gotten this far and for understanding intuitively that I deserve more. This work is the greatest act of self-love there is, and I am ready.*

Lastly (and perhaps most importantly), these experiences are not about stoking eroticism (though it's absolutely OK if that shows up), they are about breaking down and eliminating that which gets in the way of a baseline of comfort – the prerequisite to fun, playful, uninhibited, adventurous, connective sex (add or subtract any of those words depending on what you specifically are looking to glean from sex).

All Start Here: Individual Sensate Focus

Why would I engage in touch experiences on my own? With myself? That seems – wacky.

Precisely the reason it may seem wacky is precisely why it's important, that is learning how to encounter our own vulnerability and to feel comfortable within it and in our relationship to ourselves (our bodies, our sensuality, our emotions, our sexuality) is foundational to a connective, dynamic experience with ourselves and others. After all, not feeling comfortable or at ease with ourselves is kind of a big barrier. Learning how to feel safe, steady, and at home in our own experience, moving anxiety, stress, fear, and panic out of the way, will make meaningful room for possibility to come forward. It creates the space necessary for pleasure, desire, and arousal to surface – whatever that might look like for you on any particular day. It's a reclamation story, a new beginning, an opportunity to understand and then rewrite your relationship to yourself.

Building a foundation of comfort with your sexual self (i.e. yourself), eases the transition into the relational realm where we level up in terms of the quality and brand of vulnerability we encounter. *If any of the individual experiences feel inaccessible or challenging due to disability, body size, or any other variables that might affect physical comfort, feel free to use props (pillows, wedges, etc.) to help your body into release, or simply skip to the partnered experiences. This is your body and it's invited, all bodies need help and support.*

Getting Started: Pelvic Floor Awareness Training

The information that follows includes bits of an interview with Michelle Thibeault, PT, founder and owner of Diversified Physical Therapy. Michelle graduated with a B.S. in physical therapy from the University of Hartford, specializing in treating pelvic floor dysfunction. In 2012 she graduated from the Sex Therapy Postgraduate Institute of New York as a Sex Counselor.

Our pelvic floor muscle group plays a central role in our sexual functioning, while also being yet another place where our bodies hold anxiety, pressure, stress, and fear. Without immunity from the physical tension that accompanies these feelings, it is very much a gatekeeper, granting us access to our arousal and sexual functioning when released, and impeding or blocking arousal when activated (clenched). Our conscious awareness of this tension becomes undetectable with the familiarity we keep with it, in the pelvic floor and in the body at large. When we understand what full release in this muscle group feels like, when we visit the corresponding sensations in the body on a regular basis, we can start to notice as soon as tension has entered the body (i.e. the mind), and release it, allowing blood to move back through, occupying the tissues, lighting up sensory nerve endings. The way to understand what full release feels like is to practice full release, and also to explore the different levels of tension to varying degrees. Familiarity with both tension and release not only allows for identification of anxiety in the body, but also paves the way for greater connection to arousal.

Fun Fact: A commonly known fact among midwives and birthing professionals is that the jaw and pelvic floor are profoundly connected! Releasing the jaw releases the pelvic floor, something we can use to our advantage in our work with sex, but also when birthing babies!

So How Do We Practice?

For People with Vulvas

To begin:

- Lie down and rest your hand gently over the vaginal opening, then squeeze up and in (as if you can imagine holding a small blueberry inside your vaginal canal that you need to keep in place), hold, and release. Take a beat, then release even further (or simply release again). Notice if you're holding your breath or clenching the muscles of the buttocks.
- Alternatively, while seated in a chair, release the muscles in your thighs, abdomen, and buttocks while relaxing your jaw. Squeeze up and in as if trying to move that blueberry further up into the vaginal canal while hugging it.
- When releasing your pelvic floor, it can be useful to image a flower blooming, petals unfurling in a slow, gentle bloom rather than a "bearing down." No significant effort should be expended here.

Imagine closing your labia, as if your labia were butterfly wings and you want to gently close them in. Alternatively, imagine you're in a crowded room and you have to pass gas and don't want to. Practicing pulling that in. We're not using your legs, nothing else should move. Lastly, you can put a finger inside the vagina and that way you'll really feel the lift. If you don't want to put a finger inside, you can put a finger on the perineal body, so the place between the vagina and the rectum or between the scrotum and the rectum.

(Michelle Thibeault, April 2023)

For People with Penises

To begin:

"*Oh, so it's like when I twitch my penis!*" Although you won't find this described in any formal literature, many people with penises describe this experience as very helpful in assisting them as they isolate and practice tensing and releasing their pelvic floor muscles. "If you have a scrotum, it's like you're lifting that scrotum up towards you, lifting and pulling it up" (Michelle Thibeault, April 2023). Again, you should be able to breathe freely with no muscle tension in the abdomen or buttocks.

Note for all (people with penises, vulvas, and intersex genitals): Locating the pelvic floor muscles using the "stop–release" method while urinating is not advised!

> You don't want to be doing these exercises on the toilet because there is actually a reflex where you contract your pelvic floor muscles and it tells your bladder to tell your brain, "not time to go." It's one of the shut-offs we use for people with urinary urgency: do Kegels (PM exercises). So, I don't want people practicing on the toilet because they've trained their brain that that's the place they go to the bathroom.
>
> (Michelle Thibeault, April 2023)

The goal of our practice with contracting and releasing is not about trying to beef up or strengthen the pelvic floor muscles (PM), although there are great benefits to strengthening (longer, firmer erections into old age; more forceful and complete ejaculations = less prostate enlargement problems; tones the vagina; prevents the leakage of urine and incontinence as we get older). How to properly exercise the PM is something to consult with a pelvic floor physical therapist around. In fact, these therapists and sex therapists often team up in favor of holistic client care. The pelvic floor physical therapists are able to directly interact with, learn from, and treat what is happening with the body, or pelvic floor, while the sex therapist is able to address the emotional/psychological origins and maintenance of the struggles, while only able to provide verbal instruction with regard to the behavioral aspect of the work.

We can move through the initial exercises as described above in "To begin" and then after getting a feel for where this muscle group exists and how to isolate it, we want to move move along in our practice using the suggestions described below.

Practice Regimen

Once familiarity with this muscle group has been achieved, simply begin with 15 "squeeze, release" repetitions once or twice daily. Play with a quick rhythm to the hold and release (hold for a second or so, and then immediately release), and also a slower pace (big slow breaths while maintaining the squeeze), followed by slow, focused release as you exhale. Pause, then release even further.

Scale Exploration

As you become increasingly familiar with the experience of tension and release in your pelvic floor, imagine the levels of tension existing on a spectrum, from 1 being no tension, to 10 being the greatest amount of tension. Can you tighten up to a level 6, breathe for six seconds, then release to the count of six? Can we squeeze up to a level 7, hold to the count of 3 seconds, then release down to a level 3, hold to the count of three seconds, then release all the way to 0? Release even more. Explore the scale, fine-tuning your ability to understand the different levels of tension, and the sensations involved in release.

Releasing the Pelvic Floor for Easy Circulation (People with Penises and their Partners)

Start by taking off all of your clothes, including underwear. Take a few moments to simply lay with one another, one big spoon and the other little spoon, releasing into the bed, releasing the jaw, slowing your breathing, leaving the day behind. See if you can synchronize your breathing, feeling the rise and fall of each other's breath (back to chest and chest to back), release even more deeply into the bed. After a few minutes, the person with the penis looking to expand their practice (you) will move onto your back, facing up, and your partner will begin slowly caressing your stomach, thighs, and genitals with their hand for 10–15 minutes very slowly and gently. As you become aroused, if they feel or notice tightening of the pelvic floor, they will lightly tap your lower abdomen and then wait for you to release the muscle before beginning again. After your partner has pointed out your unconscious tensing a handful of times (or so – it's OK if it takes a while), you will begin to recognize it yourself and gain the ability to keep your PM released without feedback or prompting from your partner (Keesling, 2006).

Signs of tightening or clenching of PM:

- Clenched buttocks (body raised slightly off the bed).
- Tense thighs.
- Tight or tense abdomen.
- Shallow breathing.
- Others?
- It is common for partners to be able to feel or see blood flowing into the shaft of the penis when PM is released, and then to watch or feel it flow back out when clenched.

(Keesling, 2006, p. 209)

If this experience is challenging, it's information! What is it like having your partner interact with your penis in this entirely different (for most of us) way? Without penetration, "sex" according to your typical script, or "performance" on the table? If you find the number of reminders isn't diminishing, ask yourself if there are aspects of the experience that feel challenging to you. Are you trying to accomplish anything? Are you hoping your partner experiences you a certain way? Is any nervousness or anxiety following you into the experience? If the felt sense of tension and anxiety doesn't diminish with practice, it may be useful to begin with the Back Caress for Couples, and then return to this experience once a foundation of release and ease has been cultivated there.

Sensate Focus Basic Practice Progressions

With the exception of the narrating touch progressions, the sensate focus experiences described below were adapted from *Sexual Healing: The Completest Guide to Overcoming Sexual Problems* by Barbara Keesling (2006).

We've gained a sense of connection and familiarity with our pelvic floor, now we're ready to move on to some basic practice SF progressions! Now, remember: the slower you go, the faster you go. These experiences will provide useful information only insomuch as we're tuned in and engaged, which requires understanding why it's useful to attune to our sensation and experience in this way in the first place. If you find yourself struggling with the method to the madness, refer back to the "buy-in" section at the beginning of this chapter, and add any reasons that feel meaningful of your own from the reading and learning you've done thus far.

What Is This Again?

In a nutshell, touch experiences that progress from seemingly basic "non-erotic" (even though if that shows up, that's completely OK), sensory-focused exploration with specific parameters and boundaries spelled out, to increasingly "sexual" or erotic experiences where we move from sensory focus, deeper into sensory immersion. All experiences directly target and address the anxiety and tension in our bodies and mind and create and deepen new associations that make room for our sexual functioning, while also paving the way for emotional and psychological freedom, comfort, and play.

Set-Up

For all of the basic practice progressions described, we want a comfortable environment that allows for focused awareness and attention. This means that music and TV are off, phones on silent, lights dim (not too bright or dark), and any animals or pets are out of the room. Right now, we are also keeping unintended expectation or pressure at bay by avoiding attempting to create a "romantic" ambiance with candles, rose petals, silk sheets (you get the point). These experiences are not meant to elicit any specific feelings or set the stage for any particular kind of tone. It's almost as if we want the environment to act as a comfortable but neutral container, where the internal elements of our experience are able to be witnessed and felt without external distraction.

The Touch

While participating in the experiences, in either the passive or active roles, have front-of-mind the following. This touch is:

- **For your own interest or curiosity, or "non-demand"**: we are coming fully into our own experience – our own thoughts, emotions, sensations, and instincts and getting to know intimately what they are made of. This is our training in absorption in our own sensory landscape, the portal into sexual responsiveness and surrender.
- **A sensory exploration**: Thoughts? Come back to sensation. Anxiety? Release the body and come back to sensation. Sensation is simultaneously our point of focus or grounding mechanism and also an element of exploration and learning in and of itself, in the same way that we anchor ourselves in, and also get to know the breath in meditation.
- **A caress**: The quality of the touch we're exploring with is slow, soft, and gentle – a true caress! We are not using pressure (unless a bit is needed) the way we would with a massage. A massage is about an outcome, particularly pleasure or relief; the caress itself is our vehicle for slowing down and coming further into ourselves in reaction to exploring the visual, emotional, psychological, and tactile realm of our bodies, or the "other" (if applicable).

- **Very slow:** The touch is so very slow. Think slow and then slow that down some more. The slowness allows for us to understand and experience the nuance and finer details of our exploration, it allows those deeply buried emotions or memories room to surface, and it also potentially activates the release of oxytocin, or the "cuddle hormone" to allow for even deeper release and connection.
- **Mindful:** The touch is here to help us return to the present moment, with everything it brings for us, over and over again. We are noticing when we've left the present moment, when we've become unhooked from the tether of sensation, and simply coming back, slowly and gently.

How will I know when I'm/we're ready to move on to the next progression/experience?

It is critical that we not move on before we're ready as we will work against ourselves and the foundation of release we're cultivating, the new associations being carved out and reinforced, the quality of connection and exploration we're inviting in, alongside the important discovery of clues that live in the details of our experience, pointing us in the direction of aspects of our healing calling for our attention. So how can we be sure? Unfortunately, it's more of an art than a science, but we do our best to understand readiness through our ability to return to sensation with relative ease, to notice the thoughts and return rather than getting lost, to move through feeling, rather than feeling stuck in it (*this agitation just won't lift!*), and to discover ease and release in our musculature (or identify tension and release when it arises). In other words, we look to our experience of mindfulness, attunement, release, and learning to assist us in our determination.

Experience Check-In: "But I have ADHD!"

Sensate focus compliments all bodies, all sexual orientations, all gender expressions, all abilities, and makes room for and celebrates neurodiversity as a direct reflection of and profound learning experience of and with *you* uniquely. If partnered, sensate focus provides rich understanding: about our sensory experience, our relationship to emotion, to our executive functions, to the complexity of us, and then illuminates possibilities for greater connection within that complexity. Moving further in, getting to know the intersections between our ADHD or autism spectrum disorder, for example, and our past, or our wounding, or our training in intimacy and closeness, opens doors for greater precision in how we navigate the kind of intimacy we're searching for today. When to back off, when to come closer in, what connection looks like for me, and how I can understand how it works for you. Sensate focus removes categories (although they inform our process), and asks the question: "*What is this like for you uniquely? How will we work with it?*" And then it shows us the ways.

Sequence Overview

Recommended Progression Sequence for Couples

- Back caress;
- Front caress (no breasts or genitals);
- Front caress with breasts and genitals;
- Genital caress;
- Narrating touch;
- Mutual caress;
- Peaking;
- Plateauing;
- Advanced or Diagnosis specific progressions (Erectile Dysfunction and Vaginismus are explored in Chapter 22).

Recommended Progression Sequence on Your Own

- Front caress (no breasts or genitals).
- Front caress with breasts and genitals;
- Genital caress;
- Narrating touch;
- Peaking;
- Plateauing;
- Advanced or Diagnosis specific progressions (Erectile Dysfunction and Vaginismus are explored in Chapter 22).

The suggested sequences above may imply a linear path in terms of our progress, or a build towards specific elements. Again, our sexual experience is complex, deeply personal, and unique to who we are and how we live, love, and express ourselves. There is no one way to be sexual and to create the kind of sexual life that fits us. SF allows us to find the progress we're looking for and skip or edit out aspects that are not meaningful or desirable. In other words, the progressions may end after time spent with the front caress if your goal is greater embodiment and you found it there. The progressions may end after peaking practice with a partner, if those experiences freed you of the performance anxiety that inhibited authentic expression. Your healing starts and ends where you determine.

The Progressions: Let's Get Started!

Recommended frequency: 1–2 times a week. Regular experience with sensate focus is critical for reinforcement of new ideas, sensations, learning, and experience.

Read the instructions and then place them aside and watch what unfolds in the moment. There is no such thing as a "wrong" way to do these experiences - in fact, it is useful to understand how our brains fill-in-the blanks around what is retained from these pages. Memorization will only lead to performance.

Front Caress (Individual)

Set up your space with comfort and focused awareness in mind: lights not too bright or too dark, comfortable temperature, phones on silent, and no distractions or external stimulation. Before coming into the bed, take off as many articles of clothing as you feel comfortable with right now, not the amount you think you "should" remove, and determine if any parts of the front of your body are off limits today. Give yourself permission to identify these spaces in the moment as well, and caress around them. Check in with yourself:

How does it feel to consciously set aside time just for me?
What's it like to consider that I'm preparing to spend time touching my own body for my own sake, without an outcome in mind?

You are about to have an intimate experience with yourself. How does that land within you? Are you inclined to reframe it at all? If so, that's OK, simply be mindful of the adaptations you make and the reasoning behind them.

Can you give yourself permission to look however you're going to look, feel however you're going to feel, experience whatever you're going to experience without judgment from yourself? Can you unhook yourself in this moment from the "shoulds" that you either feel and cannot articulate, or can very much identify and name?

When you're ready, come into the bed and lie on your back, making your body as physically comfortable as is available in this moment. Give yourself a few minutes to settle in: releasing the weight of your body into the support of the mattress, feeling the coolness of the sheets or blankets against your skin, closing your eyes (or holding a soft gaze in a general area – not fixed or targeted spot) and taking a few deep breaths, releasing your shoulders, jaw, and pelvic floor as you exhale. Take a moment to notice any sounds that are passing through.

When you're ready, place your hand on any part of the body that feels most available for you and slowly begin caressing the surface of your skin. Move slowly, breathe, release. Notice the buzziness or trickling in of any thoughts that surface as you touch, allow them to come forward, note them, and then return to the point of contact between your hand and your body. Do any emotions reveal themselves? Can you notice the sensations in the body that accompany the emotions? Allow the feelings to stay, don't try to push them away or encourage them along; simply stay with sensation as you continue to slowly explore your own body, your own skin, for your own interest or curiosity.

(**If emotion becomes overwhelming,** please pause or stop at any point. Notice your context: remind yourself you are safe as you release your jaw, shoulders, and pelvic floor. Check in with yourself: *what do I need to take care of myself in this moment?* If answering this question feels hard or unavailable, simply stand and bring movement to your body. This can help reorient you and process through the feeling in a different way. If the sensation passes, check in and notice if simply thinking about continuing the experience brings the intense emotions back up in any capacity. If this is not your experience, slowly and gently resume the caress.)

Move very slowly over your shoulders, arms, elbows, all the way down to the other hand and back up, making your way slowly toward the chest. In this first caress, we are going to move around breasts and genitals, so do so slowly, paying attention to sensation and thoughts as you move towards the belly. Breathe, release your shoulders, release any muscles that hold noticeable tension. Continue the caress, allowing your own interest or curiosity to lead. Notice the temperature of your skin and the different textures you encounter in this slow, steady pace. Bring awareness to the pressure of your hand against your skin. Notice thoughts as they come and go as you might notice a faint sound in the air, gently and without resisting or attaching to them. When you recognize that you've been carried away by a thought (which will happen and is OK!), simply and gently return to sensation, return to the feeling of your hand against your skin, against your body. Observe the thoughts as they come and go, taking note of what they do and don't have in common. Let thoughts go, let emotions be, notice and follow sensation in the body.

Stay with this experience for ten minutes, give or take. Once finished, simply rest on the bed and notice what is with you: sensation? What is the quality and rhythm of the breath? Any emotion? What has shifted since you began?

Post-Experience Recommendation

After finishing each experience, it can be extremely helpful to grab a notebook and simply write out, stream-of-consciousness style, what was noticed: thoughts, feelings, sensations, interpretations. Do this with no consideration for grammar, complete sentence structures, correct spelling, simply jot or even draw it out how it surfaces in your brain and body. Do similar themes, memories, and/or sensations show up as you return to this experience? How might you makes sense of this? Is it an opportunity for a conversation with and within oneself? A lesson from the past in need of attending to or editing in order to make room for openness or ease?

Basic Back Caress (Couples)

We're going to treat this like a date night: put the phones down, give each other your undivided attention, chat and get to know one another (because we're always getting to know one another) – keep it light and friendly! No politics or other potentially challenging or heavy topics, including trying to problem solve about that issue the two of you had last week. Easy, friendly conversation and connection. Have a snack, like fruit and cheese, something relatively light. Limit your alcohol intake to one drink and only if you *absolutely* must (we all know the toll alcohol can take on circulation, and we want to be as clear headed and tuned in to undisturbed sensation as possible).

After spending a good amount of time talking and connecting emotionally together through conversation and shared time, head into your bedroom. Make sure it feels comfortable: light on but not too bright, but not so dark you can't see one another; temperature feels good; TV is off; dogs are outside. Next, you will both undress as much as you're comfortable, including the choice to have underwear on or off (notice any inclination or sense of pressure to mirror your partner's choices here – what's it like to make a choice in the context of intimacy for yourself? We can be in our own choices, together. A practice!). Come into the bed, and one of you is going to be big spoon, the other will be little spoon as you lay together and just allow yourselves to sink into the bed. Feel the temperature of the sheets against your skin, notice any sounds in the air, feel the warmth of your partner's body against yours, see if you can synchronize your breathing to theirs. You're putting the day behind you and arriving fully in this moment together.

After about five minutes, one of you will be the active partner, and the other will be the passive partner. The passive partner will lay on the front side of their body with their back side facing up. Once comfortable, the active partner will begin slowly caressing the back side of the passive partner's body for their own interest. Each part you will caress slowly, paying particular attention to temperature, texture, pressure. Remember, this is a caress: slow, mindful, and for your own interest or curiosity. You may use your palm, fingers, back of the hand, or arm. As you touch, check in with your body: breathe, notice any tension, and release it, come back to the point of contact between your skin and your partners. Focus on sensation. If any thoughts emerge, simply notice them – don't try to resist or pursue them, just notice, and come back to the point of contact between your skin and your partners – resume the touch.

Passive partner, your job is to simply receive the touch, noticing the thoughts and feelings that emerge, releasing any tension in the body, breathing. If any emotion surfaces, notice it, and let it be, releasing into its accompanying sensations, passively allowing it to move through or come to fruition as it will – return to the touch. We will not be communicating unless any big discomfort shows up. In that case, you want to verbally let your partner know that you will need to pause. The task here is to stay connected in the midst of complex emotion. How might you do that in a way that feels comfortable? Would that mean having them hold you while you steady yourself? Hold your hand as you turn away to attend to the emotion? Think about this in advance.

If you return, do so very slowly, breathe. Check in with the body, release the jaw, release. If arousal occurs, we will treat it in the same spirit as everything else: passively receive the sensation, notice, breathe – don't try to encourage or build on it, don't try to push it away. If orgasm happens, passively receive the sensation, if clean up is required, simply do so and come slowly back to the experience.

Active partner, you will continue to touch for your own experience, checking in with the body, noticing sensation, emotion, and thought as you slowly move along in your caress. If, however, you notice tension in your partner's body as you touch (simply if you happen to notice, this is not your job), we're going to tap that part of the body very lightly with our pointer and middle finger and that is our signal, passive partner, to release that part of the body.

After 10–15 minutes, we will stop, come back to that spoon breathing we did in the beginning and recalibrate. *What am I feeling now? How has it shifted since we began? What am I noticing in my body?* Breathe slowly, and release the weight of your body into the bed. After a few minutes here, we will switch! Passive partner, you're now active, and active partner is now passive. At the end of the final 10–15 minutes, return to the spoon breathing position, release into the bed, and notice what is with you.

- A timer is a great way to assure our brains don't get hung up on time but be strategic about the sound you use! A very light, subtle chime is great – just perceptible enough to notice. Last thing we need is to be jolted out of the experience with alarm bells!
- When you're finished with the experience, take 5–10 minutes to debrief together. We will only be sharing aspects that were interesting, surprising, or informative in a neutral or positive way about *your* experience. From here on out, we are protecting your intimate life and bedroom from creating new or reinforcing old negative or challenging associations. This part of your life we want to treat as a sanctuary. If the experience was challenging or very uncomfortable, that must be brought to

therapy, not because that's "bad" but because it's important information that is being revealed! A trained therapist will be able to help make sense of the discomfort and plan the next experience accordingly.

Examples of neutral or positive feedback might look like:

- *"I noticed some tension in my chest when we began touching, then noticed it started to dissipate as we moved along."*
- *"I was super agitated and anxious when my chest was being caressed, but I was able to bring myself back to the touch."*
- *"I kept trying to predict where you might go next, which was interesting."*

Experience check-in: "That sucked!"

You may find that this experience feels awkward, pointless, uncomfortable, agitating, like a puzzle to figure out – all important ways our brains and bodies are working to cope with the vulnerability we feel! This is the beginning! *What was the "awkward" about? Putting myself out there? Being exposed? What's with pointless? Why is my brain deciding that I have better places to be? Things to do? Am I approaching this clinically, from my intellectual brain because this is the main place I live and operate? Is being with feeling too hard?* If we find ourselves talking through the entire experience, are we filling the silence, trying to distract from our feelings? Every reaction has information to look at, all the pieces! If the experience was uncomfortable, that is precisely why we will do it again. To cultivate comfort. Why?

Because all that was asked of you was to touch each other's skin. That's it! Look at all it brought up! How might all of the feelings that surfaced as a result of simply slowing down to touch and be touched have everything to do with the sexual struggle you're contending with? Because it does. This is the beginning, you're on your way!!

Front Caress Excluding Breasts (If Applicable) and Genitals: Couples

Come into the bed and just like last time one of you is going to be big spoon, the other will be little spoon as you lay together and allow yourselves to sink into the mattress. Feel the temperature of the sheets against your skin, notice any sounds in the air, feel the warmth of your partner's body against yours, see if you can synchronize your breathing to theirs.

For this caress, the passive partner will lie on their back facing upwards, eyes closed or holding a soft gaze. Active partner will begin caressing the whole front of the passive partner's body, from head to feet, for their own interest or experience, excluding breasts and genitals.

Caress as slowly as possible, moving as you're inclined around the body. Maintain contact with your partner's skin so as to avoid the possibility of a startle response. Touch for your own interest, exploring parts that are interesting to you in the way that feels most comfortable for you. You can choose to use your palm, fingers, back of your hand, or arm. **Remind yourself that your partner will let you know if they experience any discomfort**, now is the time to explore for yourself. Breathe, release, slow down even further.

As the passive partner, simply receive the touch. Notice the thoughts and feelings that accompany sensation, allow them to be. Breathe, release your body. Focus on the point of contact between your skin and your partner's skin. Speak only if you experience any discomfort during the experience. If you feel yourself tensing up, slow your breathing down even further and imagine your leg muscles sinking into the bed.

In the active role, if you notice any signs of anxiety or stress during the caress (muscle tension, rapid breathing, rapid heart rate, quivering stomach), lightly tap on that part of the body with your index and middle fingers to signal your partner to release. Remember, our main task is to move deeply into our own experience, with all of the learning and information that lives there. We will provide this signal only if we happen to notice tension as we focus on sensation.

After about 10–15 minutes, we will stop, come back to that spoon breathing we did in the beginning and recalibrate. *What am I feeling now? How has it shifted since we began? What am I noticing in my body?* Breathe. After about five minutes here, we will switch! Passive partner, you're now the active one, and active partner is now passive. End with the spoon breathing again, come back into the moment, and engage in the quick debrief as last time.

Expect that this experience might be different, or not! Whatever shows up is absolutely OK and invited! Facing upwards, with multiple intimate parts of the body visible can feel next-level in terms of vulnerability. Allow any feelings to surface, notice their intensity or subtlety, and come back to touch. If you need to pause or stop at any point do so! Ask yourself, what do I need from myself and my partner right now? What comes to mind even just sitting here? Our goal is to stay connected in the midst of big feelings, what might that look like?

Experience check-in: "Sensate focus feels like an intrusion. I feel like I'm being used or objectified by my partner."

If this happens, and you find yourself feeling objectified in the experience, regroup and remind yourself of who your partner is and what you know of and feel from them when it comes to the relationship. If your understanding of your partner is that they love you, care for you, and/or are respectful and attentive to who you are and how you feel, the feeling may be surfacing precisely because the context is "safe" enough for it to reveal itself. The feeling or feelings may be linked to the past in a way that is emerging in the present, alerting you to their presence as a barrier to intimacy, a factor in the anxiety tied to closeness and sexuality.

If this rings true, see if you can remind yourself of who your partner is as the anxiety begins to surface. If comforting, ask for eye contact or to hold their hand as you let this part know that *in this relationship, I'm OK. This is OK. I can stay.* Breathe, release, and slowly return to the caress if that feels available to you.

Front Caress Including Breasts (If Applicable) and Genitals: Couples

Follow the same instructions as spelled out in Experience #3, this time including breasts and genitals. Each part of the body is to be treated similarly; shoulders are to legs are to vulva. That is our breasts and genitals aren't receiving any special attention, including no penetration with fingers as part of the caress.

Experience check-in: "That tickles!"

Many people find that the slow, gentle caress involved in sensate focus inspires ticklishness on various places of the body. See if slightly more pressure resolves this feeling, and also notice how it evolves as you move along in the experiences. Ticklishness can be attributed to sensitivity (some people are just more ticklish than others), or it can be an anxious response, and very often is! If the feeling begins to lift as you progress, you'll have your answer!

Narrating Touch

Without learning how to talk about our bodies, intimacy, and sex openly and directly, we will inevitably bump into difficulty speaking to our experience of it while in it; articulating our wants and boundaries, providing accurate and detailed instruction to eager-to-please (or explore) partners. The inability to comfortably talk about our bodies, our parts, and what we would like more or less of, means we are very frequently at best "tolerating" and at worst bracing through aspects of our experience simply because we cannot grab the vocabulary or feel frozen in our attempts at verbalization. You can imagine the associations that get created when we visit and revisit experiences of a similar nature. You can imagine the impact on our desire.

Conversely, when we learn to use our words with our partners, communicating around sex becomes normalized, making for less loaded conversations where any feedback or offering up of suggestions feels like personal rejection or an ego wound. With less silence comes more options, more nuanced exploration and understanding, more reward.

Narrating Touch for Couples

We begin in a routine manner with each experience, so after you've settled into the bed, spent a few moments breathing together in spoon position and slowing the body down, releasing tension in the jaw, shoulders, abdomen, buttocks, and so on, we will move into our active and passive roles. The active partner will begin a front caress, but in this version, they will verbalize the parts of the body they're touching, "*I'm caressing your shoulder, I'm caressing your chest, I'm caressing your thighs*" and so on. This sounds clinical (and it may or may not feel that way) but can we get curious about the other aspects of the experience? Can you notice any other feelings or sensations connected to naming the parts of the body in such an intentional, slow way? Do you (active partner) feel inclined to move more quickly past any parts of the body in the naming of them? How does verbalization effect your experience? Check in with the body periodically and release, slow down, breathe. Passive partner, what thoughts emerge as you listen and notice the sensations in your body? What emotions surface? As with the other experiences, notice the thoughts and return to sensation, allow emotions to be, experiencing them in their fullness, and passively receive all the dimensions of the experience, witnessing what your body/heart/mind do with this new input.

After 10–15 (ish) minutes, come back into your spoon breathing position and recalibrate (i.e. check in with yourselves): *how do I feel? What has shifted since the start of this experience with my partner? What sensation is with me now? Any emotions identifiable?* And then switch positions and the previously passive partner will take the active role and verbalize the parts of the body they're touching as they engage in the front caress. End back in spoon position, with one final internal check-in. Then turn towards each other and briefly debrief (remember, we're sharing information about our own experience only).

Note: It is OK to struggle! This seemingly simple exercise challenges us to say words that for many of us have been felt as "unspeakable" or even shameful. Maybe your experience of these words has been primarily in the context of humor or jokes (often how we relate to concepts that raise discomfort). If initially we are able to name a few parts as we caress them, that's a great starting point! Ease will build with practice, so there's no need to rush or push ourselves past any significant discomfort – that will only serve to undermine the foundation of release you've cultivated. Take your time and revisit the experience again and again until ease is present. Remember, rushing past or jumping ahead reinforces the anxiety or sexual struggle.

Another version of this experience, of equal importance, places verbalization on the part of the passive partner, that is "*You're caressing my neck, you're caressing my calf, you're caressing my hip.*" How does active acknowledgment of the other change the experience for you? What differences did you notice, if any?

Once you've practiced the experience as described and have noticed more release in the body, and more mindful attunement (i.e. less "checking-out" or "getting lost" in our thoughts or hijacked by big emotions), you can begin to introduce different words to more accurately describe your experience and add dimension to the touch itself. This can add a more erotic element to the touch for some, simply more practice towards ease in communication for others, or both!

Literal

"You're stroking my thigh"
"I'm leading my fingers past your navel"
"You're touching my neck"
"I'm caressing your shoulder blade"

Sensory zoom-in

"Warmth of your hand on my cheek"
"Shutter as you graze my breast"
(Bringing in "self") "My heart quickens caressing your stomach"

Pleasure/curiosity requests

"Please keep stroking my thigh"
"Use a firmer touch around my navel"
"Use just your fingertips to caress my shoulder blades"

Anticipation/tease (What are the pre-requirements?)

"I'm going to slowly graze your cheek"
"I'm moving toward your breasts, but first hips ... stomach"
"I'm touching your scrotum ... inner thighs ... perineum ... scrotum"

When participating in the pleasure and curiosity requests, keep in mind that when more time or a variation of the touch is requested in a particular area, the active partner will continue the touch for as long as they are inclined to! They are then welcome to continue to explore for their own interest, returning to sensation, emotion, and self-connection. If the passive partner would like even more time, or more pressure, they can request it again. We are moving away from anticipating or guessing what the other would like or dislike and trusting them to verbalize for themselves.

Another version of narrating touch can center the **verbalization of boundaries, or boundary practice!**

In this version, we will spend 5–10 minutes in front caress for each partner, and then when ready, the person who will be the first passive partner will periodically and intentionally instruct the active partner to either pause when on a specific part of the body that feels like a yellow zone (i.e. *I need to check in with myself to determine if a boundary is needed*), instruct them to move their hand *around* parts of the body that they don't want to have touched in the moment, or to *avoid* specific parts altogether. If a specific part of the body is not identified as in need of avoiding altogether, then the active partner can reapproach that part as they move back around and the passive partner will either set the boundary a second time, decide it is OK to go there this time, or instruct the active partner to avoid altogether should they determine that it is, indeed, off limits. This might sound like:

- *"Move around my shoulder."*
- *"Avoid my vulva altogether."*
- *"Pause (internal check-in) … approach my neck slowly."*

Alternatively, this experience can be done in "yes's," "no's," and "maybe's". The caress moves slowly enough (which is the instruction anyway) for the passive partner to determine along the way what is a "yes," a "no," or a "maybe" as the active partner approaches. If we land on a "maybe," the active partner will slow the caress even further while waiting for the "yes," or "no." A "maybe" can also mean experiencing the even slower movement of the partner's hand. It is OK to be uncertain and to explore that uncertainty!

Connection with our boundaries, the ability to verbalize them with ease, and to watch as our partner demonstrates respect for those boundaries is an exercise/practice in self and relational trust and presence. A win all around!

Experience check-in: "What if we're turned on at the end? Can we have 'sex'?"

This is an important consideration! We are in the midst of actively breaking down associations attached to your sexual script, perhaps even associations and held experience in the body that organize your sexual script entirely! What we don't want to do is take two steps forward, and two steps back: carving out new grooves and then reinforcing old ones. This can be a big ask for one or both partners! Keep in mind, any sexual "sacrifices" you make now are in favor of a sexual life that is moving and vital for you and your partners (if desired) moving forward. It is in favor of greater ease, which comes with greater possibilities. It is recommended that you hold off on your version of sex, or any aspect of your sexual menu that holds anxiety while you navigate these experiences, while exploring other ways of interacting with the arousal in the body after these experiences. Mutual masturbation? Oral sex (if this is not the version of sex we are targeting)? One person witness and supports while the other self-stimulates? This is a great opportunity to refer to your pivot playlist and expand on the options available.

Genital Caress for Couples

Come into the room, find your spoon breathing positions, let your bodies sink into the bed – into each other. When ready (after about five minutes), the passive partner will lie facing upwards as they did previously, and the active partner will begin a slow, gentle front caress. Explore the entire front side of your partner's body for your own interest. Release your pelvic floor, breathe. Passive partner, receive the sensations, noticing the warmth of your partner's hand or arm on your skin – breathe. After about ten minutes, active partner – you will slowly guide your caress down to your partner's genitals. If the passive partner has a vulva, you may choose to use lubrication to slowly move your fingers over their labia and clitoris. Pay attention to how the outer and inner labia feel, notice textures of the skin. Move your hand from exploring the vulva to their inner thighs, pubic mound, then back down. Explore for your own interest, let it guide your hand – release, breathe. For a few moments, position yourself so that you can get to know your partner's genitals visually. Take the opportunity to learn about the hairs, the colors of the skin, the entire landscape with your eyes as you continue to slowly caress the area, or rest your hand for moments at a time. If you feel yourself becoming mechanical, slow your caress, slow your breathing, come into focused awareness of temperature, texture, and pressure. If you notice your partner's body tensing up, lightly tap the hip area to signal release.

If your partner has a penis, you may (this is optional) choose to warm some lubricant in your hand and slowly caress the shaft of the penis and scrotum with your fingers. Don't try to turn your partner on, or "try" to bring any feeling or sensation forward whatsoever. Allow whatever surfaces to surface, exploring the experience that is unfolding as it is. Breathe, release, explore the area for your own interest. Take this opportunity to really get to know what your partner's genitals look and feel like. Slowly move your fingers around the shaft and head of the penis, then carefully run them around each testicle.

An erection is not an expectation for this experience. Caress your partner's penis and discover the sensations involved in whatever it feels like that day. Experience exactly what the skin feels like on the different parts of your partner's genitals. If you notice your partner's body become tense, signal for them to release with a light tap around the hip or on the thigh. Slow your breathing and release as you touch. If arousal and ejaculation happen, gently wipe them off and continue with the caress. Do the caress for 10–15 minutes.

When you are the passive partner, lie on your back with your legs slightly spread – release your pelvic floor. Place your arms at your sides, close your eyes or hold a soft gaze. As you receive the genital caress, all that is required of you is to focus, notice, breathe, release. Soak up the sensations like a sponge, release the body even further.

What matters here is our ability to leave ourselves alone, witness, and learn. Passively experience the feelings, thoughts, sensations, and breathe. Finish your time by returning to spoon breathing, then a debrief.

Identical instructions apply for intersex genitals with all the experiences! We are simply slowly exploring the genitals for our own experience, interest, or curiosity, with a slow, mindful caress. Focus on sensations, notice textures, areas of warmth and coolness, the different colors of the skin.

Experience check-in: arousal in the body

It may feel strange to be in the presence of physical arousal without "doing" anything about it – that's good stuff! We want to confront our performance narratives and shift into a different mindset; sensate focus is facilitating just that. So instead of, "*I have to do something with this!*" it's "*I get to experience and get to know this without expectation at all.*"

Peaking

Peaking is for you if: you have erectile dysfunction; early ejaculation; delayed ejaculation; difficulty reaching orgasm; you have little, limited, or very specific experiences with sexual or sensual arousal in the body; you feel disconnected from sensations associated with arousal; you just want to explore, learn, and connect more deeply with yourself!

How would you describe what sexual arousal feels like in your body? Would you say there are lots of different levels of arousal that you journey between? How much of your sexual experiences are spent within a specific quality of arousal? Does the range change when in partnered sexual situations? Most of us have never considered these kinds of questions, let alone attempted to answer them. Why does it matter? Because when working with sexual struggles or "dysfunctions" we have often attempted to distance ourselves from our arousal in order to manage emotions that come with our sexual energy, or perhaps prolong or regulate aspects of the experience. Moving away from sensation in our bodies can and often does accomplish diminished arousal, at the expense of deep pleasure, surrender, and importantly, our ability to understand what is required to enhance ejaculatory and erection control, to linger within a certain range of arousal, to understand how close or far away we are from orgasm, and to feel into the emotions that partner with the sensations.

Peaking is the practice of building our understanding of our arousal through self and then partnered (if relevant) touch, using a scale as a measure for the various levels. Through slow, mindful caress, we allow our arousal to go up and down, identifying the levels as we experience the sensations, and becoming intimately familiar with the entire range the more we practice. Over time, what can initially feel like our arousal has a mind of its own, jumping from a 2 to a 9, or hovering in one place, transforms into ease in visiting all or most of the levels in a more linear fashion or according to where we'd like our arousal to linger. Greater awareness plus greater ease, equals greater control whilst letting go (experiences that can live alongside one another when control is uncoupled from stress). This practice is foundational for treating many sexual dysfunctions including desire, arousal, orgasm, ejaculation, and erection struggles.

Use the arousal scale below as an example of how you might fill in the numbers for yourself as you learn. Everyone is different, so pay attention to what a 2, 6, or 9 feels like for you uniquely rather than searching for the specific sensations listed.

Arousal scale: 1 = no arousal, 10 = orgasm

- 2–3 = subtle glimmers of fluttery feeling in chest, warmth in body, anticipation.
- 4–5 = heart rate increases, excitement builds, breathing quickens, tingly sensations in stomach and genitals.
- 6–7 = strong desire for continued contact, urge to increase stimulation, "electric" feelings throughout the body.
- 8 = labored breathing, rapid heartbeat, build of sensation in genitals.
- 9 = nearing the "tipping point" of orgasm. Place of "orgasmic inevitability" (can but doesn't necessarily correspond with "ejaculatory inevitability" for those with penises).

It doesn't matter which numbers are reached in the initial experiences, simply that we begin to get a sense for how each level feels in its own unique expression.

Building Arousal Awareness with Self-Touch (Individual)

To begin, come into your comfortable position on your bed (or wherever you feel most comfortable) with the setting arranged to minimize external noise or distractions. Let your body sink into the bed, noticing the temperature of the sheets, releasing your jaw. Don't skip this part, really take a moment to settle in. Start caressing the front of your body as you did in the front caress, slowly. Stay here for approximately five minutes. Then allow your hand to begin exploring your genitals as you did in the genital caress, touching slowly, allowing curiosity to lead. You will stay here for the next 10–15 minutes. As you're caressing yourself, noticing the temperature of your skin, the textures that make themselves known, the pressure of your hand against your body, check in every few moments and give numbers to the different levels of arousal you feel. Every couple of minutes ask yourself *"What number would I give this feeling? This level of arousal feels like a/ an _____ "* Keep the caress slow, check in with your breathing, release the pelvic floor. The aim is not to "get to" certain numbers at this point, rather simply to notice the ones that show up. Bring yourself back to how your skin feels, how sensation feels in your body, and allow your arousal awareness to come and go as it will. Release and breathe. Keep your body as still and released as possible. If you find yourself at orgasm (again, not the goal or aim in any way – simply another aspect of the experience that can show up), try to experience the sensations without out moving your body or tensing up. Passively allow them to move through you.

But what if I am only able to notice and name one number on the scale? That is great! Get to know that number thoroughly. As you continue to come deeper and deeper into connection and familiarity with what arousal at that level feels like, you will start to notice the finer distinctions. For example, say you can only identify level 6. As you continue to revisit 6, can you start to notice what 6.5 feels like? 5.5?

Peaking practice (individual)

Begin as you did in the previous arousal awareness experience, slowing down, releasing your jaw, pelvic floor, shoulders, breathing. Spend approximately five minutes with a full front caress, then move to a genital caress, release your pelvic floor. Stay here, release again, and slowly explore non-demand touch (i.e. without striving or goal orientation) of your genitals, inner thighs, lower abdomen and pelvis area for another five minutes, give or take. Release the pelvic floor, notice the sensation in your penis/vulva/ genitals as you come back to this part of the body, giving it your focused but gentle attention. As you caress, when you feel you're at (around) level

4, stop caressing and notice the arousal drops back down a couple levels. Slowly begin the caress again until you're around arousal level 5 or 6. Again, stop the caress and allow arousal to go down a couple levels, to a 3. Continue through all identifiable levels, stopping at each one to allow arousal to drop a level or two. Keep the caress, your rhythm, as slow as possible, focusing on touch, release your jaw, notice your pelvic floor. Spend as much time as is required to allow arousal to rise and fall a few levels with each peak. Don't rush, take plenty of time.

Notes:

- The phase in which you allow and feel into the arousal going down is just as important as being attuned to the phase in which it goes up.
- Allow whatever time it takes for arousal to fully drop back down several levels.
- When you begin to re-engage in the caress to begin a new peak, start very slowly and gently.

Plateauing

Plateauing is for you if: you have erectile dysfunction; early ejaculation; delayed ejaculation; difficulty reaching orgasm; you have little, limited, or very specific experiences with sexual or sensual arousal in the body; you feel disconnected from sensations associated with arousal; you just want to explore, learn, and connect more deeply with yourself!

Plateauing is an advanced form of peaking in which we identify an arousal level and hover within that range by first stopping, then pausing, then slowing our touch.

Plateauing Practice (Individual)

Begin slowly with a front and genital self-caress for about five minutes (don't skip this part). Focus on sensation in the body, release, breathe. Increase stimulation slightly and do a few low-level peaks (levels 3 and 4), breathe, take your time, release the pelvic floor. When you reach level 5, stop the caress and allow your arousal to go down, but only to level 4. Then start to caress again and go up to level 6. Hover between levels 4 and 6 by stopping and starting the caress, releasing your jaw, breathing slowly. After a while, see if you can recognize finer distinctions (levels 4.5 and 5.5).

Explore plateauing at higher levels (6, 7, 8, 9) by stopping and starting your caress. Take your time, allowing 15–20 minutes for the experience. End however you feel inclined, including orgasm if desired/available.

Keep in mind throughout that there is no pressure and no one way to define progress. For example, it doesn't matter which numbers you plateau between or if plateauing versus peaking is not available today. The most critical ingredient is our ability to remove pressure and allow ourselves to learn to recognize the arousal levels that reveal themselves in the experience now. Watch for pressure or goal orientated mentality. It can sneak in undetected and undermine the foundation of release that is central to the resolution of sexual challenges.

Experience Check-in: Partner Involvement

Once a sense of ease has been cultivated with peaking and plateauing on your own, you can include your partner if applicable. Involving your partner directly targets any relational anxiety that might play a role in the struggle, allowing your progress to fold itself progressively into the relationship. This might look like having your partner witness, lay alongside, and/or engage in a chest and arm caress as you explore peaking and plateauing for and with yourself. You can also provide instruction around the touch you have been exploring in these experiences, demonstrating, and then having them use their hand, communicating when to slow down and speed up to peak or plateau. This not only addresses the relational anxiety but provides an opportunity to practice giving and receiving active instruction and learning.

Mutual Touch (Partnered)

The version of mutual touch described below is adapted from Linda Weiner and Constance Avery-Clark's, *Sensate Focus in Sex Therapy: The Illustrated Manual* (2017).

Begin with a front caress, about 5–10 minutes each.

In this experience we will lie down facing one another. Close your eyes and hold each other's hand (the hand you have available) for a moment, breathe and feel into this point of contact. Release into the bed, notice the sensations already surfacing or simply the sense of stillness. Notice the emotions beginning to percolate or the sense of spaciousness (or lack of emotion) that may be present. Open your eyes, holding a soft gaze, and begin to touch each other at the same time for your own interest or curiosity, exploring your partner's shoulders, chest, neck, abdomen, and hips with your hand. We are excluding genitals for this experience, and breasts are optional until we determine we're ready. Move slowly, release the jaw, release the pelvic floor, release. This experience asks us to take in sensation from two sources simultaneously: where we are touching and where we are being touched, so be patient with yourself as you acclimate to this back-and-forth dance for your attention. Also, this is the first time we are turning towards each other, facing each other in our experience. What is it like to continue to touch for your own interest, be in your own experience, and not attempt to "do" anything to "please" the other in this position? Let your attention go where it will, but if you notice yourself primarily focused on where you are touching, move your attention to where you are being touched and vice versa. We are now learning to focus alternatively on each source of stimulation, attending to this back and forth until sensation landscapes merge into absorption. This practice allows us to move into and appreciate differentiation, or that space between self and other, alongside the many elements that inspire connection (touch, emotion, interaction, learning, growing).

Explore alternating between touching simultaneously and taking turns.

Things to Consider

Mutual touch can feel like a "leveling up" in terms of our experience of vulnerability – or not! We are facing each other, and therefore potentially face to face with another version of performance concerns, and often the less obvious ones. This can show up as:

What is my face doing? Should I smile? Will they think I'm having a bad time if I don't? Should I make eye contact? Look away?

This progression is another opportunity to put learning and new understanding to practice. Do you dare drop the "sexy" face you think they want to see for the real thing? Your authentic expression? Will you risk allowing any and all emotion to be in the room, even if it's discomfort? Can we remember to make room for us, that this *is* our practice?

Basic Practice Wrap

Congratulations! Finding yourself at the end of this section means important strides have been made and a deeper, more connected relationship to your sexuality (e.g. your vulnerability, your emotion, your sense of self, your physiology, and your boundaries) has been cultivated, and a greater sense of ease in sharing and letting go has emerged in your relationship (if applicable). Amazing!

As you journeyed through the experiences, was there information that surfaced that seemed to weave itself throughout? A memory that continued to visit? Feelings that seemed to surface consistently? It is important to reflect on this information and take a critical and compassionate eye to its wisdom. Your body, heart, and psyche will continue to communicate areas in need of healing, learning, and being attended to. These elements are the building blocks that make up our barriers to intimacy, and are therefore details we don't want to miss or bypass or minimize. We will be in communication with ourselves in this way forever if we continue to make our own vulnerability approachable, and if we continue to cultivate individual and shared intimacy. And we want to! No more collecting ghosts, shame, and traumas to live frozen in our sex, in our bodies and spirits, stirring up anxiety, depression, and distance with others.

Visit and revisit these experiences as needed when tension and anxiety surface in your experience, and reinforce and strengthen new associations – learn, explore, and connect. Although the experiences listed in this chapter comprise the "foundational" progressions of the sensate focus approach, they are the most powerful in terms of confronting and helping us move through our sexual anxiety, creating a foundation of release that moves our conscious (or self-conscious) mind out of the driver's seat.

22 Advanced Practice
Erectile Dysfunction and Vaginismus

In this chapter we will elaborate on the learning we did in Chapter 21 and go into greater depth with two common sexual struggles: erectile dysfunction (ED) and vaginismus. Although we're only focusing on these specific challenges, the experiences described for ED can also benefit those who are struggling with early or rapid ejaculation, while the experiences described for vaginismus can also provide benefit for those with sexual pain (originating from tension in the pelvic floor), or sexual aversion. Move slowly and stay with each experience until ease and mindful attention have been cultivated (again, this need not be perfect, but we want to feel like we are noticing and releasing tension in the body, letting our emotions be without resistance or encouragement, and are able to catch and then bring ourselves back to sensation when the mind drifts).

Pre-requisites

Before beginning your advanced practice, it is strongly recommended that you get an examination with your obgyn, pelvic floor physical therapist, or urologist – depending on your anatomy and the nature of the challenge. Not only is it important to understand if the body is trying to communicate a very real medical concern or issue, but it is also critical to be able to rule this out so that your anxiety doesn't have this worry to work with. Understanding what is and isn't going on with your anatomy and physiology can effectively scratch one, or many very common sources of anxiety off the list.

What If I know My Challenge Is the Result of a Medical Issue?

There are still possibilities for healing. When we uncover a diagnosis, we invite anxiety in alongside it in two forms: larger scale questions about life moving forward (e.g. *What does this mean for me? My sexuality? My pleasure? My relationship(s)?*) and logistical questions during and about

DOI: 10.4324/9781003369080-26

sex itself (*Will this hurt like last time? Probably, so I better start bracing. Will I gain an erection at all? Oh god, it's not responding. Can I reach orgasm today? Will my body let me?*). Understanding the role anxiety plays in your relationship to yourself as a sexual person now, as well as how it impacts what your body is capable of, and what possibilities sensation holds, will prevent the issue or diagnosis from being more limiting than it needs to be.

Sexual Struggles Involving Penises

Anxiety at Baseline

Just a reminder that we walk into sexual experiences having learned a multitude of harmful ideas from the world about what it means to have a penis and to be having sex with a penis. Some common ideas include:

- Penis must look the part: circumcised vs. uncircumcised (depending on the person experiencing it), girthy, long, smooth, _____ (add any ideas you received).
- Must always be "ready to go": i.e. arousal and sexual functioning are on demand and available despite how we feel, the day we've had, our relationship to the person on the other end.
- Erections must last long enough, but not too long.
- Rock hard erections only.
- Must ejaculate (and potentially inside partner) and _____ (what expectations do you have for the role ejaculation and ejaculate play in the experience?).
- Plays central if not primary role in great sex (for people who have sex with penises): if something "goes wrong" or not as expected with the penis, then the experience is "ruined," or a "failure," or "bad sex."

These ideas are in the background (or perhaps the foreground), exerting an influence to varying degrees based on the person. They are the ingredients that make up a baseline experience of anxiety that each person with a penis must contend with as they approach sex. They comprise some of the base layers of our anxiety pyramid, with the other aspects of our larger systems and relationships building and elaborating on our anxiety stories, and their power, from there. How are these ideas shaped by culture, race, religion, and background for you uniquely? For example, *An Asian person with a penis? what ideas did you learn about being a black person with a penis? A Christian or Muslim person with a penis? A "jock" in high school with a penis? A non-binary person with a penis?*

What is your response to the narratives above? Your answers inform your sexual values, and are important to carry with you and access when anxiety places you in direct contact with these sources of pressure in our sexual experiences. Some sample responses could include:

- Penis must "look the part": *My penis is a part of my body, unique and specific to me. All penises look different, just like all people look different. If I am judged by the appearance of my penis, just another part of my body, that reflects poorly on the person I'm with.*
- My penis must be "ready to go" and I must feel desirous all the time: *I am a human being, and my sexuality is informed and influenced by a multitude of complex factors, from my history to my self-worth, to the quality of my relationships, to the kind of day I just had, to the feelings I'm currently sitting with. My sexuality doesn't exist separately from me.*
- Erections must last long, but not too long: This is an impossible bullseye to hit, as it is entirely subjective and varies person by person. *My arousal will unfold in its own time, at its own pace, as a reaction to the experience, rather than an expectation. If I try and exert control, I will disconnect from the experience. I choose to be "in" and to let go of outcome because I know I can always pivot. My erection is one aspect of the experience among many.*
- Rock hard erections only: Erections vary in firmness throughout the course of an experience, especially a dynamic one. *When I lose my erection, it is likely to come back if I continue connecting and exploring. Either way, sex will still be rich and intimate. I don't need an erection to have a hot, or connective, or rewarding experience.*
- Must ejaculate: *My ejaculate is just that: fluid that comes from my body. It is not a reflection of my masculinity, for example, or the only expression of a good time. I can use my words, sounds, and body language to convey what is/was exciting or erotic or pleasurable in an experience. Ejaculation and orgasms aren't always the most rewarding aspects of a sexual experience.*
- Plays central role: *"I" play the central role, my partner(s) play the central role. People are having sex with me, not my penis. There is so much more to having sex with me than just interacting with a penis or any one body part. I want my partners to feel that from me also.*
- How might you counter some of the narratives that reflect the identities you occupied growing up and/or occupy currently? Ideas you internalized based on *your* culture, race, religion, background, and what the world told you it meant to be "you" with a penis?

For help navigating "premature" or rapid ejaculation, I recommend read-ing Metz and McCarthy's, *Coping with Premature Ejaculation: How to Overcome PE, Please Your Partner, and Have Great Sex* (2003).

For help navigating delayed ejaculation, I recommend reading Barbara Keesling's *Sexual Healing: The Complete Guide to Overcoming Sexual Problems* (2006).

Erectile Dysfunction

Once we've cleared any physiological or biological struggle that might be causing or contributing to the issue, we need to think of ED as being less about the loss of your erection, and more about your reaction to it. We will address both the panic reaction at the prospect (and reality) of the loss of your erection, as well as cultivating connection to your arousal in a way that allows for a greater sense of connection with (which translates to a sense of control in relationship to) the levels of arousal you hover between. We will learn how to help rather than hinder ourselves when the brain kicks our sympathetic nervous system into action, while holding in mind our practice with pivoting to prevent "show-stopping" or "record-scratch" moments that only serve to strengthen ED.

Where to Begin?

It is recommended that you begin with the following progressions indi-vidually. The quality of anxiety we contend with on our own can be a little or a lot different, illuminating the role relational anxiety plays in the strug-gle, so starting on your own can ease the transition into partnered experi-ences, not to mention the added benefit of getting to know your solo sexuality in a new and more expansive way.

With the exception of experiences for those with same-sex anatomy, the sensate focus progressions described below were adapted from Sexual Healing: The Complete Guide to Overcoming Sexual Problems by Barbara Keesling (2006).

Let's Review

- Stress/anxiety/concern = sympathetic nervous system response: blood flow is moving away from the genitals and to large muscle groups/vital organs. In other words, if I worry about my erections, I will likely lose them without return.
- Clenching the pelvic floor or moving into "strive" or "power-through" mindset causes the blood that was already in the shaft past

the pelvic floor muscle to be pushed into the penis creating a harder erection momentarily, while the tension introduced in the pelvic floor creates a sort of "seal" at the base, preventing easy blood flow from continuing to move into, fill, and flow through the penis – and the erection is lost.

- During the plateau phase of arousal, many people with penises will lose their erection temporarily. Loss or the decrease in firmness of erections is common throughout an experience.
- Many people with ED are very familiar with the lower levels on the arousal scale; intimate familiarity with all levels via peaking and plateauing will increase the ability to stay within a desired range at any place on the arousal scale.
- Low desire accompanies most sexual challenges and ED is no exception. Expect avoidance to be a constant companion in your healing, learn from it, and know it is normal. The revival of desire has its own trajectory (described at the conclusion of this section).

Arousal and Erection Scales

When working with ED, we will be exploring two different scales: an arousal scale and an erection scale. We will begin with the arousal scale which asks that we pay less attention to the firmness of our erections as an indicator of level of arousal, and tune in instead to the feelings of arousal in the body. This can be hard to define. Below you will find a vague and hypothetical description of the levels. As you make contact and become increasingly familiar with your own, add more detail to the descriptions. Remember, the more familiarity, the better.

Arousal Scale: 1 = no arousal, 10 = orgasm

- 2–3 = subtle glimmers of fluttery feeling in chest, warmth in body, anticipation.
- 4–5 = heart rate increases, excitement builds, breathing quickens, tingly sensations in stomach and genitals.
- 6–7 = strong desire for continued contact, urge to increase stimulation, "electric" feelings throughout the body.
- 8 = labored breathing, rapid heartbeat, build of sensation in genitals.
- 9 = nearing the "tipping point" of orgasm; place of "orgasmic inevitability" (can but doesn't necessarily correspond with "ejaculatory inevitability").

The arousal scale can include emotional and psychological indicators of arousal level as well as the sensory information. The arousal scale is utilized to understand our arousal experience outside of erections.

Erection Scale: 1 = flaccid penis (no erection), 10 = intensely hard erection

- 2, 3, 4 = stages of "filling": penis becomes increasingly engorged and warm.
- 5–9 = "degrees of rigidity" (Keesling, 2006, p. 67): penis has a "locked-in" feel.
- 10 = extremely "full and rigid" erection, uncomfortably hard.

The erection scale is used to determine the degree of erection and its accompanying sensations, not to rate how "great" the erection is (a major distinction), with all levels being meaningful and important. We can learn how to work with our penises to have a meaningful experience at every level. We will learn not to fear a 3 or a 4 (a huge part of the problem), while "working" for a 7 or 8. Use your experience to add detail to the specific levels on the scale. Place these scales to the side and visit them in the order they arrive in the sequences spelled out below.

Suggested Sequence of Experiences

Remember to reference the progressions listed in Chapter 21 (front caress, genital caress, etc.), and take your time with each one. We will work against ourselves if we're rushing past or "pushing through," bypassing or eroding the foundation of release (in both body and mind) that is so pivotal to our progress.

Begin on your own, skipping past any partnered experiences. Once you have finished all individual experiences, begin from the beginning (yes, step #1) with your partner. And lube, lube, lube!

You will notice that the progressions that follow seem to build toward anal or vaginal penetrative sexual or sensual experiences, targeting the anxiety that can surface when interacting with these parts of our partner's bodies in particular. This is not meant to suggest that sex should progress in any particular way, that any one kind of sex is centered over another, and that sexual experiences need to culminate in penetrative sex with genitals whatsoever. This is simply an example of one path, inspired by a common presentation of ED. You may find resolution of your particular expression of ED at any place in the progressions (often the basic progressions are the most effective as they directly target anxiety and performance narratives in a generalized way), each experiences holds the potential for change if we truly and meaningfully engage.

Sex is so much more than one menu item (i.e. penetrative sex). Allow the experiences that follow to reveal the richness that lives beneath your skin, woven into the exploration, and within the connection we have with ourselves and our partner(s).

1 Front caress.
2 Genital caress.
3 Releasing the pelvic floor for easy circulation (people with penises and their partners).
4 "Come and go" erections (partnered):

- Spend the first few moments in spoon breathing, then 5–10 minutes of front caress for each partner (optional genital or oral caress for your partner – all still non-demand, exploring for your own interest). You will then find a comfortable position on your back with eyes in a soft gaze or closed, while your partner begins a front caress, slowly leading into a genital caress. Breathe slowly, release your jaw, check-in with and release your pelvic floor. Your partner will increase stimulation to your penis ever so slightly, and when they notice an erection (levels 3 and above), they will stop the touch and wait until the erection goes back down to 1. They will then slowly begin the caress again, allowing the erection to return, then stopping to allow it to go back down to 1. Repeat this process for 20 minutes. If your erection only happens once or twice or even not at all, that's OK! Maintain release in the pelvic floor, in your jaw and abdomen, and continue to breathe and track sensation. This is progress.

- This experience can be a challenge, and an aggravating one. Expect your brain to kick into high gear at the prospect of "wasting" an erection, and consciously, willfully allowing it to subside. The come-and-go instruction places us in direct contact with our inclination to "worry" about erections and whether they will show up, and then our struggle to keep them around. You may (and will very likely) find yourself defaulting to old processes that you now know don't serve you (tensing the pelvic floor, squeezing your thighs, quickening, or holding your breath). Release, breathe, and remind yourself of morning or nocturnal erections, the ones we gain without conscious input, free from tension, absent any "striving" or struggle. What goes down, comes back up if we can pave the way for it to do so. Take your time, watch the frustration come and go as the brain begins to understand that *I will not be resisting any longer, I'm making room for my natural functions, I'm getting out of my own way.* You are teaching your brain a new reaction to a formerly panic inducing experience, a critical step in your practice! You are ready to move on when you feel completely at ease with the feeling of your erection subsiding.

5 Peaking:
  a Peaking experience #1: building arousal awareness with self-touch.
  b Peaking experience #2: peaking practice.
  c Peaking experience #3: peaking with the erection scale:

- Begin with a front caress, moving to a genital caress. Move slowly, breathe, squeeze, and release your pelvic floor a few times to make contact with this part of the body. Release even further. Increase stimulation ever so slightly and this time allow your *erection* to build to a level 4, stop, breathe, and allow your erection to subside to a level 2 or 3. Slowly begin the caress again, stopping at each peak (or whatever peaks are available) and allowing the erection to subside one or two levels each time.
- The first few times will be challenging, and truly it doesn't matter how many peaks you identify. If each time you return to the caress, your penis peaks at a level 5, get to know that 5 just as we did for arousal awareness; 4.5 and 5.5 will reveal themselves over time if we stay released, move slowly, and get to know sensation without pressure to move more quickly along (keep an eye out for it).
- Explore doing several peaks at one level, or with exclusively the lower, then middle, then higher levels. Repetition is extremely effective, so the more you practice peaking at a level 5, for example, the more ease and knowing is cultivated, and the body understands how to visit and revisit that experience, that level or realm of arousal.
- Keep in mind: all aspects of this experience are important. Tune into sensation as erections build, and also tune into sensations as they subside. Notice the thoughts that surface, do not resist them, simply and gently return to the touch. Notice any tension in the body, release. Notice any emotions that emerge and let them be (*they can stay, I'm not "doing" anything with them*). Be patient and allow for plenty of time for erections to build and subside.
- Stay with this practice until you can move through the scale in a more linear way, for example, stopping at a 3 to let the erection subside two levels, then a 5, then an 8. Once a sense of ease, release, and control has been cultivated, it's time to move on to plateauing.

6 **Plateauing**
   a **Plateauing experience #1: plateauing practice.**
   b **Plateauing experience #2: plateauing for erections:**

   - This experience is identical to peaking with the erection scale described above, but rather than stopping and starting, you will slow and speed up your touch to hover between levels of erection. Spend a few seconds to a minute on each plateau, moving through various ranges on the scale. Breathe, release, take your time. In this experience, experiment with different movements of the body, including *slight* thrusting, to help you plateau. See if you can explore alternating between slowing and speeding up touch, changing your breathing, and incorporating movement to plateau.

- The more ways you can play with variation in your practice, the better. In one experience, try plateauing only in the lower levels, and then the higher levels the next.
- As always, stay patient and resist the urge to want to move quickly to the next progression. Remember, "goal orientation" is a part of the problem, a mindset that risks moving our physiology into sympathetic response. Take your time and check in if progress feels elusive: Am I putting pressure on myself? Am I needing to address pressure in the relationship? Am I carrying more tension than I realize into the experience? Play it safe and add more time in the front caress to your progressions, and/or tune into and fully release the pelvic floor a few times before beginning the experience.

7 **Partnered intimacy:**

a If you have made it this far (first off, YAY! Congratulations!), it is time to begin from Step #1 with your partner, if partnered. Follow the exact steps as described, with a few additions:

   i When engaging in peaking and plateauing with a partner, when using the arousal scale, you will let your partner know when you've reached a peak, and they will stop the stimulation until you notify them to begin again (i.e. arousal has gone down sufficiently). They will begin with stopping and starting, and then move to slowing. With plateauing, your partner will notify *you* when you've reached a specific level of erection, and they will slow and speed up their touch to help your body hover in the desired range.

   ii After practicing peaking and plateauing with manual stimulation from your partner, see if you can incorporate oral stimulation, alternating between hand and mouth. This is optional but another way to expose the brain and penis to different sensations and erotic stimuli. Once plateauing becomes familiar, see if you can practice plateauing using your own hand but placing your hand and penis up against or very near the part of the body you wish to penetrate (anus or vagina). This allows us to take our learning and apply it to what might be an area of your partner's body linked to anxiety or pressure, pairing ease with the approach and proximity.

b **Flaccid or semi-erect insertion.**

Spend 5–10 minutes in front caress. When ready, invite your partner to lie on their back at a right angle to you, in a sort of side-by-side "scissors" position, where your penis is near their anus or vagina (i.e. most easeful position that allows for penetration). Scoot up against each other so that your genitals are in contact, or close to it, your partner's left leg on top of yours, and their right leg in between your legs. Your partner will begin caressing their vulva and vaginal opening, or anus and surrounding area with lubricant. If we're making contact with a vagina, it doesn't matter the degree of your erection, your partner will gently fold or guide your partially erect or flaccid penis into their vagina, using plenty of lubricant. If we are working with an anus, we want to achieve around a level 6 or 7 erection (level of erection required may vary) before you gently insert your penis, using plenty of lubricant. Do not "stuff" for either (ouch!). You will remain as motionless as possible, focusing on the sensations in your penis enveloped in your partner's vagina or anus/rectum Release your pelvic floor, release your jaw, and breathe. If your penis slips out, or an erection is unavailable in this experience for anal insertion (which is absolutely ok and not required), either re-place it, or allow it to rest against the vaginal opening or near the anus (resting against the buttocks or in-between butt cheeks), and releasing. Notice any thoughts that emerge, and gently return to sensation. Allow emotions to be, while releasing your jaw, abdomen, and pelvic floor. Breathe slowly and release any tension you may notice in your legs, let go into the bed. Do this for approximately 10 minutes.

i We are building familiarity with sensation and this part of our partner's body in an entirely new way. Confronting and unraveling performance pressure, pairing release with penetration at all (or varied) levels. Remember, all experiences provide an opportunity to practice a new response to a formerly anxiety or panic inducing situation. Release your jaw and pelvic floor even as/if anxiety reveals itself or as you notice the moving and shifting of sensation in your penis. Stay in the connection, and allow your brain and body to understand safety via the pairing of release with penetration or when nearing penetration (often the greatest source of anxiety for some). If interacting with an anus/rectum, remaining motionless in the way the experience describes may cause your erection to diminish or to go down entirely. Again, breathe and release, allow the body to do as it will and then rest your penis as close to where it may "slip out" as feels comfortable, staying in the experience for the allotted amount of time.

ii Explore this experience multiple times, incorporating slightly more movement each time. See if you can very slowly practice a few peaks, and then move into plateauing. At first, you can stop at each peak and simply stay, resting inside of your partner's vagina or anus (higher level peaks only - option to explore peaking at lower-mid levels near the anus or using oral or manual stimulation from partner, and then slowly insert at higher levels) until arousal has diminished. Alternatively, you might want to start inside, incorporate movement until you've peaked at the desired level, and then pull out to allow arousal to diminish before inserting again. Check in to assure your partner's comfort along the way. It is recommended that you do not ejaculate or finish inside of your partner until peaking and plateauing is experienced with ease. This allows us to work with penetration first, without the added internal pressure to ejaculate and/or "watching for" ejaculation and/or orgasm. Once ease with penetration and arousal explora- tion has been achieved, these elements will unfold on their own.

Additional Practice

What you've just experienced are many of the sensate focus progressions designed to address ED. If you've made it this far, that means you've come deeply into your body, into sensation, and have unraveled challenging asso- ciations and predictions along the way. This is huge! If progress isn't notice- able, you may have moved too quickly through a specific part of your journey. Back up and slow down. Squeeze and release your pelvic floor a few times before each experience, then release some more. Can you identify any performance narratives that haven't been shook? Any sources of pressure? A sex therapist will assist in identifying these elusive and often hard-to- recognize elements with proficiency should a sense of being "stuck" remain.

Variations of Experience

There are many ways of incorporating different colors of eroticism into the experience. As you move into the more advanced experiences, try incorpo- rating different kinds of touch sensation, different levels of eye contact, and even verbalization to understand the impact of variation on arousal, sensa- tion, and immersion. For example, *what happens if my partner uses their words to describe the touch they're doing while watching arousal increase and then quiets the conversation in order to allow it to decrease during a plateau experience? What happens if I use one hand to stimulate myself to a level 6 in a plateau experience while my partner caresses my body, incor- porating light scratching or pressure sensation until I ask them to pause while I hover?*

Outlook Forecast

I've resolved my ED, now where's my desire?

It can take a little while for desire to resurface. Why? Because of the strong associations that have been formed and then reinforced, links like sex = shame, or sex = embarrassment. For desire to come back online, we need a meaningful series of "wins," and that doesn't mean consistently hard erections. "Wins" means that the heart and mind understand in an embodied way that *"my sex life is a place I can show up and know that, erection or not, I am OK. We are OK."* A new association has been formed and the brain predicts a different experience/outcome. If we no longer fear losing our erections, and can truly throw away that concern, then a context has been created that is safe enough for desire to come back online. An added bonus is that when that kind of sexual environment has been achieved then erections are much more likely to come around and stay around.

Sexual Problems Involving Vulvas

Anxiety at Baseline

It is important to consider the many ways sex might be characterized by distrust or feelings of anxiety for people with vulvas. Of primary consideration are two factors:

• Fear of sexual violence;
• Socialization around bodies, beauty, and worth.

People socialized female are taught from a young age that their sexuality can be a danger to them, simply for having the genitals that they have, and that male sexuality is uncontrollable and therefore threatening. We understand from an early age that violence is primarily perpetrated by males and that all people with vulvas should be vigilant about their surroundings, always on guard, and looking over their shoulder. We are taught that cisgender men in particular "only want one thing" and are willing to do what it takes to get it. With these ideas informing our understanding of sex and "male" people, even when we come to understand our sexual orientation as gay, asexual, or bisexual (among others), fearful ideas around sex are directed primarily at people with vulvas, and follow us into the bedroom, affecting the ease with which we explore, let go, exercise boundaries, and play. The kind of fear associated with violence is different from the fear we are all exposed to around pregnancy and STIs, it simply goes much deeper.

Additionally, people socialized female are exposed to the confusing double message of *"dress and look the part to attract a man"* and *"your sexuality can be dangerous to you, men are lustful and boundaryless in their pursuit of sex. So ... sexy but not too sexy? High skirt but not too high or I'm inviting in uncontrolled sexual advances and unhinged sexual behavior? I am nothing if I'm not noticed, but I can't be too visible or else I'm in danger."* And those aren't the only problematic messages. A few (of many) others, centering different themes, include:

- Offer sex but not too soon or they won't respect you; wait too long and he'll leave (i.e. don't be a slut but don't be a prude).
- Feign excitement and pleasure so I don't disappoint his ego; it's my job to make sure his self-esteem is attended to, or else.
- After a certain point in a sexual experience, you must proceed or else you'll give him "blue balls," which is painful and unfair.

This in mind (and it's only a sliver), is it any wonder that those who were socialized female disproportionately present with low or no desire in therapy? Is it any wonder that in the sex = something to fear versus "tons of fun" double message we receive, one wins out over the other? Is it any wonder that all genders struggle with sex?

What is your response to the narratives above? Your answers inform your sexual values, which are important to carry with you and access when anxiety places you in direct contact with these sources of pressure in our sexual experiences. Some sample responses could include:

- *I will share myself: my heart, mind, spirit, body, sexuality when I choose according to what feels right for me. I am always learning to trust myself and my instincts, though it isn't always perfect. I am not afraid to "weed out" those who do not respect my timeline, my feelings, and the respect I hold for myself.*
- *Sex is and will be an expression of my authenticity. I am here to feel, to express, to connect, and to be profoundly me. It is not my job to be what someone else wants me to be for their ego. My partners will know that what they witness and what is being shared is sacred and personal and therefore deeply intimate.*
- *At any point I have the option to stop doing anything that no longer serves me, and the same goes for anyone I am being sexual with. I understand that by pivoting when I'm tired, or bored, or uncomfortable, I am actively protecting my sexual desire and willingness to show up for my shared sexual life. I am protecting my relationship to sex as self-care versus a task among others.*

Vaginismus

To Review

Vaginismus is the involuntary contraction of the vaginal walls, prohibiting penetration (with a finger, tampon, speculum, penis, and/or Q-Tip). This can happen in a way that feels aligned with our emotional experience (e.g. *I'm feeling very nervous, and my body is prohibiting penetration*) or completely outside of what we register experiencing emotionally (*I'm feeling desirous, yet my body is prohibiting penetration*). Why does this happen? A few things come to mind:

- Many people with vulvas have learned to separate themselves from this part of their anatomy. Many of us have no sense for what they look like, *really* look like. Many of us try to distance ourselves from the goings on of this part of the body: the vaginal mucus, secretions, dryness, smells, and textures. In deciding these things are "gross" rather than the body doing its job to keep us healthy, rather than indications of physiological processes at work or warning signs when something is off, we've effectively distanced ourselves from more information about who we are. We've decided this source of learning and connection is not valuable, or worse. Despite the experiences below being focused on the vulva in a lot of ways, it is important to understand this part of the body as existing alongside the others, as part of a whole. All you.
- "Good girls don't" and/or "abstinence until marriage": When we learn to say "no" to sexual concepts, sexual feelings, and sexual experiences we train our body in that "no." It gets meaningfully digested, not only in the mind, but in our musculature as well. These messages don't simply vanish when we want them to (often after having gotten married): our bodies continue to respond to their initial training, the association, the prediction (*"sex is dangerous"* – it doesn't care about the "before marriage" part).
- Lack of sex education and shame: How do we know what is "normal" if we're not taught what "normal" is? In other words, *how do I know my vulva looks like it should? How do I know it's natural to queef, or for things to make squishing sounds? How do I know vulvas can ejaculate too?* If we don't know, if we're not taught or lack self-experience, all of the above might be startling, confusing, overwhelming, or embarrassing, even just to ourselves. Shame and disgust are repelling, our body will do its own version of recoil in response to these super charged feeling states.
- Sexual trauma: Of course our bodies will work to protect us from the threat of danger. The panic alarm that the mind transmits to the body is a prediction of threat, and an attempt at a shield. It is a beautifully wise adaptation that has simply overstayed its necessity.

The great news is – vaginismus can be very responsive to healing. Take your time, listen to yourself, and be patient as you work to unpair panic from your sex, effectively freeing yourself from the control of the past.

The following progressions we will simply number rather than name, as they all build off each other in mostly nuanced ways. Remember to take this slow! Stay with each number until you feel a sense of ease or release in the body and mind and are noticing thoughts and feelings rather than getting lost in them. With particularly challenging experiences, it is recommended that you grab a pen and paper and simply write in your journal afterward, stream-of-consciousness style. This need not look pretty or grammatically correct: we are allowing our brain, inner voice, memories, other versions of ourselves that get stirred up, unexpressed emotional experience, and so on, to move through us and onto the paper. Stay with that experience if the discomfort is not too great (like a 4 or 5 on a scale of 1–10), or back up to the previous number if you find yourself towards a 7–8. Keep in mind everything you've learned while engaging in these experiences: our bodies are learning to let go of old messaging and allow in new ideas, which can be hard. It might be helpful to prepare by writing down a list of four ideas or sexual values you're hoping to embody as you bump into anxiety and tension (e.g. old messaging, or memory) on your path towards progress. These could be counter-points to hypothetical statements like *good girls don't* (if you identify or have identified as "girl") or *sex isn't about me*, as we did above. How might *you* counter those two statements at this point in your process, given your learning this far? What others can you add? Don't overwhelm yourself with too many, three or four is a good starting point.

In these experiences, we will be using our fingers, another part of who you are. Our fingers are soft, moveable, and can feel more intimate than a dilator (although dilators are our friends and can or will be amazingly helpful as well). The vaginal canal exists at an angle inside our bodies; fingers can understand this without jabbing or poking. We start with fingers and then move to dilators or toys with increased familiarity and ease. If you have a partner with a penis, you will advance to incorporating this part of their body if desired.

If pain or discomfort occurs with any of the experiences below, or if locating the pelvic floor is challenging, please seek the assistance of a pelvic floor physical therapist. In fact, working with such a therapist is just an all-around good idea. They can help facilitate this healing in ways a sex therapist cannot, with knowledge of the pelvic floor and the ability to interact with this part of the body in a trauma-informed way.

The number of progressions or experiences found below can feel overwhelming. It is important to move very slowly when we encounter any amount of resistance, anxiety, discomfort, or tension. However, it is likely that you will pick up momentum if you have indeed paced yourself where it matters. Once that momentum really picks up, you can determine to skip a number or two and see how that feels. We can always back up again if needed.

As you move through the experiences, it can be helpful to expose yourself to sex positive learning and information to help reinforce new messaging you're hoping to embody. Run to your library or bookstore and grab a few of these important titles, taking note of places of discomfort as you read:

- *The Body Is Not an Apology: The Power of Radical Self Love*, by Sonja Renee Taylor (2021).
- *Come as You Are: The Surprising New Science That Will Transform Your Sex Life*, by Emily Nagoski (2015).
- *Sex for One: The Joy of Selfloving*, by Bettie Dodson (1996).

All of the following sequences begin in the same way. Each number builds on #1 and *will only describe the differences to incorporate*. Stay with each experience until the body experiences release, emotion is met without resistance, and the mind can notice thoughts rather than getting lost in them. Remember to talk to your body/brain if it's helpful when anxiety surfaces to deliver its warning. Use grounding reminders that resonate, such as: *"This body is mine, it is OK for me to be here, I'm letting go."* Keep in mind the younger parts of you that are trying to understand safety in this experience, honor their effort with patience, tenderness, and care.

- A word about language: If the word "penetration" has any challenging associations attached to it, if the word feels aggressive or threatening in any way, change to "insertion" or another word of your choosing. We want to convey that this experience is one we're inviting in, rather than something that is happening "to" us. Also, for many, practicing relinquishing control and letting go into our arousal, sensation, connection, emotion, and so on, feels scary. Many liken it to being "out of control." Rest assured, when we let go we are doing so with our consciousness, and therefore ability to communicate, make choices, and act on our own behalf, available to us. The same goes for our partners. We are not "out of control" when we step into our arousal or eroticism, we are letting go within the safety we've cultivated in our sexual self-knowledge and connections (to self and other). We are in a dance that permits movement into transcendence, sensation, connection, play, and then back into present-moment awareness and negotiation/articulation of boundaries and/or wants, when needed.

1 Prepare your environment to assure focused attention and awareness (no television, place your phone on silent, find a comfy temperature, dim the lights). Perhaps place objects nearby that can be comforting or grounding, like a calendar, to remind us of the day and year and

paintings or pictures that you care for. When you're ready, take off your clothing with the exception of your bra (if you have one) and underwear (if you need to start with a shirt or pants on, or both, that is absolutely OK – begin where you feel comfortable not where you think you should begin). Come onto your bed and allow your body to sink into the mattress, releasing your weight into its support. Breathe deeply and slowly, releasing more tension with each breath. Release your jaw, release your shoulders, release your pelvic floor. Notice external indications of safety: *I'm in my room. I live with people I trust (if that feels applicable to you). My door is closed and locked, I am in control of this environment.* Release, breathe, and remind yourself that you are in charge of the experience itself. *I can stop, pause, slow at any point and will listen to my body's signs and signals to do so as/if they reveal themselves. Doing so is progress.* Breathe, release – release even further. When you're ready, close your eyes or maintain a soft gaze (whatever works best in terms of focus), and begin caressing your hands, arms, shoulders, and upper chest. Move very slowly, breathe, release. From there you will move around the breasts (if you have them) and caress the upper part of the abdomen and then move around the lower abdomen and genitals and caress the places on your upper legs that you can comfortably reach. Continue caressing your body with the exception of breasts and genitals for your own interest or curiosity. Notice thoughts as they emerge and gently, slowly, return to sensation. Allow emotions to surface without resistance or encouragement, simply let them be with you. Breathe. Listen to your body and pause if/when needed. See if you can keep your hand in contact with the body as you pause, check in, and give yourself care. If you return to the touch, do so slowly and stay in the experience for 10–15 minutes (or as long as you're able – working up to 10 minutes is an option). When finished, take a moment to check in: *what sensation in the body can I identify now? What has shifted? How do I feel emotionally? What did I notice?* Only proceed if this experience was not overwhelming or immensely troubling in any way. If this was the case, that is important information and deserves to be understood and worked through in a safe, therapeutic context. Pushing past our alert system can cause us more harm. Listen to your instincts, and give yourself the opportunity to experience the kind of care you deserve with a skilled sex therapist if called for. We all should've had it long ago.

2 Begin with the front caress for around 10 minutes, and then move the caress towards the lower abdomen, and rest your hand right before the pubic mound or the place where pubic hair often begins. Notice the warmth of your hand as it rests on this part of your body. Breathe, release your jaw, release the pelvic floor, release. Allow feelings to surface, release your shoulders, release your jaw. Notice the

thoughts that make themselves known, notice and come back to the warmth of your hand on your skin, the sensation in the body. After 3–5 minutes here, take another minute or so with the full front caress (excluding the vulva) and finish with full release into the bed, a brief check-in, and optional journaling time.

3 Front caress, pause with hand on pubic mound. Breathe, release, rest here for 3–5 minutes, noticing sensation.

4 Front caress, pause (3–5 minutes each time) with fingers resting gently over vaginal opening (upper part of hand sits on top of the pubic mound, fingers laying softly over opening).

5 Front caress, pause with pinky finger resting over vaginal opening. Release, breathe.

6 Front caress, apply generous amount of lubricant to the pinky finger and pause with pinky finger inside the vagina, up to the first knuckle.
   Checking-in: What has my experience been like thus far? What emotions have been with me? What thoughts surface with regularity? Is there something for me to address within them? Are they simply my brain's effort at providing distance or space from my experience, attempting to protect me? Can I appreciate that wisdom as I gently guide my awareness back to my experience? How am I relating to my body? Am I approaching myself tenderly? What am I learning about myself with and through my body?

7 Front caress, pause with pinky finger inside the vagina, up to the second knuckle.

8 Front caress, pause with pinky finger all the way inside the vagina.

9 Front caress, pause with the ring finger one knuckle inside the vagina.

10 Front caress, pause with ring finger inside the vagina, up to the first knuckle (same for second knuckle, then all the way in).

11 Front caress, pause with two fingers resting over the vaginal opening.

12 Front caress, pausing with two fingers inside the vagina, up to the first knuckle (same for second knuckle, then all the way in).

13 In this experience, we're going to begin folding in very slight movement of the fingers inside the vagina. You get to determine how much movement feels approachable for you, checking in with your body as you go to determine if you need to slow down. Begin with a front caress as always, and once both fingers are resting inside the vagina, if a starting place is invited, you can begin by just slightly moving both fingers forward and back about an inch (or up and down, if that visual makes it clearer), slowly. Breathe, release, stay here, and continue with movement for 3–5 minutes, notice.

14 Front caress, two fingers inside vagina incorporating more movement (can be up and down a bit more, or you can include a sort of side-to-side or circular movement). Release the jaw, breathe slowly.

15 Front caress, two fingers inside vagina, moving slowly and freely, allowing your own curiosity to lead where you touch. Notice sensations, textures, temperatures as you explore this part of your body, of who you are. Can you begin to tap into a sense of empowerment or care (or grief or emotionality) as you connect to all of yourself and parts that have only been separated from the whole because of people and/or systems that exist outside of us: memory, story, messaging, and/or trauma. *This body is mine and I will live freely within it.*

For some, this point may represent the end of your movement through the progressions. For those who would like to experience easeful penetrative sex with a sex toy (dildo) or penis, move through as many of the remaining numbers that apply.

If possible, this is the time to purchase an average-sized dildo or a larger dilator. There is a world of options here, so a good sex toy store is a great place to start. Most are staffed by knowledgeable and highly trained employees who can assist in helping you locate the toy that feels most comfortable to you. If this feels challenging, check in and ask yourself what the discomfort might be made of. *Do I have ideas about who sex toy stores are generally for? Does going to a sex toy store make my sexuality a reality in a different way than exists within the walls of my home? Do I feel uncomfortable or shy about advocating for myself in this way?* Any place you're at with your responses is absolutely OK. Options are available online as well as you continue to grow increasingly comfortable in your relationship to your sexuality and sexual expression.

Begin this experience with a front caress, making sure to give yourself the full ten minutes or more to connect with sensation, release your musculature, breathe, and feel the presence of yourself in your body: "*I am here.*" Move slowly, attending to thoughts, returning to sensation, and allowing emotion to surface and do as it will. Once you are ready to move on, allow yourself to slowly caress your pubic mound, feeling the textures of any hair that may be present there, or the smoothness or roughness of the skin if without hair. Slowly caress the labia, both inner and outer (not to be confused with "internal" and "external," some people have inner labia that are visible externally and others do not), noticing temperature, textures, sensations that live in this part of the body. Breathe, release your jaw, release. After a few moments here, place some lubricant at and around the opening of the vagina and on the dildo or dilator. Be generous in the amount. Lay the toy lengthwise on the labia, feeling into the contact that it's making with your body. Notice any thoughts that surface, return to sensation, release your pelvic floor, slow down, breathe. When ready, slowly insert the toy no deeper than an inch into the vagina. Rest it there, continuing to gently support the toy as it rests. Check in with the body: *Do I feel any tension anywhere? My legs? Shoulders? Buttocks?* Release. Breathe slowly, deep, full breaths. After several minutes (3–5), gently remove the toy, place your hands where you feel inclined (alongside the body, folded on your abdomen, over your chest), and take a moment to check in. *Is there emotion with me? What sensation do I notice in the body? What has shifted since I began this experience? How do I know I'm OK?*

Also, if it feels true to you, this might be a great time to recognize how far you've come. Even if this particular experience/number was a struggle, even if it brought up a whole lot (which, thank you body!), you are at a major point in your process. A lot of growth had to happen to get here, which required a ton of bravery and healthy challenge/risk-taking. How does it feel to acknowledge it?

16   Front caress to genital caress, place lubricant on vaginal opening and dildo, insert two inches in, rest it there and release the pelvic floor. Breathe.
17   Front caress to genital caress, insert dildo as far in as feels comfortable (not as far in as you think you "should" bring it, play it safe), rest it there, notice sensation, thoughts, feelings emerge, release the body, breathe.
18   Front caress to genital caress, insert dildo, rest for a moment, and then slowly incorporate slight movement forward and back. Move slowly, breathe, release the pelvic floor, release the jaw. Continue to slowly move the toy within the vaginal canal for a few minutes, resting again for a beat at the end, recalibrating, breathing.
19   From here, continued experience with the toy is important. With continued exploration and practice comes increasing amounts of ease and comfort. If you've made it to this point, a new understanding has already been communicated to the body, a new line of trust has been established. This is huge! (Now is the time to give yourself an enormous "pat-on-the-back" as we did in school. Time to get proud and/or acknowledge yourself, your bravery, your persistence. This is a turning point in your relationship to yourself, to your body, to your sexuality. Yay!).

If partnered, now is the time to include them in the experience. What this entails is beginning at #1 (or 2 or 3, depending on how you feel – again, play it safe), but this time your partner will be caressing your body. Your partner will be resting their hand on the pubic mound, their fingers resting over the vaginal opening, their pinky finger entering up to the first, then second knuckle, then all the way in. If your partner has a vulva and you use a strap-on or toy for penetration, your partner will be holding the toy or

having it on their body as they insert one inch, rest, then two inches, rest, and then all the way in, rest. If your partner has a penis, follow the numbers below.

20 Front caress to genital caress, resting penis over the vaginal opening without going "in." Feel the sensations of the penis against your skin, notice emotions that surface and let them be, letting go of tension in the jaw as you exhale. Release the pelvic floor, breathe.

21 Front caress to genital caress, active partner will stimulate themselves to a 5 or above on the erection scale (see beginning of chapter), or to a half-to-full erection. They need not be fully erect for the experience. Once erect, they will apply a generous amount of lubricant to the vaginal opening and their penis, focusing on the tip. They will then slowly insert the tip of the penis about an inch into the vaginal canal, and simply rest it there for a few minutes. Breathe, notice the sensation of your partner's penis inside of your vagina, allow thoughts to come and go, release.

22 Front caress to genital caress, insert semi-fully erect penis halfway in, rest (3–5 minutes). Release your jaw, breathe.

23 Front caress to genital caress, insert semi-fully erect penis all the way into vaginal canal, rest.

24 Front caress to genital caress, insert semi-fully erect penis all the way into the vaginal canal, incorporate slight, slow thrusts (just two or three shallow thrusts).

25 Front caress to genital caress, insert semi-fully erect penis all the way into the vaginal canal, incorporate moderate movement: slow but slightly longer thrusts.

26 Front caress to genital caress, insert semi-fully erect penis all the way into the vagina, incorporate full movement.

Incredible work! If you've made it here, or halfway through, or a quarter of the way, I hope you're tremendously proud. You have just participated in guiding your body and mind carefully into new understanding, you have just untied yourself from associations that have limited your sex, placed barriers in your intimacy, and the penetration aspect was only one. Continue to hold to your values and your body, heart, mind, and sexuality will continue to thank you.

For more expansive healing and a deeper dive into the origins and physiology of Vaginismus, refer to *10 Steps: Completely Overcome Vaginismus* (Books 1 and 2), by Mark Carter and Lisa Carter (2015).

Conclusion
Trust Fall

How challenging is it to be human, to have made and felt a million mistakes, and then to trust yourself and risk trusting others? How hard is it to surrender when trauma, heartbreak, and struggle teach us to hold on, manage, and control? How impossible can it feel to share yourself when we find ourselves and our bodies landing somewhere on the "not good enough" spectrum multiple times a day/week/month? We don't escape our own rough edges and tender bruises with sex, we are profoundly in the presence of them. And yet, sex is frequently talked about as either joyous and transcendent or dangerous and harmful. It can be either/or, black or white, *and* more frequently, it is a swirly, blurry, gray universe in-between.

Anxiety alerts us to some of the reasons why sex is hard, why intimacy is unsafe or even dangerous, whether that danger has anything to do with today or our ghosts from the past. The good news is we always have a choice: to close ourselves in and control, or to open ourselves up and let go. If your home was destroyed by a tornado, stealing beloved possessions, everything you hold dear, leaving behind trauma and confusion, how might you rebuild your home? Would you board up the windows? Lock the doors? Keep yourself confined and "safe"? Or would you want to run in the fields, smell the flowers, let the sunshine in and sing?

Therapists receive several calls a week from individuals looking to pursue sex therapy for themselves alone, without their partner's participation. When asked why, the responses are often *"This is just too personal,"* *"I feel too vulnerable,"* *"This is a 'me' problem."* Can something that *is* personal be too personal? Can something that *is* vulnerability be too vulnerable? If sex isn't these things, what does it become? Is therapy about sex, about intimacy, at all? Or are we actually just trying to fix our performance?

Learning to be with and trust ourselves, to feel comfortable and at home within our bodies and psyche, not only helps resolve our erectile dysfunction, rapid ejaculation, low desire, sexual pain, or vaginismus, it connects us to our emotions, our history, our ongoing learning about who we are

DOI: 10.4324/9781003369080-27

and what we want. It is healing, the kind of healing that reverberates out and impacts the whole person. Learning to befriend sex's asks to share, reveal, connect, express, play, exercise, and respect boundaries, means greater ease in these areas in our day to day. How then could depression survive? Addiction? Eating disorders? Many if not all of our struggles as humans find their origins in the difficulty we have in relationship to these aspects of our humanity. When we lose sight of who we are, we suffer; sex is the same.

Our nervous system lets us know that our sexual functioning is in favor of homeostasis, our sense of balance and well-being, just like its neighbor, sleep. It offers experiences in real time that straddle the line between reality and fantasy, waking mind and dream space, in order to take us into an abstract realm where we meet ourselves in a new way, and release all that we're not. Our bodies know when we deny that opening, when we stand too far in our reality thinking space, fearful of jumping for precisely all of the reasons we should.

This is forever work, a practice in understanding how to love and be loved, see and be seen, invite in and release, every day as we will never not contend with our conditioning, with the rules of the world, with hatred and violence, with ignorance and fear. We have a million reasons to hide, to hold back, to perform, and to armor up. As Dr. Candace Hargons discussed, to let go, to love, to express how we feel, to share, to be vulnerable – requires bravery. It was an act of bravery sitting down with this book. If we want connection, healing, and sexual vitality, bravery and risk will be our constant companions. What else could be more important? The world can be *the* great distancer; sex brings us back to ourselves, back home.

Thank you, sex, for asking me to fully embrace my humanity, to love and accept myself despite, and even because of, my shame. And to dare to show that to others.

Thank you, anxiety, for revealing a deeper wisdom, for showing me the lessons I no longer wish to house and carry with me into my intimate life and relationships. I'll take it from here.

Sex is vulnerability.
Sex is connection.
Sex is play.
Sex is sharing, revealing, surrender.
Sex is us – in all our complexity.

So good riddance, let's dance.

Works Cited

Anderson, J. (2024). Gender Dysphoria as an Expression of Disconnection. https://southshorefamily.com/staff/jordon-anderson/

Brewer, J. (2022). *Unwinding anxiety: New science shows how to break the cycles of worry and fear to heal your mind*. Avery, an imprint Penguin Random House.

Carlan, H. (2020, November 23). *Fearing the black body: The racial origins of fat phobia*. Sabrina Strings, NYU Press, 2019. Center for the Study of Women. https://csw.ucla.edu/

Carter, M., & Carter, L. (2015). *10 Steps Completely overcome vaginismus (Book 1 & 2)*. M. & L. Carter.

Cohen, Siggie. (2024) Have you noticed that anxiety and fears in our kids have skyrocketed lately? *Instagram*, March 15.

Colier, N. (2016, May 4). When it's time to let go of control and surrender. *Psychology Today*. https://www.psychologytoday.com/us/blog/inviting-monkey-tea/201605/when-its-time-let-go-control-and-surrender

Corinna, H., & Turett, C. (n.d.). *Yes, no, maybe so: A sexual inventory stocklist*. Scarleteen. https://www.scarleteen.com/

Davidson, E. (2021, September 3) The myth of confidence. *Loose Lips Magazine*. Retrieved from https://looselipsmag.com/essays-columns/the-myth-of-confidence/

Davis, K. (2022). Book Review: Fearing the black body. The Racial Origins of Fat Phobia by Sabrina Strings. *European Journal of Women's Studies*, 29(1), 190–192. https://doi.org/10.1177/13505068211065599

Dodson, B. (1996). *Sex for one: The joy of selfloving*. Three Rivers Press.

Donaghue, C. (2015). *Sex outside the lines: Authentic sexuality in a sexually dysfunctional culture*. Benbella Books.

Duclos, S. (2023). Death, sex, and older partners: moving to pleasure. *Generations Journal*. https://generations.asaging.org/death-sex-and-older-partners-moving-pleasure

Feldman Barrett, L. (2018). *How emotions are made: The secret life of the brain*. Mariner Books.

Feldman Barrett, L. (2021, April 29). Your brain predicts (almost) everything you do. *Mindful.org*.

Garbes, A. (2018). *Like a mother a feminist journey through the science and culture of pregnancy*. Harperwave.

Haines, S. (1999). *Healing sex: A mind-body approach to healing sexual trauma*. Staci Haines.

Hargons, C. N., Thorpe, S., & Gilbert, T. O. (2022). Black people's constructions of good sex: Describing good sex from the margins. https://journals.sagepub.com/doi/abs/10.1177/13634607221101854

Hargons, C. N., & Thorpe, S. (2022). #HotGirlScience: A Liberatory Paradigm for Intersectional Sex-Positive. https://journalofpositivesexuality.org/wp-content/uploads/2022/04/10.51681.1.811_HotGirlScience_Hargons-Thorpe.pdf

Kabat-Zinn, J. (1990). *Full catastrophe living: Using the wisdom of your body and mind to face stress, pain, and illness*. Random House.

Kaplan, H.S. (2015). *The illustrated manual of sex therapy*. Routledge.

Kaupi, M. (Host), The Six Principles of Sexual Health: Out of Control Sexual Behavior, Audio Podcast, Institute for Relational Intimacy, https://www.theharveyinstitute.com/publications/interviews-presentations

Keesling, B. (2006). *Sexual healing: The complete guide to overcoming common sexual problems*. Hunter House Inc. Publishers.

Klein, M. (2016). *His porn, her pain: Confronting America's pornpanic with honest talk about sex*. Praeger, an imprint of ABC-CLIO, LLC.

Levine, P. A. (1997). *Waking the tiger: Healing trauma*. North Atlantic Books.

Ley, D.J. (2014). *Myth of sex addiction*. Rowman & Littlefield.

Menakem, R. (2021). *My grandmother's hands: Healing racial trauma in our minds and Bodies*. Penguin Books.

Metz, M.E., & McCarthy, B.W. (2003). *Coping with premature ejaculation: How to overcome PE, please your partner & have great sex*. New Harbinger Publications.

Miller, M.V. (1996). *Intimate terrorism: The crisis of love in an age of disillusion*. Norton.

Morin, J. (2012). *The erotic mind: Unlocking the inner sources of passion and fulfillment*. HarperCollins.

Nagoski, E. (2015). *Come as you are: The surprising new science that will transform your sex life*. Simon & Schuster.

Ogden, G. (2011). *The return of desire: A guide to rediscovering your sexual passion*. Trumpeter.

Perel, E. (2006). *Mating in captivity: Reconciling the erotic + the domestic*. HarperCollins.

Pillay, S.S. (2011). *Your brain and business: The neuroscience of great leaders*. Pearson FT Press.

Real, T. (2008). *The new rules of marriage: What you need to know to make love work*. Ballantine Books.

Robertson, C.B. (2019). Why is sex associated with death? https://caffeincandphilosophy.com

Schmalbruch, S. (2015, January 28). Here's the trick olympic athletes use to achieve their goals. *Business Insider*. Retrieved from https://www.businessinsider.com/olympic-athletes-and-power-of-visualization-2015-1

Schnarch, D.M. (2009). *Intimacy & Desire: Awaken the passion in your relationship*. Beaufort Books.

Strings, S. (2019). *Fearing the black body: The racial origins of Fat Phobia*. New York University Press.

Taylor, S.R. (2021). *The Body is not an Apology: The power of radical self love*. Berrett-Koehler Publishers.

Tolle, E. (1999). *The power of now: A guide to spiritual enlightenment*. New World Library; Namaste Publishing.

Weiner, L., & Avery-Clark, C. (2017). *Sensate focus in sex therapy: The illustrated manual*. Routledge.

Index

For Product Safety Concerns and Information please contact our EU
representative GPSR@taylorandfrancis.com Taylor & Francis Verlag GmbH,
Kaufingerstraße 24, 80331 München, Germany

Printed and bound by CPI Group (UK) Ltd, Croydon, CR0 4YY
08/06/2025
01897006-0005

"*Overcoming Anxiety in Sex and Relationships* is a refreshing resource that teaches readers how to build a more compassionate, mindful, and empowered relationship to the very human experience of anxiety so they can make more space for play and pleasure in their lives – something we all need and deserve more of."

Anne Hodder-Shipp, CSE, *award-winning sex and relationship educator, instructor, and author of Speaking from the Heart: 18 Languages for Modern Love*

"*Overcoming Anxiety in Sex and Relationships* is a right-on-the-mark resource at a couldn't-be-more-perfect time! In a post-quarantine, COVID world with volatile, global, geopolitical violence, a domestic epidemic of daily shootings, and an unprecedented erosion of reproductive rights and sexual freedoms, it seems anxiety, stress, and worry have become the societal norm, impacting individuals and couples in profound ways. This easy-reading book is invaluable – not just a great resource for sex therapists and counselors, but for anyone looking to understand how emotion, physiology, and socialization combine to create obstacles to the kind of sex we want – and most importantly, it helps us find our way through them. Paula has taken her years of training in sex therapy and deftly condensed and simplified complex therapeutic topics, making her advice to readers approachable, relatable, and actionable."

Dr. Richard Siegel, PhD, *sex therapist and supervisor, educator and trainer, author and researcher, and Co-Director of Modern Sex Therapy Institutes*